CLINICAL ENDOCRINOLOGY

An Illustrated Text

This book has been developed in conjunction with the **Slide Atlas of Endocrinology**, sponsored and distributed by Sandoz Products Ltd.

Sandoz Pharmaceuticals
A division of Sandoz Products
98 The Centre
Feltham
Middlesex TW13 4EP
England

Sandoz Pharmaceuticals Corporation
59 Route 10
East Hanover
New Jersey 07936
USA

Gower Medical Publishing Ltd.
Middlesex House
34–42 Cleveland Street
London W1P 5FB
England

CLINICAL
ENDOCRINOLOGY

An Illustrated Text

Editors:
G Michael Besser MD DSc FRCP
Professor of Endocrinology
Physician in Charge
Department of Endocrinology

Andrew G Cudworth MD PhD FRCP
Late Professor of Human Metabolism
Consultant Physician
Department of Diabetes and Immunogenetics

St. Bartholomew's Hospital
London, UK

Editorial Assistant:
Pierre-M G Bouloux BSc MBBS MRCP
Research Fellow
Department of Endocrinology
St. Bartholomew's Hospital
London, UK

Foreword by:
Jean D Wilson MD
Professor of Internal Medicine
The University of Texas Health Science Center at Dallas
Dallas, Texas, USA

J.B. Lippincott Company · Philadelphia

Gower Medical Publishing · London

Distributed in the USA and Canada by:
J.B. Lippincott Company
East Washington Square
Philadelphia, PA. 19105
USA

Distributed in all countries except the USA, Canada and Japan by:
Chapman and Hall
11 New Fetter Lane
London EC4P 4EE

Translated and distributed in Italy by:
USES, Edizione Scientifiche Spa
Via Ricasoli 48
50122 Florence
Italy

ISBN:
0-397-44550-4 (Lippincott)
0-906923-76-X (Gower)

Library of Congress Catalog Card Number: 87-80385.
Library cataloging in Publication Data is available.

Printed in Hong Kong by Mandarin Offset

Typesetting by TNR Productions Ltd., London, UK.

Typeface: Plantin Light.

Project Editors: **Melanie Paton**
David Goodfellow

Design: **Mick Brennan**

Illustration: **Mick Brennan**
Karen Cochran
Jeremy Cort

This book is dedicated to the memory of Andrew Cudworth,
a brilliant colleague and friend.

Foreword

Illustration has contributed both to the evolution and to the teaching of endocrinology. To cite a few examples: the superb drawings in Thomas Addison's *Disease of the Supra-Renal Capsules* of 1855 clearly document the association of adrenal insufficiency with *acanthosis nigricans* and with vitiligo, neither of which was recognized as a distinct entity at the time. Examination of the photographs of the eunuchs of the Chinese court make it possible to delineate the frequency and manifestations of the feminizing state that follows castration of men. Likewise, in examining early drawings and paintings of dwarfs it is possible to identify subtypes that were not originally recognized. Photographs of Robert Wadlow, the Alton Giant (both still photographs and movies), illustrate the consequences of untreated gigantism that may in fact be unique for all time. Nevertheless, in contemporary textbooks, illustrations of patients and of X-rays rarely live up to the level of the nineteenth-century drawings, not because black-and-white photography at its best is not adequate for illustrating detail, but because the usual photographic plates for printing such photographs tend to blur with use.

The present textbook of endocrinology continues in the Gower tradition to utilize two advances in the communication of science. One is color photographs that serve to illustrate the diagnostic standards by which endocrine patients are categorized and understood in the 1980's (posterity will almost certainly categorize them differently). Superb photographs of patients, excellent reproductions of X-rays and examples of state-of-the-art scans of

several types have been assembled from a multitude of sources. The second advance is the application of the graphic revolution originated by the *Scientific American* for the communication of scientific information. To this end, multicolor graphics have been designed to survey the scientific underpinning of endocrinology from the human leucocyte antigen system to neuroendocrinology. Finally, the text is lucid and comprehensive and effectively builds upon the illustrative material. The net consequence is a new standard for an endocrine textbook and for the teaching of endocrinology, one that should have special appeal for students, house staff and endocrinology fellows.

Although extreme examples are sometimes chosen for illustrative purposes this serves to fix in the mind of the student disease patterns that are more than the sum of the individual parts (acromegaly and myxedema, for example). However, such photographs can also have a distorting effect on education. It does not take a physician or even a student of medicine to recognize that something is wrong with a patient with florid thyrotoxicosis, whereas the separation of subtle endocrine disease from normal variants is one of the perpetual challenges of medicine. Perhaps the next graphic revolution will make it possible to illustrate consistently the spectrum of changes between the normal and the abnormal.

Jean D Wilson MD
Dallas, Texas, USA

Preface

Of recent years there has been dramatic advance in the understanding of the normal physiology of human endocrinology and, as a consequence, of its pathological processes and their management. This has largely been as a result of improvements in analytical techniques and in specificity and sensitivity of hormone assays, based usually on radioimmunoassay. These innovations have allowed separation and accurate measurement of the relevant endocrine factors in blood, CSF and tissues, and also new immunocytochemical procedures for cellular localisation of hormones. Neuroendocrinology has become a clinical science with elaboration of profound new concepts of the relationship between mind and body, and the mechanisms governing the body's homeostasis and its disturbances in disease. These developments were behind the design of this textbook originally planned with my late colleague Andrew Cudworth, who tragically died so young and unexpectedly soon afterwards. The text is highly illustrated using the new techniques developed by the publishers. It was initially produced as a slide atlas and the principal messages of the book which have developed from it, are conveyed in the diagrams and pictures, explained and expanded by the text. Normal physiology is the starting point of each section so that the

pathological and clinical features of the disorders, their investigation and management can be based on this fundamental knowledge. Special attention has been given to radiology and neuroradiology of endocrine diseases, and the inter-relationships between the behavioural and emotional features of the disorders and the chemical changes which have induced them. Diabetes mellitus and its closely related topics are not dealt with here as there will be a sister book devoted to this subject, to appear shortly.

Many colleagues have contributed to this work and my thanks go to them for making it possible, and for their tolerance. Especial appreciation is owed to Professor Israel Doniach, who acted as the expert advisor on histology and Dr Pierre Bouloux for his dedicated work as editorial assistant. The staff of Gower Medical Publishing have been long-suffering during the production of the atlas and this textbook, and I wish to extend my gratitude to them for their expert attention and help, especially to Melanie Paton and David Goodfellow.

G.M.B.

Contributors

Peter H Baylis BSc MD FRCP
Consultant Physician and Senior Lecturer in Medicine, Royal Victoria Infirmary and University of Newcastle-upon-Tyne, Newcastle-upon-Tyne, UK

Paul E Belchetz MA MD MSc FRCP
Senior Lecturer in Medicine and Honorary Consultant Physician, University Department of Medicine, Royal Liverpool Hospital, Liverpool, UK

Charles GD Brook MD FRCP
Consultant Physician, Department of Paediatrics, The Middlesex Hospital, London, UK

Timothy Chard MD FRCOG
Professor of Reproductive Physiology, St. Bartholomew's Hospital, London, UK

Janet E Dacie FRCP DMRD FRCR
Consultant Radiologist, St. Bartholomew's Hospital, London, UK

Israel Doniach MD FRCPath FRCP
Emeritus Professor of Morbid Anatomy, University of London and Honorary Lecturer in Histopathology, St. Bartholomew's Hospital, London, UK

Paul L Drury MA MRCP
Consultant Physician, Department of Diabetes, King's College Hospital, London, UK

Christopher RW Edwards MA MD FRCP
Professor of Clinical Medicine, Western General Hospital, Edinburgh, UK

Reginald Hall BSc MD MB BS FRCP
Professor of Medicine, University of Wales College of Medicine, Cardiff, UK

David A Heath MB ChB FRCP
Reader in Medicine, University of Birmingham, Queen Elizabeth Hospital, Birmingham, UK

Vivian HT James PhD DSc FRIC FRCPath
Professor of Chemical Pathology, St. Mary's Hospital Medical School, London, UK

Derek PE Kingsley FRCS DMRD FRCR
Consultant Radiologist, The National Hospital for Nervous Diseases and The Hospital for Sick Children, London, UK

Richard J Lilford MRCOG MRCP PhD
Professor of Obstetrics and Gynaecology, St. James's University Hospital, Leeds, UK

Vincent Marks MA DM FRCP FRCPath
Professor of Clinical Biochemistry, University of Surrey and Consultant in Chemical Pathology, St. Luke's Hospital, Guildford, UK

Lesley H Rees MSc MD FRCP
Professor of Chemical Endocrinology and Honorary Consultant Physician, St. Bartholomew's Hospital, London, UK

Seymour Reichlin MD PhD
Professor of Medicine, Tufts University School of Medicine and Senior Physician and Chief, Endocrinology Division, New England Medical Center Hospital, Boston, Massachusetts, USA

Edward O Reiter MD
Professor of Pediatrics, Tufts University School of Medicine and Chairman, Department of Pediatrics, Baystate Medical Center, Springfield, Massachusetts, USA

Louis M Sherwood MD
Baumritter Professor and Chairman, Department of Medicine and Professor of Biochemistry, Albert Einstein College of Medicine, New York, USA

Michael O Thorner MB BS FRCP
Professor of Medicine and Head, Division of Endocrinology and Metabolism, Department of Internal Medicine, University of Virginia, School of Medicine, Charlottesville, Virginia, USA

W Michael G Tunbridge MD FRCP
Consultant Physician and Senior Lecturer in Medicine, University Department of Medicine, Newcastle General Hospital, Newcastle-upon-Tyne, UK

John AH Wass MD FRCP
Reader in Medicine and Honorary Consultant Physician, St. Bartholomew's Hospital, London, UK

F Elizabeth White MRCP DMRD FRCR
Consultant Radiologist, Freeman Hospital and Newcastle General Hospital, Newcastle-upon-Tyne, UK

Contents

1 Neuroendocrine Control of Pituitary Function

Seymour Reichlin, MD,PhD

Among the most important advances in endocrinology has been the unravelling of the mechanisms by which the pituitary is regulated by the brain. Each of the known pituitary hormones is controlled by one or more hypothalamic releasing or inhibitory factor. With the elucidation of human pancreatic growth hormone releasing hormone (GHRH) in 1982, the major hypophysiotrophic hormones have been isolated and their structures identified. Synthetic peptides have now been used to diagnose endocrine disease, and several have already been used for treatment. These advances have made the need to understand the anatomical and physiological basis of hypothalamo-pituitary control even more relevant.

The concept of neurosecretion which underlies our understanding of the way in which neural information is converted into chemical messages results from the work of Scharrer and colleagues in the 1930's. They recognised that certain nerve cells in the brain of insects, fish and the neurohypophyseal system of mammals resembled gland cells. Scharrer introduced the term neurosecretion to describe this phenomenon, recognising that the histological findings suggested the possibility that some nerve cells were capable of acting like secretory cells.

The contemporary view of neurosecretion which is now recognised to be a general property of almost all nerve cells involves three different types of neurosecretory neuron: (i) neurohypophyseal; (ii) hypophysiotrophic; (iii) neuromodulatory (Fig. 1.1).

ANATOMY OF THE HYPOTHALAMO-PITUITARY UNIT

The neural lobe of the pituitary gland (posterior pituitary or neurohypophysis) consists mainly of endings of nerve cells whose origins are in the hypothalamus. The principal secretions of the neurohypophysis are oxytocin (uterus contracting hormone, milk let-down hormone) and antidiuretic hormone (ADH or vasopressin); both are synthesised as part of prohormones that include distinctive neurophysins (Fig. 1.2). The complexed neurophysin-oxytocin and neurophysin-ADH are transported down the axons in the form of granules, which are stored in the nerve endings and subsequently released in response to appropriate physiological signals. ADH release is related to the osmolality of the blood and the effective blood volume, while oxytocin is released during labour and in response to suckling. Both reactions are mediated by neural reflexes.

The anterior pituitary (adenohypophysis) is also controlled by the brain but, unlike the neural lobe, does not have a direct nerve supply. Instead, impulses from the brain are translated into chemical messages by specialised hypothalamic cells and then released into the specialised blood supply of the pituitary tuberoinfundibular neuron system (see Fig. 1.2). In turn, the tuberoinfundibular cells are influenced by neural influences from outside the hypothalamus (e.g. those influences which integrate homeostasis, stress responses, mating and reproductive functions) and also by feedback effects of both pituitary hormones and those of target glands (e.g. thyroid, adrenal cortex and gonadal steroids). The anatomical distribution of the tuberoinfundibular cell system has been elucidated by methods involving retrograde tracing of markers injected into the median eminence (Fig. 1.3), and by immunohistochemical staining of neurons containing hypophysiotrophic peptides (Fig. 1.4).

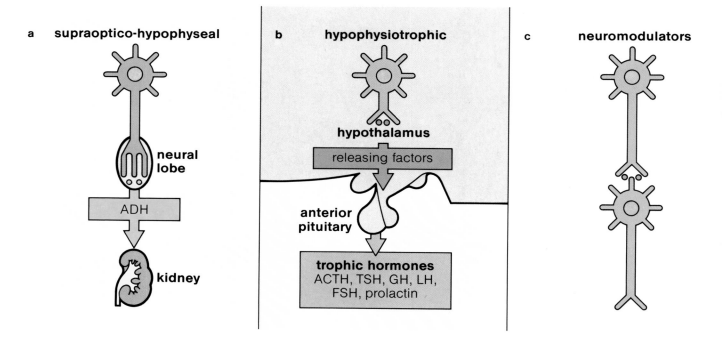

Fig. 1.1 Diagram of the neurosecretory peptidergic neurons involved in pituitary regulation and neuromodulation. View (a) illustrates the classical neurohypophyseal system. Nerves project from cells of origin in the supraoptico-hypophyseal and paraventriculo-hypophyseal nuclei, and end in the neural lobe. Oxytocin and ADH are synthesised on the endoplasmic reticulum as part of a larger prohormone (which includes the specific oxytocin- and ADH-related neurophysins), and are then packaged into granules where they are stored in nerve endings and subsequently released into the peripheral blood. Because they affect tissues at a remote site, they are classified as neurohormones. The secretions of the hypophysiotrophic neurons in (b) are also neurohormones because they are secreted into the blood and travel in the hypophyseal-portal vessels to the anterior pituitary. Some entirely analogous neurosecretory neurons do not terminate at a blood vessel, but at the endings of other nerves, and there the neurosecretory substances act as neurotransmitters or neuromodulators (c). A neuromodulator can be considered as a substance that modifies neuronal responses to neurotransmitters. Redrawn from Reichlin (1977), by courtesy of the publishers, Raven Press.

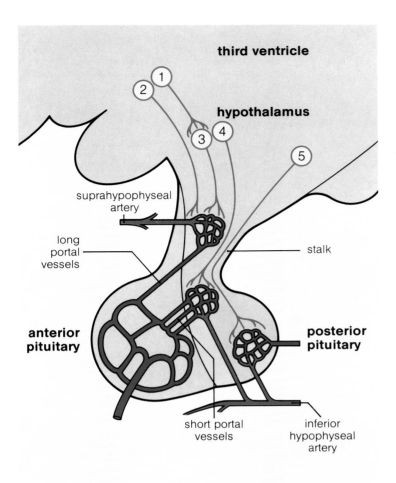

third ventricle

hypothalamus

suprahypophyseal artery

long portal vessels

stalk

anterior pituitary

posterior pituitary

short portal vessels

inferior hypophyseal artery

Fig. 1.2 Diagrammatic representation of the hypothalamo-pituitary regulatory system. The products of the posterior pituitary are synthesised in the supraoptic and paraventricular nuclei (5). After packaging, they are transported as granules, by axoplasmic flow, to the nerve terminals in the posterior pituitary, where they are released directly into the circulation to act as classical neurohormones on distinct target sites. The mechanism of anterior pituitary hormone secretion is entirely different. The pituitary hormone releasing or release-inhibiting hormones of the hypothalamus are synthesised within the nuclei of the hypothalamus (1-4) and transported to the median eminence from where they travel to the anterior pituitary via the dense capillary network and the long portal veins. These hypothalamic factors occupy specific receptors in the pituicytes and either lead to the release of the pituitary trophic hormones or inhibit their secretion. Redrawn from Gay (1972), by courtesy of the publishers, the American Fertility Society.

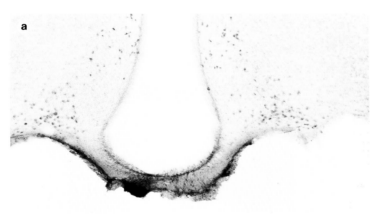

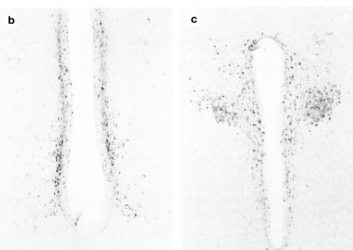

Fig. 1.3 Anatomy of the tuberoinfundibular system in the rat, demonstrated by retrograde transport of a tracer compound. A tracer compound, wheat germ agglutinin, was injected under direct vision into the median eminence of a rat. Several hours later, the animal was killed, and the brain sectioned and stained immunohistochemically with an antibody to wheat germ agglutinin. The tracer is found in cell bodies located in three main areas: (a) the arcuate nucleus, (b) the periventricular nuclei which comprise a rich plexus several cells deep that hug the third ventricle and (c) the paraventricular nuclei. Most of the arcuate cells are dopaminergic; most of the periventricular cells are somatostatinergic. The paraventricular system, however, is more complex, and includes cells that secrete ADH, oxytocin, TRH, somatostatin, neurotensin and many others. Projections from cells within all of these nuclear groups to other regions in the brain cannot be identified using this technique. From the paraventricular nucleus, TRH fibres, among others, project to the brain stem and spinal cord. By courtesy of Dr. R. Lechan.

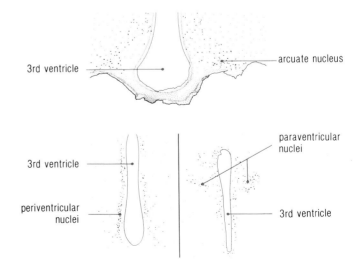

3rd ventricle

arcuate nucleus

paraventricular nuclei

3rd ventricle

3rd ventricle

periventricular nuclei

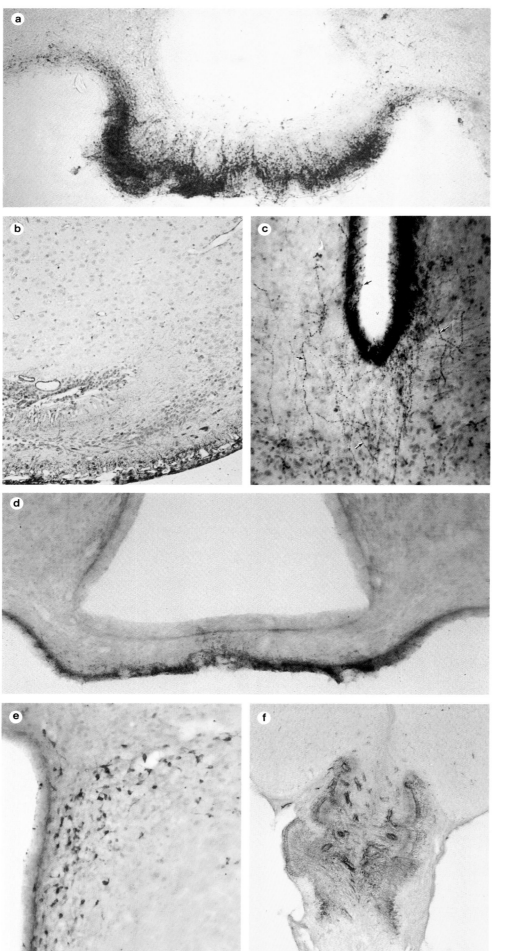

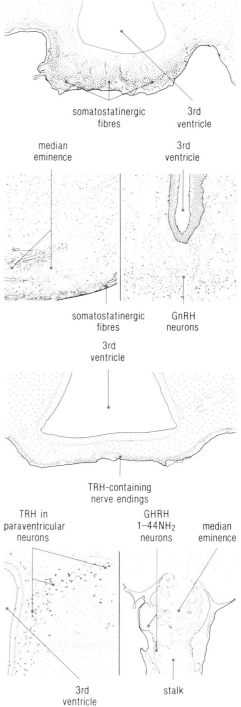

Fig. 1.4 **Hypophysiotrophic neurons in the hypothalamus demonstrated by immunohistochemical techniques using the Sternberger PAP method.** The following views are shown: (a) immuno-histochemical appearance of somato-statinergic fibres in a frontal section of the hypothalamus of the rat at the level of the median eminence; (b) sagittal section of the hypothalamus of the rat showing somatostatinergic fibres; (c) GnRH peptidergic pathways in a horizontal section of the rat hypothalamus; (d) TRH-containing nerve endings in the median eminence of the rat (frontal section); (e) TRH-containing neurons in the paraventricular nucleus of the rat in frontal section; (f) anatomical localisation of GHRH 1-44NH₂ in stalk and median eminence of the rhesus monkey. By courtesy of Drs. R. Lechan, L. Alpert and J. King.

Each known anterior pituitary hormone is regulated by one or more hypothalamic hormones, and, sometimes, a single hypothalamic hormone (a so-called 'releasing factor' or hypophysiotrophic hormone) can influence more than one pituitary hormone. All the known pituitary hormones and their regulating hypothalamic hormones are listed in Figure 1.5. The ADH and oxytocin structures were elucidated in 1954 and 1953 respectively, thyrotrophin releasing hormone (TRH) in 1969, gonadotrophin releasing hormone (GnRH) in 1971, somatostatin in 1973, corticotrophin releasing hormone (CRH) in 1981 and GHRH in 1982. New insights have clarified prolactin control. Prolactin secretion is stimulated by vasoactive intestinal peptide (VIP) and peptide histidine isoleucine (PHI, or PHM in man), and inhibited by dopamine and gonadotrophin associated peptide (GAP). GAP is a peptide identified by recombinant techniques in the GnRH prohormone. VIP and PHI are both encoded on separate exons on the same prohormone.

In general, each of the anterior pituitary hormones is regulated by the interacting influences of the hypothalamus and feedback effects from circulating hormones. However, the hypophysiotrophic hormone-secreting cells are only one class of special nerve cells in the brain that function by secreting a chemical messenger from the nerve endings. There are many other nerve cells that secrete a wide variety of other kinds of peptides or neurotransmitters, including at least five biogenic amines (e.g. noradrenaline, adrenaline, dopamine, serotonin and histamine), eight transmitter amino acids (e.g. glycine, glutamic acid, aspartic acid, taurine and gamma aminobutyric acid (GABA), cysteic acid, homocysteic acid, alanine) and more than twenty peptides. These additional peptides are also secreted by nerve cells and include the hypothalamic hypophysiotrophic hormones, the endorphins (endogenous morphine-like peptides) and the gut-brain peptides (e.g. glucagon, cholecystokinin, secretin and gastrin).

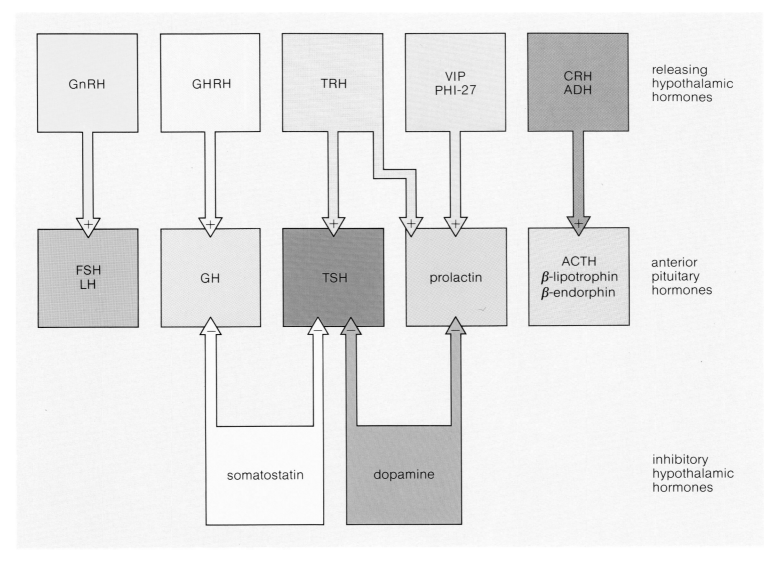

Fig. 1.5 Table of the hormones produced in the anterior pituitary and the hypothalamic hormones that regulate their secretion. Studies utilising immunoneutralisation indicate that VIP and PHI interact to release prolactin during suckling and stress. In man, an analogous peptide, PHM, appears to serve the same purpose. CRH interacts with ADH in a synergistic way in the stress-ACTH response.

Structure and Function of the Hypothalamic Hypophysiotrophic Hormones

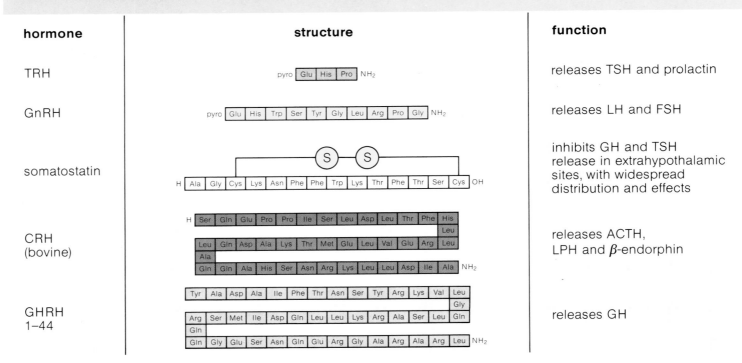

hormone	structure	function
TRH		releases TSH and prolactin
GnRH		releases LH and FSH
somatostatin		inhibits GH and TSH release in extrahypothalamic sites, with widespread distribution and effects
CRH (bovine)		releases ACTH, LPH and β-endorphin
GHRH 1–44		releases GH

Fig. 1.6 Diagram showing the structure of the hypothalamic hypophysiotrophic hormones. GHRH is the only hypothalamic hypophysiotrophic hormone which has a sole response; that is, of GH release.

Structure of Several Hypothalamic Peptides

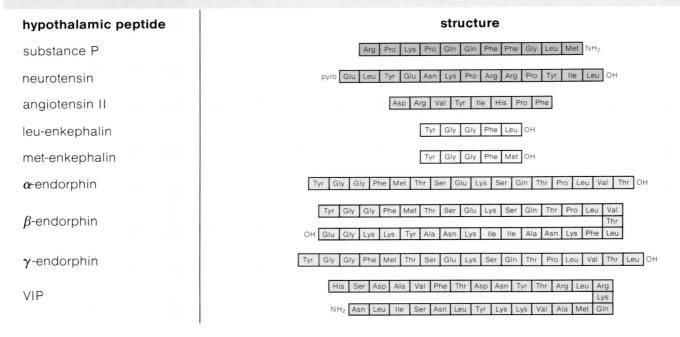

hypothalamic peptide	structure
substance P	
neurotensin	
angiotensin II	
leu-enkephalin	
met-enkephalin	
α-endorphin	
β-endorphin	
γ-endorphin	
VIP	

Fig. 1.7 Diagram showing the structure of several hypothalamic peptides. The structure and action of the peptides are known but their physiological function is not fully understood. Substance P (permeability factor) was originally found in dorsal root ganglia and is found in both peripheral and central axon projections of sensory ganglia. This peptide is probably responsible for the wheal reaction in the triple response to skin damage; it is also believed to interact with the endorphins. Neurotensin is widely distributed in the brain, and its identification in synaptosomes indicates a role as a neurotransmitter regulator of brain function. It causes a lowering of blood pressure and widespread increased capillary permeability and vasodilation. In the periphery, angiotensin II, a potent pressor agent, is formed from angiotensin I. Angiotensin II is formed *in situ* in the hypothalamus and is believed to be involved in central regulation of blood pressure, drinking behaviour and ADH secretion. The endorphins and enkephalins react with endogenous opiate receptors in various brain sites, including hypothalamus, amygdala, the dorsal root entry zone and also areas in ascending pain pathways. Their special function in the hypothalamus as distinct from a role in pain perception is unknown but they appear to modulate release of some hypophysiotrophic hormones (e.g. CRH and GnRH). VIP is found in the small intestine and in pancreatic islet cell tumours and also in hypothalamic extracts and axonal endings in brain neurons. VIP produces hyperglycaemia, acts as a hypotensive agent, stimulates water excretion by gut and also appears to be an important prolactin releasing factor.

HYPOPHYSIOTROPHIC HORMONES OF THE HYPOTHALAMUS

The search for hypothalamic neurohormones with anterior pituitary regulating properties focused upon extracts of stalk median eminence (SME) and hypothalamus. Such hypophysiotrophic materials have been called releasing factors after the first description in 1955 of corticotrophin releasing factor (CRF, now known as CRH). This term was introduced by Saffran and Schally (1955) to describe a substance extracted from hypothalamic tissues which stimulated the release of adrenocorticotrophic hormone (ACTH) from pituitary fragments maintained in organ culture. Twenty-six years later the chemical nature of this substance was elucidated by Vale and colleagues (1981). The chemical structures of the five peptide hypophysiotrophic hormones identified so far are shown in Figure 1.6. Dopamine can also be included as a hypophysiotrophic hormone because it is present in hypophyseal-portal vessel blood in sufficient concentrations to duplicate all its known inhibitory effects on the secretion of prolactin. Several hormones invoked as prolactin releasing factors include TRH and VIP. However, many other active peptides are found in the hypothalamus (Fig. 1.7). Releasing factors also stimulate other pituitary functions such as differentiation and hormone synthesis.

Certain hypothalamic factors exert significant inhibitory actions on anterior pituitary function. These inhibitory factors interact with the respective releasing factor to exert dual control of secretion of prolactin, growth hormone (GH), TSH and, to a lesser extent, the gonadotrophins. Surprisingly, the action of each of the hypophysiotrophic hormones is not limited strictly to a single pituitary hormone; for example, TRH is a potent releaser of prolactin, and in some circumstances releases ACTH and GH. GnRH releases both luteinising hormone (LH) and follicle-stimulating hormone (FSH). Somatostatin inhibits secretion of GH, TSH and a wide variety of other non-pituitary hormones. The principal inhibitor of prolactin secretion is dopamine, but this potent bioamine, acting directly on the pituitary, also inhibits TSH and gonadotrophin secretion and, under some circumstances, also inhibits GH secretion.

Thyrotrophin Releasing Hormone (TRH)

The chemical structure of TRH was elucidated by groups of investigators working in association with Schally (1969) and Guillemin (1971). Their work, which was the culmination of more than a decade of effort to identify the nature of the thyrotrophin releasing activity of crude hypothalamic extracts, made neuroendocrinology credible to the general scientific and clinical community. It also made possible the introduction of TRH into clinical medicine, vastly widened the scope of understanding of TRH in other biological systems and gave a powerful incentive to efforts to identify other biological activities in hypothalamic extract.

TRH is a relatively simple substance, a tripeptide amide (pyro) Glu-His-Pro-NH$_2$. Although some substituted forms are potent, an intact amide and the cyclised glutamic acid terminal are essential for activity. TRH is chemically stable, but is rapidly degraded in plasma by enzymatic action. Following injection of TRH in the human or in the rat, blood TSH levels rise rapidly and dramatically, a change being detected within three minutes; peak values are normally attained between ten and twenty minutes after injection in normal subjects (Fig. 1.8) and somewhat later in patients with pituitary or hypothalamic hypothyroidism. TRH is very potent, as little as 15 μg yields a detectable response and maximal effects result from a dose of 400 μg. The standard clinical dose, commonly administered as a bolus, is 200–500 μg. Transient mild nausea, a sense of urinary urgency and mild decreases or increases in blood pressure occur as side-effects of injection in an appreciable number of patients; a life-threatening reaction is rare. The surge of TSH release induced by TRH injection leads to a detectable rise in plasma tri-iodothyronine, T$_3$ (see Fig. 1.8), and also an increase in thyroxine (T$_4$) release, which is usually not large enough to produce a significant increase in plasma levels of this hormone.

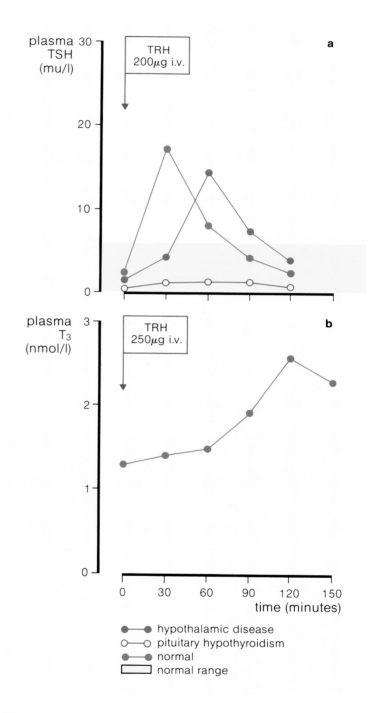

Fig. 1.8 Graphs showing the normal and diseased response to TRH. View (a) shows the delayed TSH response to TRH in a patient with hypothalamic disease. Peak plasma TSH values following exogenous TRH are reached at approximately 60 minutes compared to the normal gland, where the peak occurs at 20–30 minutes. In pituitary hypothyroidism, the TSH reserve may be severely reduced, and there may be only a slight or no response to exogenous TRH. In (b), the normal rise in circulating plasma T$_3$ following injection of TRH is shown. There is a delay before peak circulating plasma T$_3$ is reached compared to the peak in TSH.

One of the most important aspects of TRH action on the pituitary is that its effects are blocked by prior treatment with thyroid hormone. Indeed, the interaction of the negative feedback action of thyroxine on the pituitary, with the stimulating effects of TRH represents the principal mechanism of the integrated neuroendocrine control system of TSH secretion (Fig. 1.9).

In addition to stimulating TSH release, TRH is also a potent prolactin releasing factor (Fig. 1.10). The time course of response of blood prolactin levels to TRH, dose-response characteristics and suppressibility by thyroid hormone pretreatment (all of which parallel changes in TSH secretion) suggest that TRH is probably involved in the regulation of prolactin secretion. If prolactin release bioassays had been used to isolate TRH, it may have been called prolactin releasing factor (PRF).

Despite these striking overlapping effects, it is unlikely that TRH plays more than a modulatory role in prolactin regulation under normal circumstances. The prolactin response to breast-feeding (in women and experimental animals) is unaccompanied by changes in plasma TSH, thus suggesting that this neurogenic reflex does not involve TRH. However, the prolactin release stimulating actions of TRH may be responsible for the occasional occurrence of hyperprolactinaemia (with or without galactorrhoea) in patients with hypothyroidism. This finding has been attributed either to an increased sensitivity of prolactin secreting cells to TRH in the hypothyroid state, to an increase in TRH secretion, or to hypothyroidism-induced inhibition of secretion of prolactin inhibitory factors.

In normal individuals, TRH has no influence on pituitary hormone secretion other than on TSH and prolactin. However, in special circumstances it exerts a number of other effects on pituitary secretion, including the release of ACTH in some patients who have Cushing's disease and the release of GH in the majority of acromegalic patients (see Fig. 1.10). These responses are thought to result from the presence on pituitary cell membranes of TRH receptors, usually obscured by the normal regulatory processes of the pituitary. TRH also releases GH in some patients with psychotic depression. TRH inhibits sleep-induced GH release through a central nervous system mechanism, and also has other central nervous system effects.

The greatest value of TRH is in the differential diagnosis of thyrotoxicosis in borderline cases of mild thyroid overactivity. The validity of the test is based on the fact that thyroid hormones act directly on the pituitary to inhibit the effects of TRH. Therefore, if thyroid hormone is present in excess, TRH has no effect. This characteristic of TRH is evident even with minimal excess of thyroid hormone. In thyrotoxic individuals there will be no increase in TSH, and in patients with hypothyroidism the response to TRH will be exaggerated. Measurements of T_3 have been useful in determining whether the thyroid is intrinsically capable of responding to TSH. An increase in T_3 means that the thyroid is functionally normal regardless of the state of TSH secretion.

The classical response in pituitary TSH deficiency is a blockade of response and in hypothalamic disease, a delayed and prolonged response (see Fig. 1.8). However, in practice, TRH has not been especially valuable in the differential diagnosis of hypothalamic versus pituitary as causes of TSH deficiency. Although most patients with pituitary failure causing TSH deficiency will not respond normally to TRH, a few will respond, and some patients with hypothalamic disease will not respond to TRH. This degree of overlap means that an effective differential diagnosis cannot be made in individuals. Therefore, accurate radiological study and other endocrine evaluations are normally used in diagnosis.

One of the most surprising consequences of the development of specific methods for detection of TRH was its demonstration in brain tissue outside of the classical 'thyrotrophic area' of the hypothalamus. TRH has been found, using immunoassay or immunohistochemistry, in virtually all parts of the brain including the cerebral cortex, spinal cord, in nerve endings abutting upon the ventral horn motor cells and upon the intermediolateral column, in the circumventricular structures, in the neurohypophysis and in the pineal gland. TRH has also been found in pancreatic islet cells and in various parts of the gastrointestinal tract. Although present in low concentrations in these areas, the aggregate in extrahypothalamic tissue far exceeds the total amount in the hypothalamus.

The extensive extrahypothalamic distribution of TRH, its localisation in nerve endings and the presence of TRH receptors in brain tissue suggest that this peptide acts as a neurotransmitter or neuromodulator outside the hypothalamus. In particular, its distribution in the spinal cord, at nerve endings of the intermediolateral column (cells of origin of the sympathetic nervous system) and the ventral horn, may be relevant to clinical benefits claimed for TRH treatment of shock and amyotrophic lateral sclerosis.

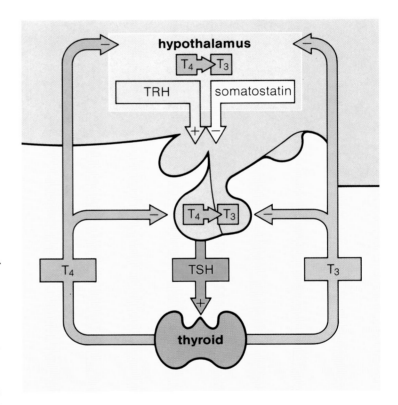

Fig. 1.9 Diagram illustrating the hypothalamo-pituitary-thyroid axis. The thyroid gland is regulated by TSH and its secretion in turn is modulated by thyroid hormones acting directly at the level of the pituitary gland. Thyroid hormones inhibit the action of TRH secreted into the hypophyseal-portal vessels by the TRH-ergic neuronal system. Somatostatin secreted by specific somatostatinergic neurons inhibits TSH release. Therefore, the rate of secretion of TSH is modulated by a positive stimulating signal from the hypothalamus (TRH) and by two negative feedback elements, one from brain, and the other from circulating thyroid hormone. The secretion of somatostatin by the brain is regulated by thyroid hormone, thus indicating that the negative feedback effect of thyroxine has two components – one directed at the pituitary, and the other indirectly through somatostatin. Both thyroid hormones, T_4 and T_3, act on both pituitary and hypothalamus. T_3 is more potent than T_4, and enzymatic mechanisms are present in both pituitary and brain (5' mono di-iodinases) to convert T_4 to T_3. The effect of thyroid hormone on TRH secretion is still controversial. Redrawn from Reichlin (1985), by courtesy of the publishers, W.B. Saunders Company.

Gonadotrophin Releasing Hormone (GnRH, LHRH)

It has been known for more than twenty years from the work of McCann (1960) and of Campbell and co-workers (1964) that extracts of hypothalamic tissue contain a biologically active substance capable of stimulating the release of gonadotrophic hormones from the pituitary. This material was isolated in almost pure form from the hypothalami of stockyard animals by Guillemin and by Schally and their collaborators and the structure finally elucidated by Schally's group in 1971. Like TRH, the amino terminal of GnRH is a substituted amide. A terminal amide group is also characteristic of a number of other small peptide hormones including ADH, oxytocin, calcitonin, gastrin and glucagon, and in all these hormones the amide group is needed for full hormonal activity.

Following intravenous injection, naturally occurring GnRH or its synthetic form triggers a prompt dose-related release of LH and FSH in man and all vertebrate species in which it has been tested. After a single bolus injection of GnRH, FSH release is delayed compared with LH secretion, the values peaking at ten to thirty minutes after injection. This is because the response of FSH to GnRH is markedly influenced by the prior GnRH secretory state, by the steroid milieu of the patient, by gonadal function, by the time course of GnRH injection (i.e. single dose, multiple pulse, or constant infusion) and by the patient's genetic sex. Through secondary effects of pituitary activation, and under appropriately defined conditions, GnRH can induce spermatogenesis and testosterone production in men with hypothalamic hypogonadotrophic hypogonadism, and ovulation in women with hypothalamic amenorrhoea (Fig. 1.11).

Most reproductive neuroendocrinologists now believe that the GnRH decapeptide is the only hypothalamic gonadotrophin regulator, and that observed dissociations of secretion of LH and FSH are due to the interacting effects of prior hormone status, steroid pretreatment, and pattern of GnRH administration. This is supported by the demonstration that antisera prepared against the GnRH decapeptide blocks ovulation in the female rat, and lowers blood levels of both LH and FSH in castrated animals. Although reports of a separate FSH releasing factor still sometimes appear in the literature, the unitary hypothesis (White 1970) is widely accepted, and there is a growing tendency to use the term gonadotrophin releasing hormone instead of luteinising hormone releasing hormone (LHRH).

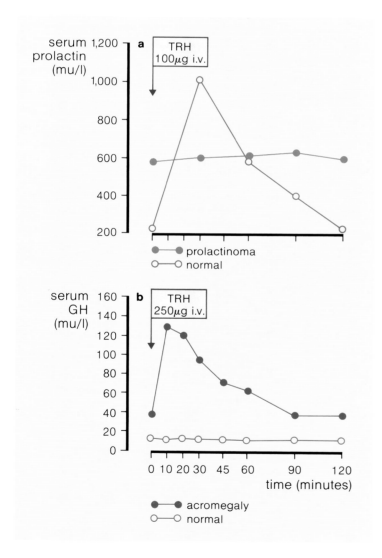

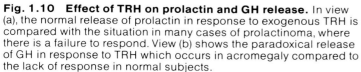

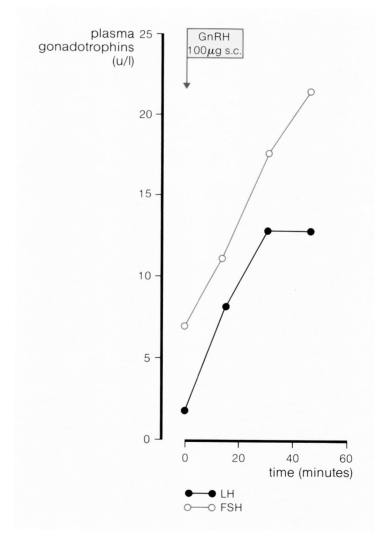

Fig. 1.10 Effect of TRH on prolactin and GH release. In view (a), the normal release of prolactin in response to exogenous TRH is compared with the situation in many cases of prolactinoma, where there is a failure to respond. View (b) shows the paradoxical release of GH in response to TRH which occurs in acromegaly compared to the lack of response in normal subjects.

Fig. 1.11 Gonadotrophin response to GnRH in a woman with galactorrhoea-amenorrhoea due to prolactinoma. This patient differs from most normal subjects in that a more brisk FSH than LH response occurs. Both the LH and FSH responses are exaggerated compared with the normal response.

GnRH has been extensively tested as a diagnostic agent in differentiating causes of hypogonadism. In patients with complete pituitary destruction, GnRH does not stimulate gonadotrophic hormone release, but in patients with lesser degrees of pituitary dysfunction associated with hypogonadism, GnRH may induce a gonadotrophin response within the normal range. Furthermore, long-standing hypothalamic dysfunction can lead to poor or absent pituitary responsiveness. For these reasons, a single bolus injection of GnRH is a poor differential diagnostic tool.

Intermittent injections of GnRH which mimic the physiological function of the hypothalamus will stimulate gonadotrophin secretion, and lead to normal pituitary-testicular and pituitary-ovarian function as inferred by sex steroid secretion, and the subsequent reappearance of fertility (Fig. 1.12). This application is the most important clinical application of the hypothalamic hormones so far. Also, it has been shown that administration of GnRH at a constant rate leads to reduced gonadotrophin secretion (Fig. 1.13). This phenomenon, attributed by some to 'down-regulation' of GnRH receptors, has been exploited for the treatment of idiopathic precocious puberty. In this disorder, the use of a 'super-agonist' of GnRH inhibits gonadal function to prepubertal levels. This approach may also prove to be useful as a highly specific contraceptive, and also in the hormonal treatment of carcinoma of the prostate.

Unlike TRH and somatostatin, almost all of the GnRH in the brain of mammals is restricted to the hypothalamus and related neural structures. Small amounts are found in the circumventricular organs, including the pineal gland. Recently a GnRH-like peptide has been reported to have neurotransmitter function in frog sympathetic ganglia. GnRH has also been found in milk, suggesting that the breast, a dermal derived structure may have embryologic origins analogous to the primitive neuroectoderm,

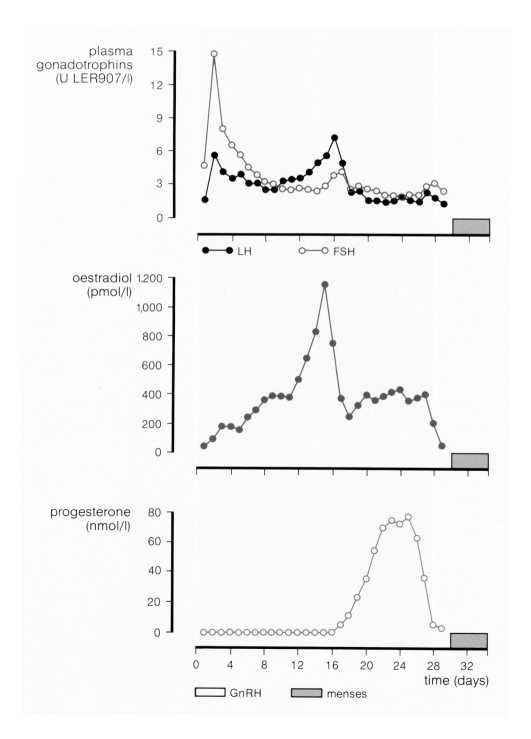

Fig. 1.12 Graph showing restoration of a normal ovulatory cycle in a woman with hypothalamic disease using intermittent GnRH. Intermittent doses of GnRH were administered at 90-minute intervals by a pump. These findings indicate that mimicking the normal pulsatile release of GnRH can restore normal cyclical function. Redrawn from Crowley and McArthur (1980), by courtesy of the publishers, Williams and Wilkins Company.

the source of neuroendocrine cells. The most important central nervous system effect of GnRH may be that involved in regulation of mating behaviour. Direct injection of GnRH into the hypothalamus has been reported to enhance female sexual responsivity even in animals without a pituitary, and hence incapable of responding with gonadotrophin-ovarian activation. Studies of the effect of GnRH on human sex drive have been unconvincing.

Growth Hormone Releasing Hormone (GHRH)
Efforts to identify the chemical nature of GHRH from hypothalamic extracts were for a long time unsuccessful. Nevertheless, a series of brilliant experiments coupled with clinical insights led, in 1982, to the elucidation of the structure of GHRH isolated from the pancreatic islet tumour of two patients with the rare disease of

acromegaly due to ectopic secretion of GHRH. Two different molecules have been identified, one consisting of forty-four amino acids, and the other forty amino acids. It has now been proven that they are identical to the hypothalamic material.

Studies on the administration of GHRH-40 have already shown a brisk release of GH in man after intravenous injection. Also, this reaction is without side-effects, since no pituitary hormone, other than GH, is stimulated by GHRH (Fig. 1.14). GHRH has been used to treat GH deficiency in hypopituitary dwarfs. Early studies show that GHRH can stimulate GH secretion from many patients with GH deficiency due to hypothalamic disease or idiopathic GH deficiency. These observations indicate that these patients do indeed have GHRH deficiency and that it may be possible, in the future, to treat such children by GHRH instead of GH to promote growth.

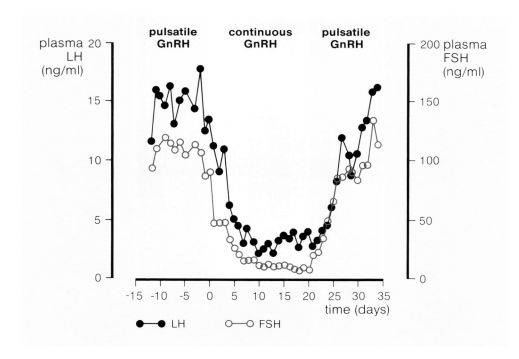

Fig. 1.13 **Graph showing the effect of constant high levels of GnRH on gonadotrophin secretion.** This data from a monkey shows suppression of secretion, the opposite effect to that achieved by intermittent GnRH administration. This phenomenon is now demonstrated in man and is used clinically: (i) to inhibit gonadotrophin secretion in children with precocious puberty, (ii) in men with prostatic carcinoma and (iii) in normal women to block ovulation. Redrawn from Belchetz et al. (1978), by courtesy of the publishers, the AAAS.

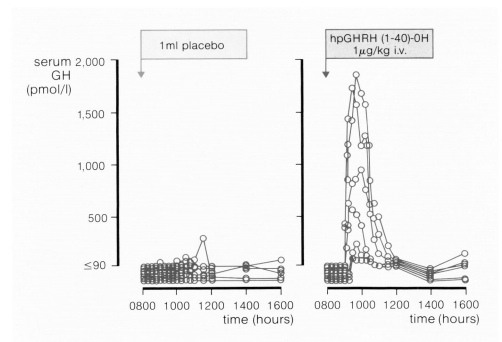

Fig. 1.14 **Graph showing the secretory response of GH to GHRH administration.** Human pancreatic growth hormone releasing hormone (hpGHRH) was injected into six normal men. GHRH has been found to stimulate the release of GH only. Redrawn from Thorner et al. (1983), by courtesy of the publishers, Lancet Ltd.

1.11

Somatostatin

During the course of efforts to isolate GHRH from hypothalamic extracts, Krulich and McCann discovered a fraction that inhibited GH release from pituitary incubates, *in vitro*. They named the factor 'growth hormone release inhibitory factor', and postulated that GH secretion was regulated by a dual control system, one stimulatory, the other inhibitory. Relatively little attention was paid to this bioactivity when first described because it was thought by most workers to be a relatively non-specific effect. Several years later, however, Brazeau and several collaborators working in Guillemin's laboratory on the attempted isolation of growth hormone releasing factor again observed the inhibitory factor, and with the background in methodology gained from earlier studies of TRH and GnRH were able in a relatively short time to isolate and identify a potent peptide from hypothalamic extracts that inhibited GH release. The material, to which the name 'somatostatin' was applied, is a fourteen amino acid peptide, lacking the amide and pyroglutamic acid termini which are characteristic of GnRH and TRH, but containing a disulphide bridge similar to that of ADH and oxytocin. More recently, other molecular forms of somatostatin have been isolated including a twenty-eight amino acid peptide (the last fourteen amino acids are identical with somatostatin-14) and a still larger form, the prohormone, with a molecular weight of approximately 15,000 daltons.

Somatostatin has been demonstrated as an important physiological regulator of GH release by studies in which the somatostatinergic pathways are damaged, or endogenous somatostatin neutralised by treatment with antisomatostatin antibody (Fig. 1.15).

Shortly after chemically synthesised somatostatin became available for study, it was found to inhibit the secretion of TSH, glucagon and insulin. Subsequently, somatostatin has been shown to inhibit the secretion of many other secretory structures in the body, including virtually all the glands of the gastrointestinal tract (Fig. 1.16). Studies of somatostatin content of body tissues, using radioimmunoassay and immunohistochemistry, show that almost every tissue that is acted upon by somatostatin contains this peptide in specialised neurosecretory cells. Thus, somatostatin, originally isolated from the hypothalamus, has been shown to be widely distributed in tissues, and in certain conditions acts as a paracrine secretion (i.e. control of one cell by secretions of an adjacent tissue) and in others as a neuroendocrine secretion (e.g. as in the tuberohypophyseal neurons of the hypothalamus).

Of the hypophysiotrophic hormones isolated so far, somatostatin has the most extensive extrahypothalamic concentration in both the other parts of the central nervous system and in extraneural structures, especially the gastrointestinal tract. In general, the major direct effect of somatostatin on nerve cells is to depress spontaneous activity; however, in some sites somatostatin seems to increase nerve activity. Applied locally to the brain, somatostatin has a sedative effect as shown by extension of barbiturate-sleeping time. It also has a hypothermic effect. In dorsal root ganglia it appears to modify centrally directed pain impulses by regulating substance P release in this dorsal root entry zone of the spinal cord. This physiological role of somatostatin in brain function remains to be elucidated. Somatostatin analogues are now being used to treat acromegaly, bleeding ulcers, hypersecretory tumours of the gastrointestinal tract and carcinoid tumours.

Corticotrophin Releasing Hormone (CRH)

Although CRH (previously known as CRF) was the first of the releasing factors to be recognised and named (by Saffran and Schally), its chemical nature was not determined until 1981 by Vale and collaborators. Patients injected with CRH responded with increased ACTH and plasma corticosteroid levels (Fig. 1.17), as well as the peptides β-lipotrophin and endorphin synthesised in the corticotrophs with ACTH as part of the precursor molecule pro-opiomelanocortin (POMC).

The availability of synthetic CRH has made it possible to clarify several classical questions about hypothalamo-pituitary-adrenal control. CRH effects on the pituitary are inhibited by cortisol, thus confirming a direct pituitary feedback effect (Fig. 1.18). ADH, which was previously thought to have CRH-like activity, has now been shown to act by potentiating CRH action.

Extrahypothalamic distribution of CRH, suspected from the results of bioassay studies, has now been confirmed by immunohistochemical methods. Its distribution in the gut now confirms that CRH is a gut-brain peptide.

Prolactin Regulating Factors

Prolactin Release Inhibiting Factor (PIF)

In keeping with the observation that the hypothalamus exerts an inhibitory effect on prolactin secretion is the finding that crude hypothalamic extracts inhibit prolactin release. This bioactivity has been termed 'PIF' by Meites (1966). PIF has been identified in portal vessel blood by Kamberi and colleagues (1971), thus

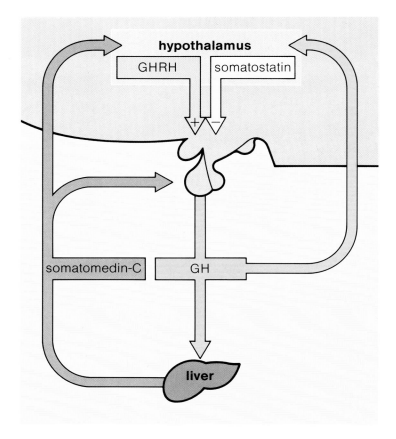

Fig. 1.15 Diagrammatic representation of the regulation of GH secretion. The secretion of GH is stimulated by GHRH from the hypothalamus, and inhibited by somatostatin release. Each of the hormones is secreted by a distinct population of tuberoinfundibular neurons. At the level of the pituitary, the stimulating effect of GHRH is modulated by somatomedin-C, a peptide formed in the liver under the influence of GH; thus somatomedin-C becomes part of the negative feedback loop control of GH secretion. The release of somatostatin by the hypothalamus is stimulated by both GH and somatomedin-C, thus comprising the hypothalamic part of the negative feedback loop for GH regulation. Redrawn from Reichlin (1985), by courtesy of the publishers, W.B. Saunders Company.

satisfying one of the critical requirements for proof of physiological significance of a hypophysiotrophic hormone.

Extensive efforts to determine the chemical structure of PIF have been undertaken in several laboratories. Dopamine is an important prolactin release inhibiting factor. This biogenic amine, the secretory product of the tuberohypophyseal dopaminergic pathways, is present in hypophyseal portal vessel blood in sufficient concentration to inhibit prolactin release. Other prolactin release inhibiting factors are GABA and GAP.

Prolactin Releasing Factor (PRF)

Although stalk section and transplantation experiments indicate that the predominant effect of the hypothalamus on prolactin secretion is inhibitory, the acute release of prolactin seen after suckling and acute stress have raised the possibility that there may also be prolactin releasing factors. Indeed TRH is a potent PRF. VIP is also a potent PRF and is synergistic with a co-secreted peptide PHI and there may be others in addition. Using neuropharmacological analysis PIF functions are generally

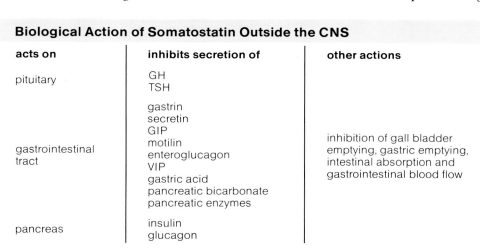

Biological Action of Somatostatin Outside the CNS

acts on	inhibits secretion of	other actions
pituitary	GH TSH	
gastrointestinal tract	gastrin secretin GIP motilin enteroglucagon VIP gastric acid pancreatic bicarbonate pancreatic enzymes	inhibition of gall bladder emptying, gastric emptying, intestinal absorption and gastrointestinal blood flow
pancreas	insulin glucagon	

Fig. 1.16 Table listing the biological actions of somatostatin outside the central nervous system.

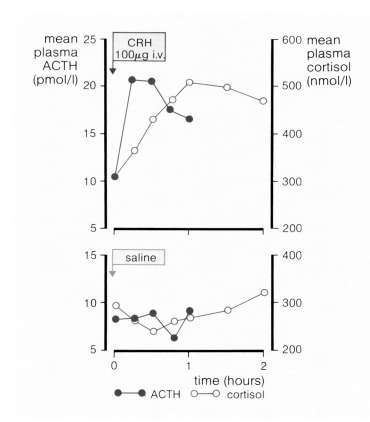

Fig. 1.17 **Graph showing ACTH release in response to synthetic corticotrophin releasing hormone (CRH).** Six normal men were injected with 100μg of CRH. The initial rise in mean plasma ACTH was followed by an increase in mean plasma cortisol. Control values after saline injections are also shown. Redrawn from Grossman et al. (1982), by courtesy of the publishers, Lancet Ltd.

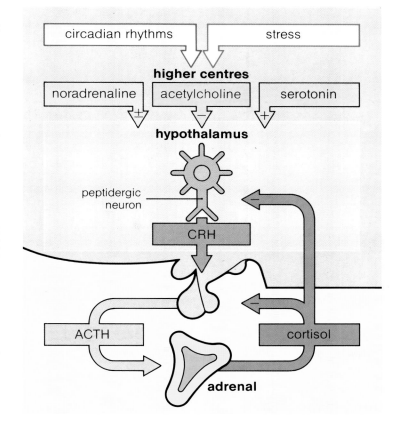

Fig. 1.18 **Diagram illustrating the regulation of ACTH secretion.** The secretion of ACTH is stimulated by CRH, and inhibited by the feedback effects of cortisol exerted directly at the level of the pituitary. The effect of cortisol on the secretion of CRH has not been elucidated, but a negative feedback effect on the hypothalamus may also be involved. Redrawn from Martin et al. (1977), by courtesy of the publishers, F.A. Davis Company.

thought to be under dopaminergic control, whereas PRF influences are thought to be mediated via serotoninergic systems.

NEUROPEPTIDES AND THEIR ENDOCRINE SIGNIFICANCE

In addition to the enkephalins and the hypophysiotrophic peptides, several other peptides have been demonstrated to occur in neurons distributed to the hypothalamus and other brain regions. Almost all are represented in characteristic glandular cells of the gastrointestinal tract, and are believed to arise in embryological life from the primitive neuroectoderm (APUD system).

Substance P is present in high concentration in the hypothalamus as well as other brain areas. Little is present in the median eminence, suggesting that there is no direct tuberoinfundibular input, but the rich innervation of most hypothalamic nuclei nevertheless suggests a regulatory role for this peptide.

Other neuropeptides with hypothalamic distribution of nerve endings are met-enkephalin (an opioid peptide), angiotensin II, neurotensin, gastrin and cholecystokinin. The presence of met-enkephalin-containing cell bodies in the hypothalamus with a median eminence distribution supports the hypothesis of an intrinsic hypothalamic control system for this peptide, as well as a system with projections from other parts of the brain.

These neuropeptides have been found to exert changes in part in hindbrain regions but there are also smaller bioaminergic systems which are self-contained in the hypothalamus. Secretion of several pituitary hormones is also affected by the neuropeptides.

NEUROTRANSMITTER REGULATION OF HYPOTHALAMIC HORMONES

The hypophysiotrophic neurons themselves are regulated by hormonal, neuropeptide and neurotransmitter influences, the latter arising from well-defined bioamine pathways that rise in the hypothalamus, and elsewhere in the brain (Fig. 1.19). One of the neurotransmitters, dopamine, is also a hypophysiotrophic hormone. It arises in the hypothalamus from a group of tuberohypophyseal neurons, is secreted into the portal vessel blood, and inhibits prolactin secretion. Biogenic amines (including dopamine) influence other pituitary secretions by their effect on hypophysiotrophic neurons.

Secretions of the hypothalamic neurons control the anterior pituitary gland. These neurons are in turn influenced by neuropeptides, neurotransmitters and the feedback effects of various hormones. These various influences are integrated with other mechanisms for control of visceral and homeostatic function.

The central adrenergic pathways are important, not only for regulation of pituitary function but for a number of important visceral and homeostatic functions. Ascending noradrenergic fibres stimulate gonadotrophin, ACTH and GH secretion, regulate the level of alertness in the reticular activating system and have important effects on eating and drinking behaviour. The ascending serotoninergic system stimulates GH, prolactin and ACTH secretion. Central dopaminergic, noradrenergic and serotoninergic systems are involved in determination of affective state, and may be involved in the pathogenesis of the major psychoses. Drugs used in clinical psychiatry that modulate this system may also influence endocrine function; for example, dopamine agonists inhibit prolactin release, and dopamine antagonists stimulate prolactin release.

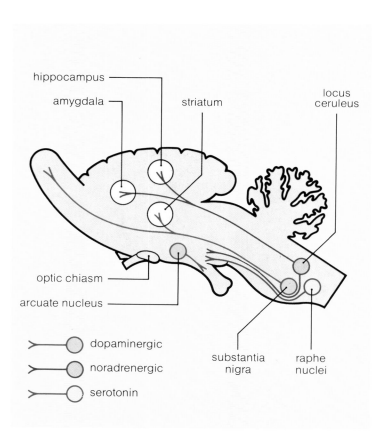

Fig. 1.19 Diagram showing the ascending bioaminergic tracts involved in hypothalamo-pituitary function in the rat.
Dopaminergic fibres comprise one group whose origin is in the *substantia nigra* in the midbrain, and projection in the basal ganglia; this serves as part of the extrapyramidal system. An intrinsic tuberoinfundibular system is responsible for dopamine secretion into the hypophyseal-portal system which regulates prolactin secretion. Not shown is the mesolimbic system that innervates the visceral brain. Ascending fibres from the *locus ceruleus* bring noradrenergic influences into the hypothalamus, and fibres from the raphe nuclei carry serotoninergic signals into the hypothalamus and elsewhere. All these neurotransmitter pathways are involved in the regulation of the anterior and posterior pituitary, in addition to other important visceral and behavioural effects. Redrawn from Martin et al. (1977), by courtesy of the publishers, F.A. Davis Company.

2 Hypopituitarism

John A H Wass, MD, FRCP

Hypopituitarism means the partial or complete deficiency of anterior and posterior pituitary hormone secretion. It occurs frequently in clinical endocrine practice and causes a wide variety of symptoms and signs which are influenced by the aetiology and rate of onset of the disorder. When hypopituitarism is slow in onset, the diagnosis may be delayed, often for many years. Hypopituitarism may be associated either with pathological processes which destroy the pituitary itself, or with those that destroy the hypothalamus and thus interfere with the hypothalamic hormone control of the pituitary gland.

Causes of Hypopituitarism

pituitary and
parapituitary tumours

trauma

radiotherapy

infarction
(pituitary apoplexy)

infiltrations
e.g. sarcoidosis,
histiocytosis and
haemochromatosis

infections
e.g. tuberculosis,
abscess, syphilis

Sheehan's syndrome

Fig. 2.1   Table of the causes of hypopituitarism. Hypopituitarism is most commonly caused by the presence of a pituitary tumour.

Pituitary and Parapituitary Tumours

anterior pituitary		**parapituitary**
FUNCTIONING	NON-FUNCTIONING	pinealoma (ectopic)
prolactin-secreting		craniopharyngioma
	adenoma	
GH-secreting		chordoma
ACTH-secreting	carcinoma	optic nerve glioma
TSH- or gonadotrophin-secreting		reticulosis
	sarcoma	sphenoidal ridge meningioma
posterior pituitary		
ganglioneuroma	astrocytoma (very rare)	secondary deposits e.g. from breast and lung

Fig. 2.2   Table of pituitary and parapituitary tumours. The anterior pituitary tumours which produce hormones (i.e. prolactin-, GH-, ACTH-, TSH- and gonadotrophin-secreting) are called 'functioning' tumours.

Characteristics of the Functioning Anterior Pituitary Tumours

tumour	staining characteristics		mean granule diameter (nm)
	H and E	**PAS-OG**	
GH-secreting	acidophil	yellow	450
prolactin-secreting	acidophil	yellow	550
TSH-secreting	basophil	magenta	135
LH-secreting FSH-secreting	basophil	magenta	200
ACTH-secreting β-LPH-secreting	basophil	magenta	360

Fig. 2.3   Table of the staining characteristics and granule size of the functioning tumours of the anterior pituitary. The periodic acid Schiff-orange (PAS-OG) staining technique is less subjective than haematoxylin and eosin (H and E) staining. Evaluation of the size of intracellular granules by electron microscopy may also be useful.

CAUSES OF HYPOPITUITARISM

Hypopituitarism is most commonly caused by the presence of a pituitary tumour (Figs. 2.1 and 2.2). These are usually benign and most frequently arise from the anterior lobe. Pituitary carcinoma is very rare indeed. Pituitary microadenomas, tumours

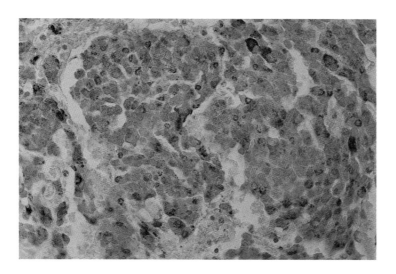

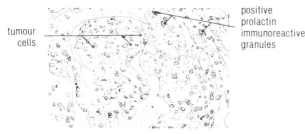

Fig. 2.4   Immunostaining of a histological section of a prolactinoma. The majority of the tumour cells contain fine, brown cytoplasmic granules thus indicating a positive immunoperoxidase reaction with anti-prolactin antibody. Immunoperoxidase and haematoxylin stain, magnification x 100. By courtesy of Prof. I. Doniach.

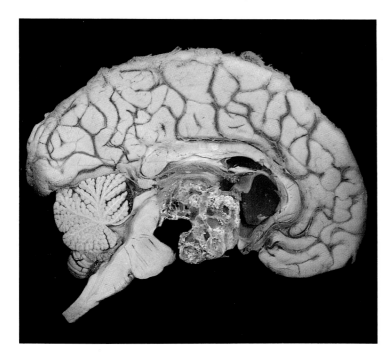

Fig. 2.5   Macropathology of a craniopharyngioma. This photograph shows a large, cystic, calcified craniopharyngioma in a hemisected brain. The lesion extends into the substance of the brain.

less than 10mm in diameter, the size of the normal gland, have a surprisingly high incidence and are present in approximately one quarter of all patients examined at autopsy. Their clinical significance is currently unknown, and because of their small size they are only very occasionally associated with hypopituitarism. Pituitary tumours range widely in size and may extend outside the pituitary fossa to compress surrounding structures.

Pituitary Tumours

Pituitary tumours account for ten per cent of clinically significant intracranial tumours. Currently, they are most frequently classified as 'functioning' or 'non-functioning' depending on whether a hormone is produced (e.g. prolactin, growth hormone-GH and adrenocorticotrophic hormone-ACTH). They are also classified according to the immunohistochemical staining characteristics of the pituitary tumour (Fig. 2.3). Since interpretation of tumour sections may be extremely subjective using the haematoxylin and eosin (H and E) stain, current practice is to use the periodic acid Schiff-orange G stain (PAS-OG). Evaluation of the size of the intracellular granules by electron microscopy is also useful since prolactin-secreting and GH-secreting adenomas have the largest intracellular granules (prolactin granule mean diameter is 550nm).

Lactotroph cell tumours or prolactinomas (Fig. 2.4) are one of the most common pituitary tumours, accounting for approximately sixty per cent of all pituitary tumours. For many years, these tumours were considered to be non-functioning; however, with the discovery of human prolactin and with the development of radioimmunoassays, it has become clear that most of these so-called non-functioning pituitary tumours are prolactinomas. The incidence of truly non-functioning adenomas varies, but is usually approximately twenty per cent.

Somatotroph cell adenomas (approximately fifteen per cent of pituitary tumours) are usually associated with gigantism before epiphyseal fusion or acromegaly after epiphyseal fusion, or occasionally both. Acromegaly is the commoner manifestation, as pituitary tumours occur most frequently in middle-age and only rarely in childhood. Large tumours or macroadenomas are often locally invasive, rendering complete surgical removal difficult or impossible. Many pituitary tumours have mixed cell populations, for example, somatotroph and lactotroph cells are associated with both increased GH and prolactin secretion. However, with 'mixed cell' tumours, the same cell is only rarely found to contain both hormones.

Corticotroph cell adenomas (around five per cent of pituitary tumours) are the cause of Cushing's disease. They may be as small as 2mm in diameter and are usually located in the centre of the gland. It is therefore unusual for these corticotroph cell adenomas to be associated with a radiological abnormality of the pituitary fossa or with hypopituitarism.

Thyrotroph and gonadotroph cell adenomas are exceedingly rare with an incidence of less than one per cent. Large non-secreting tumours may cause hypopituitarism by compressing the pituitary stalk and interfering with the delivery of hypothalamic hormones to the anterior pituitary. If dopamine secretion is interfered with in this way, hyperprolactinaemia may also ensue. Hypopituitarism can also occur as a result of compression of secretory cells in the normal gland by the pituitary tumour.

Other Causes of Hypopituitarism

Parapituitary tumours are rare and of these, craniopharyngiomas, evolved embryologically from Rathke's pouch, are the most common (Fig. 2.5). They occur above or more rarely in, the sella turcica and may be solid or cystic. The majority (70%) show calcification above the sella turcica (Fig. 2.6). These tumours may contain an oily fluid in which cholesterol crystals are present, and are characteristically lined by squamous epithelial cells. Fifty per cent of cases occur in patients under the age of fifteen years. Patients commonly present with GH deficiency and diabetes insipidus, with or without visual field defects.

Other tumours may compress the pituitary stalk and cause hypopituitarism; these include meningiomas arising from the sphenoidal ridge and, very rarely, germinomas and chordomas. Metastases from lung and breast carcinomas to the hypothalamus and pituitary are well documented, but rare.

In addition, operative surgery and irradiation for the treatment of pituitary tumours can also lead to hypopituitarism. Cranial irradiation for other reasons (e.g. leukaemia) is an increasingly common cause of GH deficiency in children because of

hypothalamic damage. Very rarely, severe head trauma causes pituitary insufficiency by damaging the pituitary stalk. Previously, post-partum haemorrhage was a more common cause of hypopituitarism. The associated hypopituitarism resulted from pituitary infarction, and is called Sheehan's syndrome. This is now mainly confined to developing countries in which obstetric services are less well-developed.

Several granulomatous or infiltrative processes, including sarcoidosis or histiocytosis-X may involve the hypothalamus and cause hypopituitarism particularly diabetes insipidus. Infections such as tuberculosis are now seen only rarely but may cause hypopituitarism associated with basal meningitis.

Isolated disorders of pituitary hormone secretion can occur in the absence of structural lesions of either the hypothalamus or pituitary. Thus, GH, luteinizing hormone (LH) and follicle-stimulating hormone (FSH) deficiency can occur as isolated

Fig. 2.6 Radiograph of a pituitary fossa in hypopituitarism. A mass of amorphous calcification extends upwards from the tip of the dorsum sellae, which is typical of a craniopharyngioma.

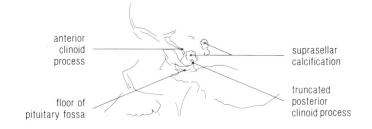

Fig. 2.7 **The development of trophic hormone deficiency in hypopituitarism.** As the disease progresses there is a characteristic order in the development of hormone deficiency. Usually GH secretion fails first, with ACTH secretion failing much later on.

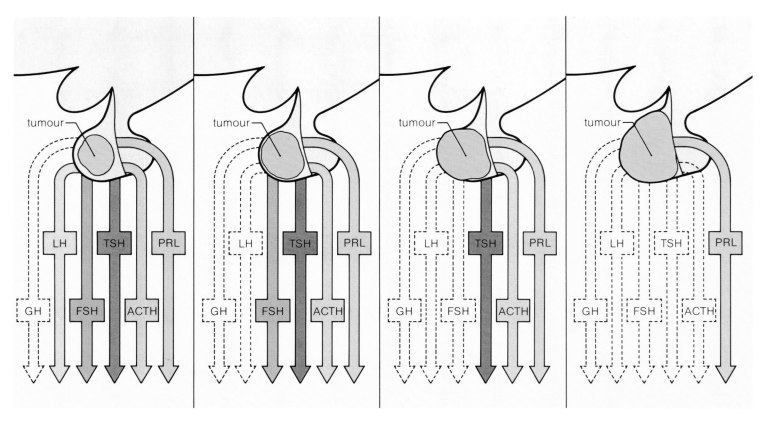

2.4

Prolactin (PRL) deficiency is rare except when associated with an early failure of lactation in Sheehan's syndrome. ADH deficiency is rare in patients with anterior pituitary tumours, but may be seen with causes affecting hypothalamic ADH secretion (e.g. head trauma).

phenomena. It is currently believed that these disorders result from isolated defects in hypothalamic hormone secretion: GH deficiency may be due to a congenital deficiency of GHRH, with LH and FSH deficiency resulting from deficient gonadotrophin releasing hormone (GnRH) secretion (i.e. Kallmann's syndrome). Isolated thyroid stimulating hormone (TSH) and ACTH deficiencies occur less commonly, and are presumably associated with deficient thyrotrophin releasing hormone (TRH) or corticotrophin releasing hormone (CRH) secretion respectively.

SYMPTOMS ASSOCIATED WITH HYPOPITUITARISM

Although symptoms may be caused by local pressure effects in patients with pituitary or parapituitary tumours, the clinical picture of hypopituitarism chiefly results from pituitary hormone

deficiency. Symptoms and signs vary widely but early symptoms of hypopituitarism relate mostly to hypogonadism in both sexes.

In progressive hypopituitarism there is a characteristic order in the development of hormone deficiency (Fig. 2.7). Usually secretion of GH and LH fails first; this is followed, later, by failure of FSH and TSH, and finally the secretion of ACTH fails. Prolactin deficiency is rare except in Sheehan's syndrome, where it is associated with a failure of lactation; when this occurs it occurs early. Antidiuretic hormone (ADH or vasopressin) deficiency is extremely uncommon in patients with pituitary tumours, although it may occasionally be seen in patients following head injuries or any other factors which interfere with hypothalamic ADH secretion. The result is diabetes insipidus. The effects of severe hypopituitarism are illustrated in Figure 2.8.

Fig. 2.8 Diagram of the clinical effects of pituitary hormone deficiency in hypopituitarism.

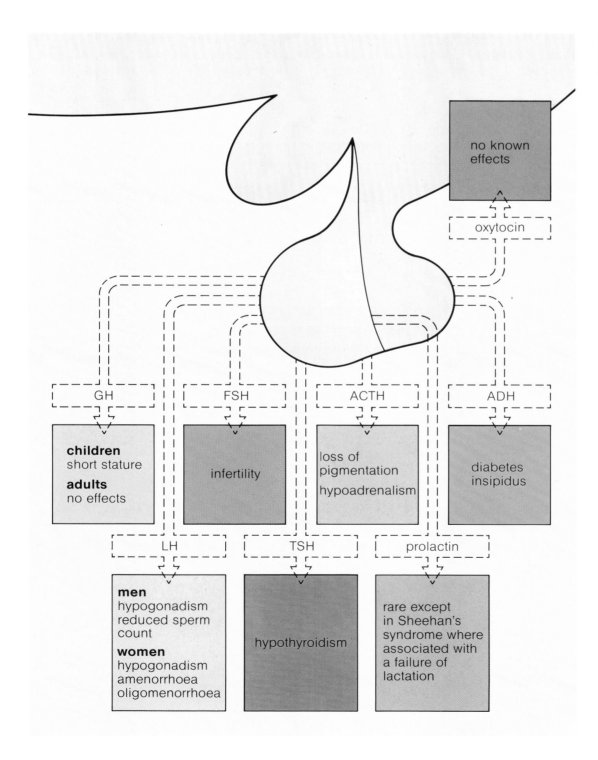

2.5

Symptoms of Deficient Anterior Pituitary Hormone Secretion

GH deficiency causes short stature in children and sometimes retarded bone development. It occurs most often as an isolated congenital defect (e.g. isolated GHRH deficiency) or in association with a craniopharyngioma, pituitary tumour or after brain irradiation for malignancy. Effective treatment with parenteral biosynthetic GH or GHRH is now available, although the potential for catch-up growth decreases as the child becomes older. Early diagnosis is therefore essential. At birth, these children look normal. Growth failure can usually be recognised between one and three years of age but may only be detected much later. Untreated, growth continues at between fifty to sixty per cent of the normal rate. Body and facial features remain immature and the patient is usually fat due to the absent lipolytic action of GH (Fig. 2.9). Body proportions and mental development are normal and congruous with chronological age. Investigation of these children shows retarded bone age in parallel with their height. GH secretion is deficient on provocative challenge (e.g. insulin-induced hypoglycaemia or arginine stimulation). There are no serious clinical sequelae of GH deficiency in adults.

Gonadotrophin deficiency also occurs early in progressive hypopituitarism. Thus patients with gonadal dysfunction should be investigated to avoid delayed diagnosis of a pituitary or parapituitary lesion. In women, gonadotrophin deficiency leads to inadequate oestrogen secretion which may result in amenorrhoea and infertility (Fig. 2.10). Oestrogen deficiency also causes dyspareunia and atrophy of the breasts. Loss of secondary sexual hair occurs in both sexes after several years (Fig. 2.11). In men, the chief symptoms of gonadotrophin deficiency are poor libido and impotence, with infertility resulting from a decrease in sperm production. The testicles become smaller and soft. Beard growth may take many years to regress and may be normal for some time after libido and sexual function have been impaired. In both sexes there is fine wrinkling of the skin, particularly around the mouth and eyes (see Chapter 10). If gonadotrophin secretion fails in childhood, while GH remains normal, there will be excessive linear growth due to failure of closure of the epiphyses. Thus a eunuchoid proportion develops, with span exceeding height.

TSH-secreting and ACTH-secreting cells are usually the last to fail in progressive hypopituitarism. TSH deficiency (Fig. 2.12) is associated with growth retardation in children. In adults, the most marked features are constipation, a decrease in energy, an increased sensitivity to cold, dry skin and weight gain; however, the features are not so marked as in primary hypothyroidism, presumably because the deficiency is usually less severe. Lack of ACTH secretion produces the symptoms of hypoadrenalism, particularly weakness and tiredness, nausea and vomiting, progressing to dizziness on standing resulting from postural hypotension. ACTH deficiency results in reduced adrenal androgen secretion and contributes to the decreased libido and loss of secondary sexual hair seen in hypopituitarism. In pituitary

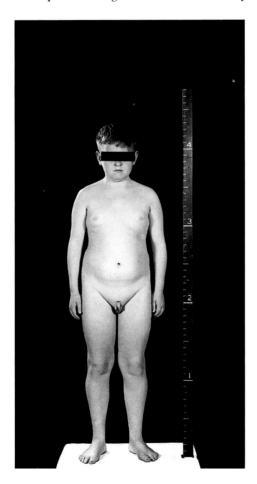

Symptoms of Gonadotrophin Deficiency

women

amenorrhoea

infertility

dyspareunia

breast atrophy

loss of secondary sexual hair

men

poor libido and impotence

infertility

small, soft testicles

loss of secondary sexual hair

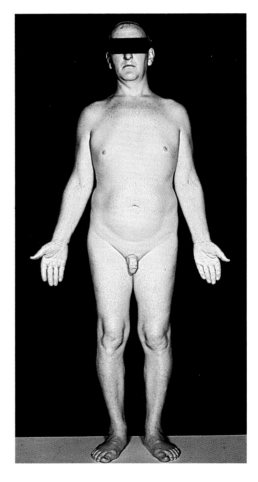

Fig. 2.9 Photograph of a fifteen-year-old boy with GH deficiency associated with hypopituitarism. This patient has short stature for his age and under-developed genitalia.

Fig. 2.10 Table of the symptoms of gonadotrophin deficiency in hypopituitarism.

Fig. 2.11 Photograph of a patient with hypogonadism resulting from a tumour. This hypopituitary patient shows regression of secondary sexual characteristics with absent pubic hair, as a result of the gonadotrophin deficiency caused by a pituitary tumour.

ACTH deficiency, there is also pallor of the skin (Fig. 2.13). Hypoglycaemia can occur in hypoadrenalism for two reasons: firstly, because of increased insulin sensitivity due to cortisol lack (cortisol is an insulin antagonist), and secondly, adrenal insufficiency decreases hepatic glycogen reserves. In advanced hypopituitarism, collapse, coma and even death are possible due to a combination of hypoglycaemia, hypothyroidism, hypothermia and hypotension. Most patients with hypopituitarism, even in the advanced stage, are well-nourished. However, severe, prolonged hypopituitarism can produce extreme weight loss and an appearance of malnutrition ('pituitary cachexia') which may be clinically indistinguishable from anorexia nervosa.

The clinical appearance of hypopituitarism may be complicated. Patients with large tumours secreting prolactin, GH or ACTH may have hypopituitarism despite over-secretion of one particular hormone. Thus, in the acromegalic patient shown in Figure 2.14, the pallor and texture of the skin is consistent with coexistent hypopituitarism.

Table of the Symptoms of TSH and ACTH Deficiency

TSH deficiency	ACTH deficiency
in children growth retardation	weakness
	tiredness
in adults decrease in energy	dizziness on standing
constipation sensitivity to cold	pallor
dry skin weight gain	hypoglycaemia

Fig. 2.12 Table of the symptoms of TSH and ACTH deficiency. As well as the symptoms listed, in advanced hypopituitarism, TSH and ACTH deficiency may lead to collapse, coma and death.

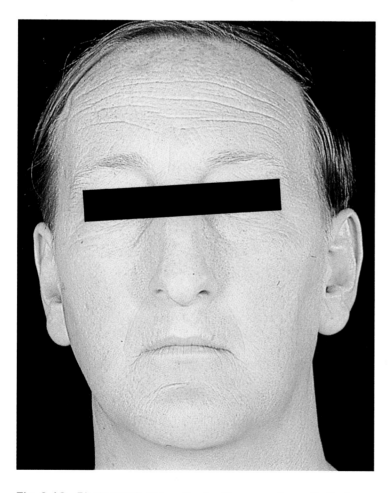

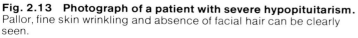

Fig. 2.13 Photograph of a patient with severe hypopituitarism. Pallor, fine skin wrinkling and absence of facial hair can be clearly seen.

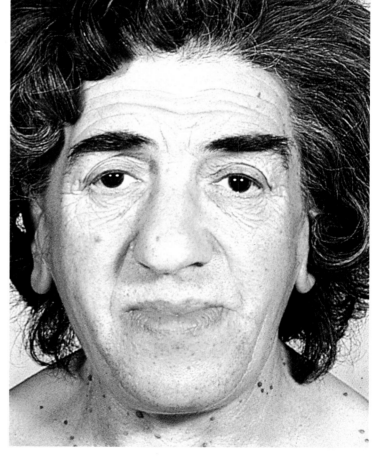

Fig. 2.14 Photograph of a patient with concomitant acromegaly and hypopituitarism. The presence of a GH-secreting pituitary tumour was the cause of the symptoms in this patient.

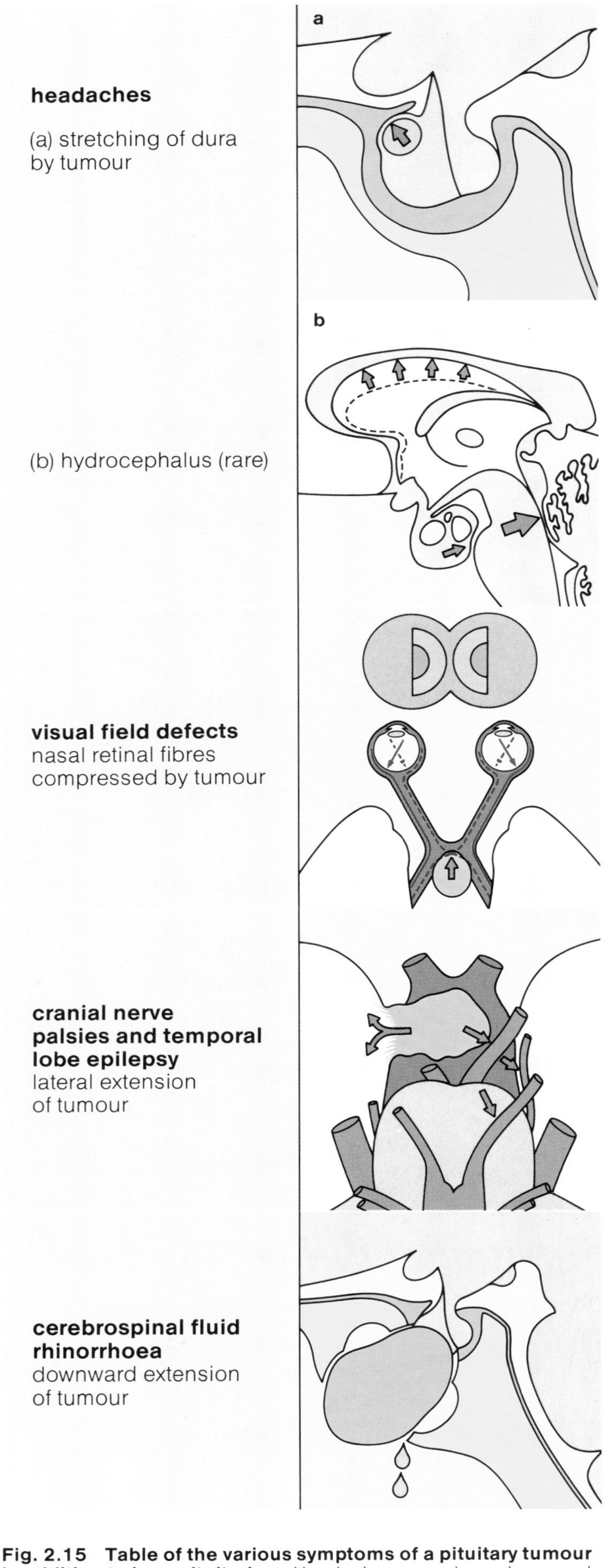

headaches

(a) stretching of dura by tumour

(b) hydrocephalus (rare)

visual field defects
nasal retinal fibres compressed by tumour

cranial nerve palsies and temporal lobe epilepsy
lateral extension of tumour

cerebrospinal fluid rhinorrhoea
downward extension of tumour

Fig. 2.15 Table of the various symptoms of a pituitary tumour in addition to hypopituitarism. Headaches are only rarely caused by hydrocephalus. Visual field defects caused by extension of the tumour are readily plotted using the Goldmann perimeter.

Symptoms Associated with Pressure Effects Due to Hypothalamic or Pituitary Lesions

Headaches are caused by local pressure from a tumour and probably result from stretching of the dura mater above the pituitary fossa in a patient with a pituitary tumour (Fig. 2.15). Rarely, they can be caused by a suprasellar tumour (e.g. a craniopharyngioma) which compresses the aqueduct of Sylvius and thus prevents the passage of cerebrospinal fluid (CSF) between the third and fourth ventricles. This results in hydrocephalus and enlargement of the third and lateral ventricles. In general, headaches caused by pressure effects are variable in location and are intermittent.

If a large pituitary or parapituitary tumour compresses the optic chiasm it may cause visual field defects. The nasal visual fields are transmitted by the temporal retinal fibres. The temporal visual fields are transmitted by the nasal retinal fibres and these fibres cross at the optic chiasm. Therefore if, as most frequently happens, a pituitary tumour grows upwards centrally towards the chiasm, the nasal central fibres become compressed causing initially an upper outer quadrant field defect. If the pressure on the chiasm continues, a complete bitemporal hemianopia may occur. With long-standing compression, this will progress to irreversible optic atrophy and blindness. The growth of the tumour and the resultant visual field defects may, however, be asymmetrical.

Lateral extension of parapituitary or pituitary tumours is less common. In approximately five per cent of patients with a pituitary tumour, there is extension into the cavernous sinus; this may cause cranial nerve palsies resulting from compression of the third, fourth or sixth cranial nerves. Very rarely, pituitary tumours extend into the temporal lobe of the brain causing epilepsy. If a tumour extends downwards, it may erode the sphenoid bone through to the sphenoid sinus and postnasal space, thus the patient may present with CSF rhinorrhoea. In contrast to the 'runny nose' of the cold, the fluid discharged contains glucose. Hypothalamic disturbance may produce disturbed consciousness, abnormal thirst, hyperphagia or abnormal temperature regulation.

DIAGNOSIS

Investigation of Patients with Space-Occupying Lesions Causing Hypopituitarism

Both anatomical and physiological aspects of the pituitary should be considered when investigating a patient with suspected hypopituitarism. From the anatomical point of view, one of the most important tests is that for visual fields, as these may indicate chiasmal compression (e.g. resulting from a pituitary tumour). For early diagnosis of such lesions, peripheral vision is assessed using a red pin, the patient informing the doctor when the colour red appears in his outer field of view (Fig. 2.16). Red colour perception is lost before other colours or white light. Visual fields should also be plotted using the Goldmann perimeter. Typical Goldmann plots showing bitemporal field defects are illustrated in Figure 2.16.

Plain radiography of the pituitary region is essential, and lateral (Fig. 2.17) and anteroposterior (AP) views of the pituitary fossa should be taken. Frequently, pituitary tumours increase the overall size of the fossa and cause blistering or ballooning of the floor of the pituitary fossa (see Chapter 21). Suprasellar calcification may be seen if a craniopharyngioma is present. The AP view is also helpful when looking at the pituitary region. Normally the floor of the pituitary fossa is flat. If there is an obvious dip in the floor of the sella turcica this may indicate a tumour (Fig. 2.18). The position of this indentation may also show the location of the tumour within the pituitary gland. The presence of a normal pituitary fossa does not preclude the presence of a pituitary tumour since ninety per cent of patient's with Cushing's disease and twenty per cent of prolactinoma patients also have normal fossae. With parasellar lesions causing hypopituitarism, the plain skull radiographs may be normal and an abnormality may only be revealed using computed tomographic (CT) scanning.

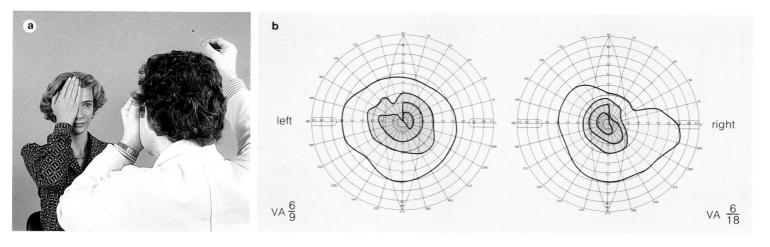

Fig. 2.16 The clinical assessment of visual field defects. Visual fields are tested accurately using a red pin, photograph (a), and the results are recorded on a Goldmann field plot shown in view (b) which also shows visual acuity (VA). In this patient, bitemporal field defects were found. Classically, this results from chiasmal compression by a suprasellar extension.

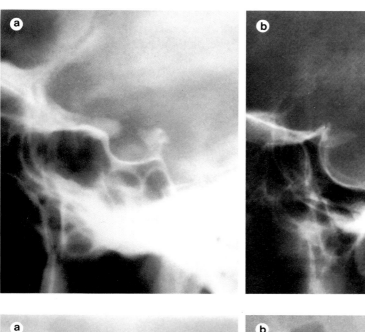

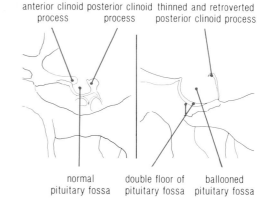

Fig. 2.17 Lateral skull radiography: comparison of (a) a normal and (b) a ballooned pituitary fossa. The ballooning of the floor of the fossa in view (b) is caused by the presence of a pituitary tumour which compresses and enlarges the surrounding fossa.

anterior clinoid process   posterior clinoid process   thinned and retroverted posterior clinoid process

normal pituitary fossa   double floor of pituitary fossa   ballooned pituitary fossa

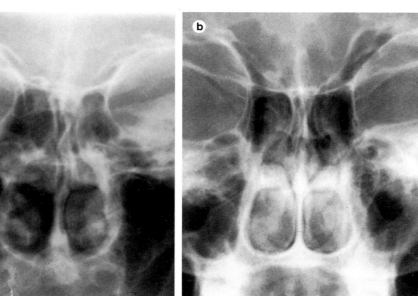

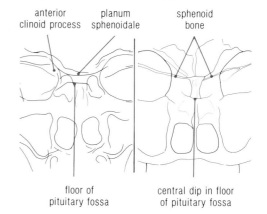

Fig. 2.18 Skull radiography: antero-posterior (AP) views of (a) a normal fossa and (b) an abnormal pituitary fossa resulting from a pituitary tumour. The depression in the floor of the pituitary fossa caused by the tumour can be seen, when compared with the normal appearance.

anterior clinoid process   planum sphenoidale   sphenoid bone

floor of pituitary fossa   central dip in floor of pituitary fossa

2.9

Contrast studies can be used to define the upper border of the tumour and its relationship to the optic nerve. In pneumo-encephalography, air is injected into the suprasellar space via lumbar puncture (Fig. 2.19). However, headaches and vomiting may be associated with this technique. Positive contrast cisterno-graphy is another means of demonstrating the suprasellar space. A water-soluble contrast medium (e.g. metrizamide) is injected into the subarachnoid space by cisternal puncture in the neck. Using this method a good outline of the suprasellar region is achieved with fewer side-effects than pneumoencephalography. However, these contrast procedures have now largely been superseded by the use of CT scanning on machines with facilities for reformation.

With CT scanning, radiographic attenuation values obtained from a scan are processed by computer to determine the density of each tissue appearing on the scan, and results are shown in the form of a cross-sectional picture on the viewing screen (Fig. 2.20). This technique is useful for delineating pituitary tumours with suprasellar and lateral extensions as well as parasellar lesions. The use of third generation scanners has greatly improved pituitary imaging and three dimensional views can be obtained.

In the 'empty sella' syndrome, an enlarged pituitary sella is usually filled with CSF. This classically occurs in obese women who have headaches, but may occur in symptom-free patients where the radiographic appearance is often found incidentally. The aetiology is unclear but may result from herniation of arachnoid through the diaphragma sellae. Pituitary function is

Fig. 2.19 Air encephalogram of a pituitary tumour.
The encephalogram shows no suprasellar extension.

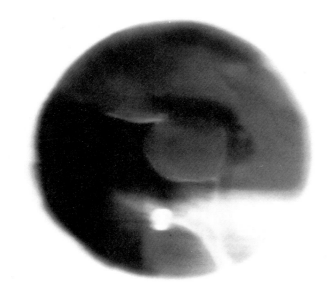

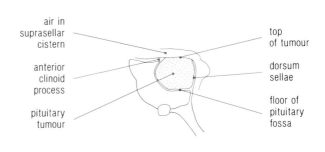

Fig. 2.20 CT scans of a pituitary tumour. View (a) shows a suprasellar extension of the tumour, and view (b) shows a lateral extension into the cavernous sinus, which may cause palsies of the III, IV or VI cranial nerves; if the lateral extension also passes inferiorly, periorbital pain may occur due to pressure on the ophthalmic branch of the trigeminal nerve.

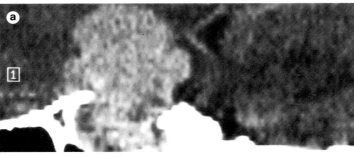

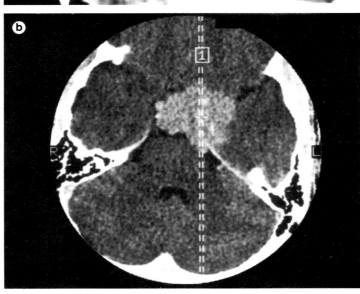

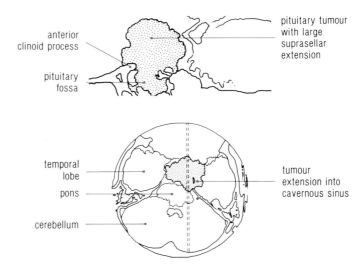

usually normal. In some patients, an enlarged sella may represent an infarcted tumour, in which case the empty sella syndrome may be associated with hyperprolactinaemia, acromegaly, Cushing's disease, a non-functioning tumour or hypopituitarism.

Endocrine Assessment of Patients with Hypopituitarism

When assessing pituitary function in the hypopituitary patient, anterior pituitary function should be tested and corrected before that of the posterior pituitary. The reason for this is that decreased ACTH secretion causes a reduction in cortisol from the adrenal gland; this subsequently decreases the glomerular filtration rate which can thus obscure the symptoms of polyuria in diabetes insipidus (Fig. 2.21).

Basal hormone levels yield much information; it is therefore important to directly measure, by radioimmunoassay, serum concentrations of prolactin, TSH, thyroxine, cortisol, LH, FSH, testosterone in men and oestrogen (oestradiol) in women. The correlation between the pituitary hormone level and the target organ hormone will help to establish the cause of underactivity in a target gland (Fig. 2.22). For example, in a patient with hypothyroidism, low or normal TSH levels combined with low thyroxine levels imply pituitary gland malfunction or pituitary hypothyroidism. High TSH concentrations combined with a low thyroxine level indicate disease in the thyroid gland itself (i.e. primary hypothyroidism).

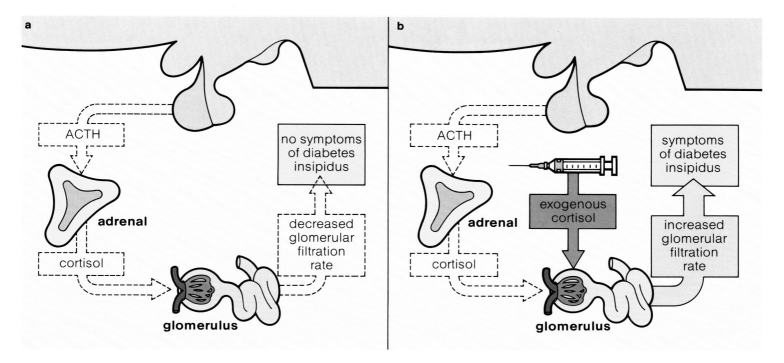

Fig. 2.21 Diagram showing the effect of decreased ACTH on glomerular filtration rate with concomitant ADH deficiency. In (a), the symptoms of diabetes insipidus are obscured by ACTH deficiency. These symptoms may appear for the first time with administration of cortisol (hydrocortisone), either orally or intramuscularly as shown in (b).

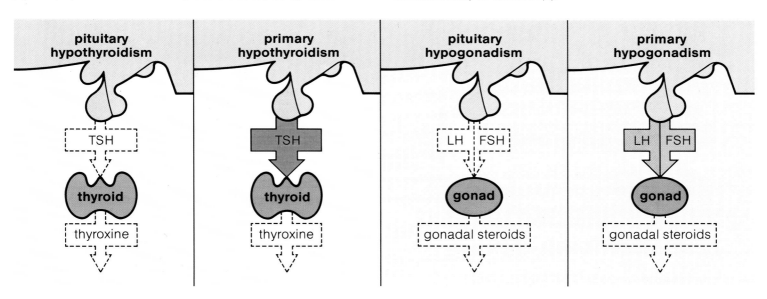

Fig. 2.22 The assessment of pituitary and target organ hormones in the diagnosis of hypopituitarism. The importance of simultaneous measurements of pituitary and target organ hormone levels should be emphasised. In hypothyroidism, low TSH in conjunction with low thyroxine implies pituitary failure in contrast to low thyroxine alone which implies thyroid failure. Similarly, hypogonadal patients have low testosterone or oestradiol in the presence of (inappropriately) low gonadotrophins.

2.11

After the assessment of basal hormone levels, dynamic tests are used to assess hormonal reserves. GH and ACTH secretion in most cases can be tested using the insulin hypoglycaemia test (Fig. 2.23), where insulin is given intravenously. Hypoglycaemia causes symptoms of neuroglycopenia such as sweating and tachycardia, with concomitant ACTH and GH release. Provided adequate hypoglycaemia is induced, cortisol levels should rise to above 580nmol/l (21μg/100ml) and GH levels to above 20mu/l (10ng/ml). If these levels are not achieved, the patient is deficient in either ACTH or GH. Intravenous GnRH and TRH may be given simultaneously to assess the secretory reserves of LH, FSH and TSH.

Patients unable to undergo insulin hypoglycaemia tests (e.g. those with a history of epilepsy or ischaemic heart disease) can be given 1mg glucagon, subcutaneously, instead. This causes a transient rise in blood glucose and during the subsequent fall cortisol and GH are released. Glucagon is a less reliable stimulus

than insulin, and in twenty per cent of patients there is no rise in ACTH or GH levels, even in the presence of normal reserves of these hormones. Arginine infusion stimulates GH secretion and may be used to assess GH reserves in some cases.

Assessment of Posterior Pituitary Hormone Secretion

The rise in plasma osmolality resulting from lack of fluid for a period of several hours stimulates ADH secretion; this forms the basis of the standard eight-hour water deprivation test which is used in the diagnosis of diabetes insipidus (Fig. 2.24). This test should be performed during the day when careful observation is possible, as severe fluid and electrolyte depletion can occur. Urine and plasma osmolality are measured for eight hours, after which a synthetic analogue of ADH, desmopressin, is given intramuscularly. The urine osmolality is then remeasured. As ADH is secreted, water is normally absorbed, with the subsequent elevation of urine osmolality. After desmopressin administration

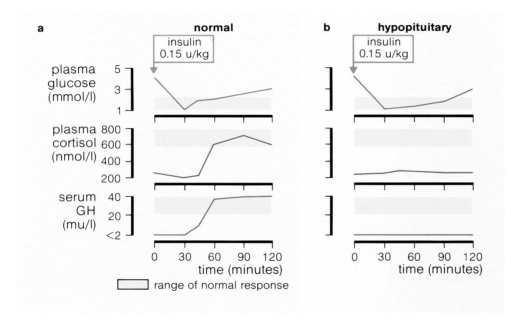

range of normal response

Fig. 2.23 The insulin hypoglycaemia test in the diagnosis of hypopituitarism. Graphs of plasma glucose, plasma cortisol and serum GH levels in (a) a normal and (b) a hypopituitary subject are shown. GH levels should rise to a minimum of 20mu/l and cortisol to 580nmol/l provided adequate hypoglycaemia is reached with blood glucose concentrations ≤2.2mmol/l.

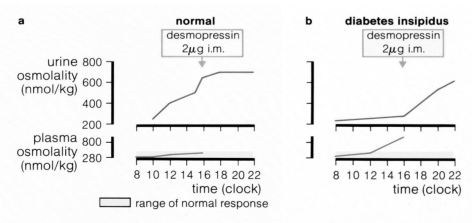

range of normal response

Fig. 2.24 The water deprivation test used in the diagnosis of hypopituitarism. Graph (a) shows the sequence of events during normal testing and (b) shows the hypopituitary response to this test. The patient with ADH deficiency fails to concentrate urine in the presence of a rising plasma osmolality.

The Water Deprivation Test

1 no water for eight hours

2 urine and plasma osmolality measured over eight hours

3 desmopressin given intramuscularly after eight hours

4 urine osmolality measured after desmopressin

there is only a small additional rise in osmolality. In diabetes insipidus, the urine fails to concentrate to twice the plasma osmolality due to lack of ADH, hence the plasma osmolality rises. The urine concentrates adequately only after administration of desmopressin. Desmopressin therefore has no effect on patients with nephrogenic diabetes insipidus, where the renal tubules are unresponsive to ADH. Diabetes insipidus may be masked in untreated hypopituitarism, sometimes only being revealed after hormone replacement, particularly with cortisol.

TREATMENT

The many causes of hypopituitarism have to be dealt with individually. Thus a pituitary tumour may be treated by surgery, radiotherapy or by medical treatment. Surgical decompression is usually required to relieve pressure effects on parapituitary structures (e.g. the optic chiasm or contents of the cavernous sinus) when the lesion cannot be shrunk medically. This occurs

with functionless tumours when radiotherapy may be given to prevent regrowth of the tumour.

Replacement Therapy

Regimens of hormone replacement therapy for gonadotrophin deficiency are shown in Figure 2.25. In women, a typical regimen is to give ethinyloestradiol (30μg daily for three weeks) and during the fourth week to administer medroxyprogesterone (5mg daily) after which a withdrawal bleed occurs. In men, depot mixtures of testosterone esters (Sustanon or Primoteston) can be given intramuscularly in doses of 250–750mg every two to four weeks. A safe oral testosterone preparation (testosterone undecanoate 40–80mg tds) is also now available. In women, libido, vaginal dryness and breast atrophy are remedied. If hypopituitarism develops at a young age, osteoporosis will be prevented by adequate sex steroid treatment. In men, strength, vigour, libido and potency are all improved.

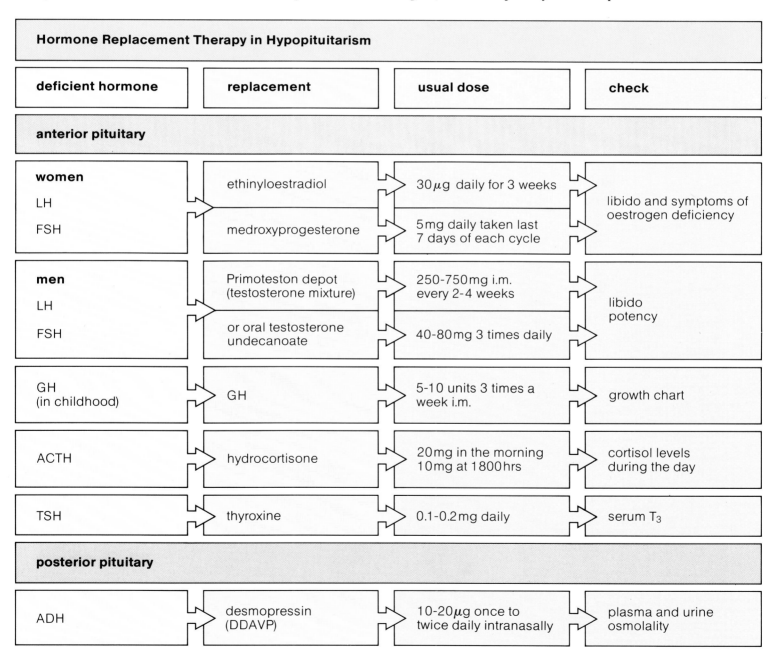

Fig. 2.25 Table of regimens of hormone replacement therapy in the treatment of hypopituitarism. The normal replacement doses for men and women are indicated. GH is only given to promote growth in children and is not required in adults.

If ovulation or spermatogenesis are required, treatment may be given either with human menopausal gonadotrophin (Pergonal) or, more recently, with GnRH delivered intermittently with a pump (see Chapter 10). If carefully monitored, these treatments result in ovulation in women and spermatogenesis in men, the latter after a minimum of three months treatment.

GH deficiency in childhood has until recently been treated by three injections per week of purified natural human GH of pituitary origin. However, there have been problems with the administration of this due to the development of slow virus infection (Jakob-Creutzfeldt disease); only biosynthetic GH should therefore be used. Alternatively, subcutaneous injections of the synthetic GHRH may be given, since this produces a rise in GH and somatomedin as well as linear growth but this is currently only a research procedure. It is unnecessary to treat GH deficiency in adults.

Replacement hydrocortisone can be administered twice daily in doses of 20mg on waking and 10mg in the early evening in patients who need ACTH replacement. The levels of cortisol obtained should be monitored, as the needs of individual patients vary from 15–60mg daily. Oral therapy should be increased during a febrile illness and, with vomiting or surgery, hydrocortisone should be given parenterally. In such situations, it is prudent to issue a blue steroid card and instruct patients to wear a Medic-Alert bracelet. Mineralocorticoid replacement is unnecessary as aldosterone secretion is not ACTH-dependent.

Thyroxine can be given to patients who are TSH-deficient. The usual dose is from 0.1 to 0.2mg daily, and it is rarely necessary to exceed this. Adequate replacement therapy is indicated by serum tri-iodothyronine (T_3) in the upper part of the normal range.

Posterior pituitary replacement is best achieved using an analogue of ADH. ADH itself has a short duration of action and may cause intense vasoconstriction; for this reason, the drug desmopressin is given ($10–20\mu g$ once or twice daily, intranasally). Recently, it has become clear that this drug is also effective orally (100mg three times daily). In partial ADH deficiency a reduction in urine volume can be achieved by using chlorpropramide which increases the sensitivity of the renal tubules to endogenous ADH. This can cause hypoglycaemia, particularly in the elderly, who should be warned to eat before retiring.

With the correct hormone replacement therapy, symptoms such as lack of libido, hair growth (Fig. 2.26) and general well-being are alleviated in most hypopituitary patients. Hypopituitarism requires early diagnosis which can be difficult unless care is taken when documenting the patient's history. Women tend to present earlier than men because of menstrual abnormalities. Once the diagnosis has been made, deficient hormones can usually be adequately replaced with complete symptomatic relief. Additionally, if a pituitary tumour is present, treatment must be directed at arresting and reversing tumour growth.

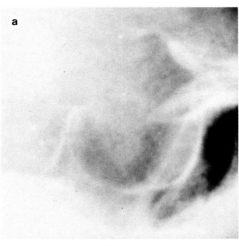
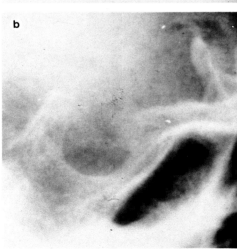
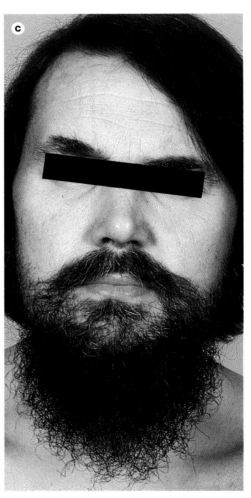

Fig. 2.26 The effects of hormone replacement therapy in a patient with hypopituitarism due to a prolactinoma. View (a) is a lateral skull radiograph of the pituitary fossa before treatment. After treatment (b) the fossa has returned to a more normal shape and has reduced in size. View (c) is a photograph of a patient after bromocriptine therapy showing extensive beard growth, which is in contrast to the lack of facial hair this patient experienced before therapy.

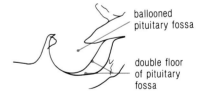

ballooned pituitary fossa

double floor of pituitary fossa

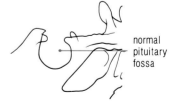

normal pituitary fossa

3 Acromegaly

John A H Wass, MD, FRCP

Acromegaly is the clinical condition which results from prolonged, excessive circulating levels of growth hormone (GH) in adults (Fig. 3.1). The rare clinical counterpart of acromegaly, which occurs in the young before epiphyseal fusion, is called pituitary gigantism (Fig. 3.2).

Acromegaly was first described in 1886 by Pierre Marie, who noted 'a striking non-congenital hypertrophy of the extremities' including the face, hands and feet. In 1891 Minkowski noted that this hypertrophy was always accompanied by an enlarged pituitary, but Harvey Cushing, in 1909, was the first to suggest that the condition was due to hyperpituitarism. This was confirmed in 1922 by Evans, who demonstrated that the parenteral injection of extracts of the anterior lobe of the pituitary gland causes true gigantism in rats, whose epiphyses never fuse, and acromegalic-like features in dogs, whose epiphyses do.

AETIOLOGY

Benign pituitary tumours are by far the most common cause of acromegaly; however, very rarely, pituitary carcinomas may be responsible. While these tumours are usually acidophil, acromegaly can also result from chromophobe adenomas. Whether the tumour results from a hypothalamic disturbance or a primary pituitary tumour is unknown at present. The secretion from pituitary adenomas usually consists of GH alone, but the tumour may also be of mixed cell types and thirty per cent of acromegalic patients are also hyperprolactinaemic. Pituitary tumours may be associated with other endocrine adenomas (e.g. multiple endocrine adenomatosis) which most commonly involve the parathyroid glands resulting in hypercalcaemia. Carcinoid tumours, usually of the lung or pancreas, may rarely be the cause of acromegaly due to ectopic secretion of hypothalamic growth hormone releasing hormone (GHRH). However, instead of a pituitary tumour, these patients have somatotroph hyperplasia in the pituitary, which nevertheless may enlarge the fossa.

DIAGNOSIS

Acromegaly is a disease of the whole organism where everything but the central nervous system enlarges. Although the diagnosis is often made accidentally, the patient usually presents complaining of a change in appearance of the face, hands or whole body, headaches, sweating, goitre or symptoms of renal stones. Early diagnosis is important but this depends upon a high index of suspicion. It often helps to look at old photographs, but a delay in diagnosis of up to twenty years may occur (Fig. 3.3). The condition is most frequently diagnosed in the third decade but may be found from the teenage years up to the seventies.

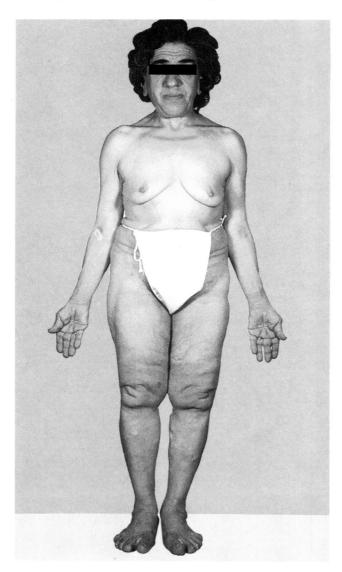

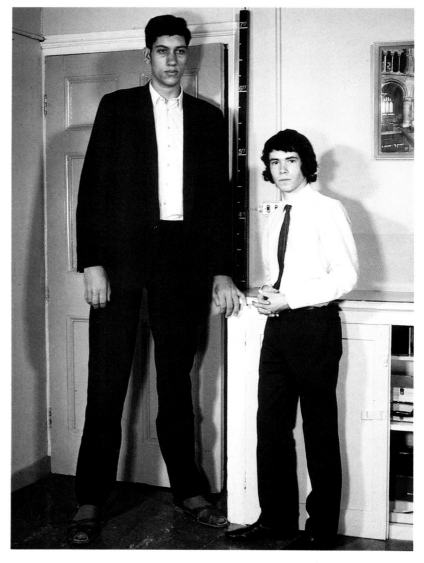

Fig. 3.1 Photograph of a female patient with acromegaly. The facial features have become coarse with progression of the disease.

Fig. 3.2 Photograph of a patient with gigantism compared with a man of average size. Gigantism is the rare, clinical counterpart of acromegaly and occurs in the young before epiphyseal fusion has taken place.

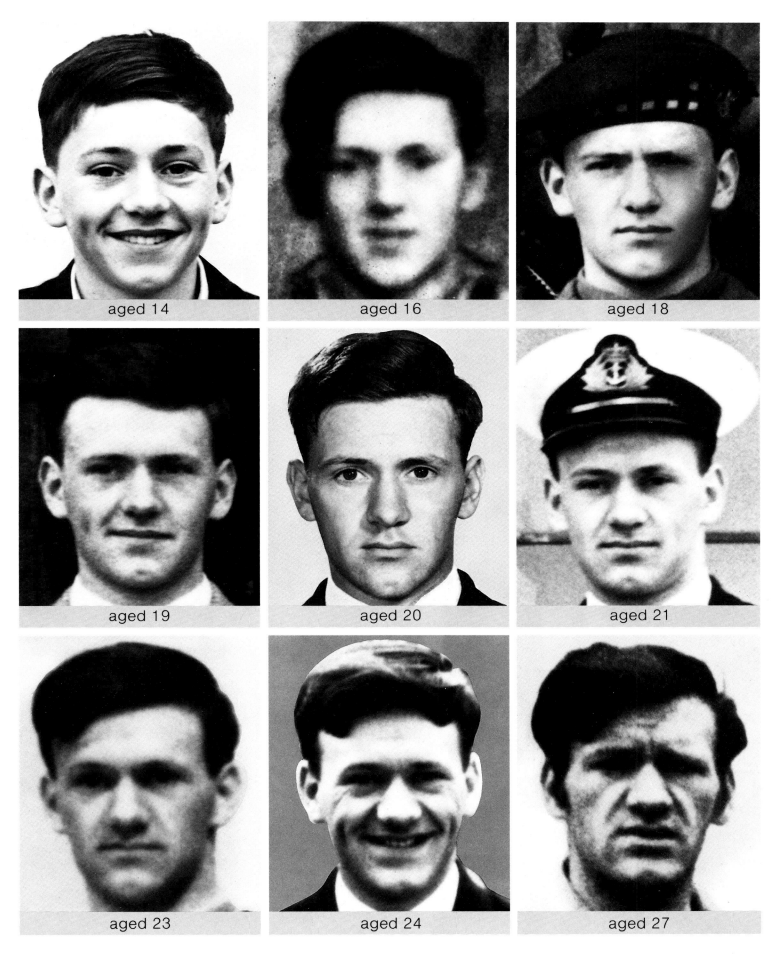

aged 14   aged 16   aged 18

aged 19   aged 20   aged 21

aged 23   aged 24   aged 27

Fig. 3.3 The change in facial appearance of a patient with acromegaly taken over a thirteen year period. The development of an acromegalic appearance is seen, with enlargement of the supraorbital ridges and nose, thickening of the lips and generalised coarsening of the features. From Belchetz (1984), by courtesy of the publishers, Chapman and Hall Ltd.

CLINICAL FEATURES

The clinical features of acromegaly (Fig. 3.4) result from (i) over-secretion of GH, which has both clinical and metabolic sequelae, and (ii) effects of the pituitary tumour which are both local and endocrine.

Clinical Effects of Growth Hormone Over-Secretion

The typical facial appearance of an acromegalic patient is shown in Figure 3.5. There is coarsening of the features with enlargement of the supraorbital ridges, a broad nose and also thickening of the soft tissues. Sweating is excessive, sebaceous activity increases, papillomas and seborrhoeic warts occur; acne and hirsuties may also be present in women. Lips thicken and prognathism occurs,

together with increased dental separation and macroglossia. Using skull radiography, prognathism (where there is loss of angle of the mandible) can be seen, as well as a thickened skull vault, enlargement of the sinuses and, in more than ninety-five per cent of patients, an abnormal and enlarged pituitary fossa (Fig. 3.6).

The hands also become enlarged in acromegaly and the fingers look short and fat (Fig. 3.7). Heel pad and skin thickness are increased, and the latter is clearly visible on the dorsum of the hand. Carpal tunnel syndrome often occurs due to compression of the median nerve and kyphosis (in long-standing acromegaly) and lumbar spondylosis may be present. Myopathy is frequent and, paradoxically, these patients are weak despite their muscular appearance.

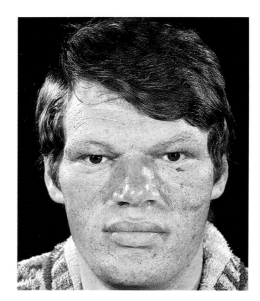

Fig. 3.5 **The characteristic facial features of a male acromegalic patient.**

Clinical Features of Acromegaly

coarse facial features	macroglossia
soft tissue thickening e.g. lips	headaches
'spade-like' hands	kyphosis
separation of teeth	excessive sweating
enlargement of supraorbital ridges	hypertension
prognathism	impaired glucose tolerance
	goitre

Fig. 3.4 **Table showing the clinical features of acromegaly.**

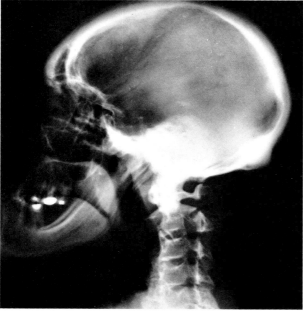

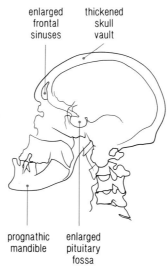

enlarged
frontal
sinuses

thickened
skull
vault

prognathic
mandible

enlarged
pituitary
fossa

Fig. 3.6 **Skull radiograph of an acromegalic patient.** The enlarged pituitary fossa and sinuses, thickened skull vault and prognathism with loss of angle of the mandible can be seen.

Fig. 3.7 **Photograph showing the enlarged hand of an acromegalic patient.** The hand is big and the fingers appear short because they are broad. There is thenar wasting because of long-standing compression of the median nerve in the carpal tunnel.

Radiographs of the hands show characteristic 'tufting' of the terminal phalanges. This may occur normally in heavy manual labourers, but the increase in the joint spaces due to the cartilaginous overgrowth typical of acromegaly (Fig. 3.8) does not. Arthritis occurs prematurely, particularly in the spine and other weight-bearing joints such as the hips and knees. The joints enlarge due to synovial overgrowth and cartilaginous thickening. The lumbar spine may also show characteristic changes with scalloping of the posterior margin and anterior new bone formation (Fig. 3.9). The heel pad thickness is usually greater than 25 mm.

Acromegalic patients may also have cardiomegaly related either to coronary artery disease, the incidence of which is increased in acromegaly, or to hypertension which occurs in thirty-five per cent of acromegalic patients. In the absence of these, cardiomegaly may be related to a primary cardiomyopathy. Hypertension is usually 'essential' but may be caused by a coexistent phaeochromocytoma or a Conn's tumour.

Diabetes mellitus occurs in approximately twenty per cent of patients and is secondary to insulin resistance as a consequence of raised GH levels. Hypercalcaemia occurs in five to ten per cent of patients usually resulting from parathyroid adenomas or hyperplasia. There is also an increased incidence of urinary calculi (five per cent) resulting from hypercalciuria, even in the absence of hypercalcaemia.

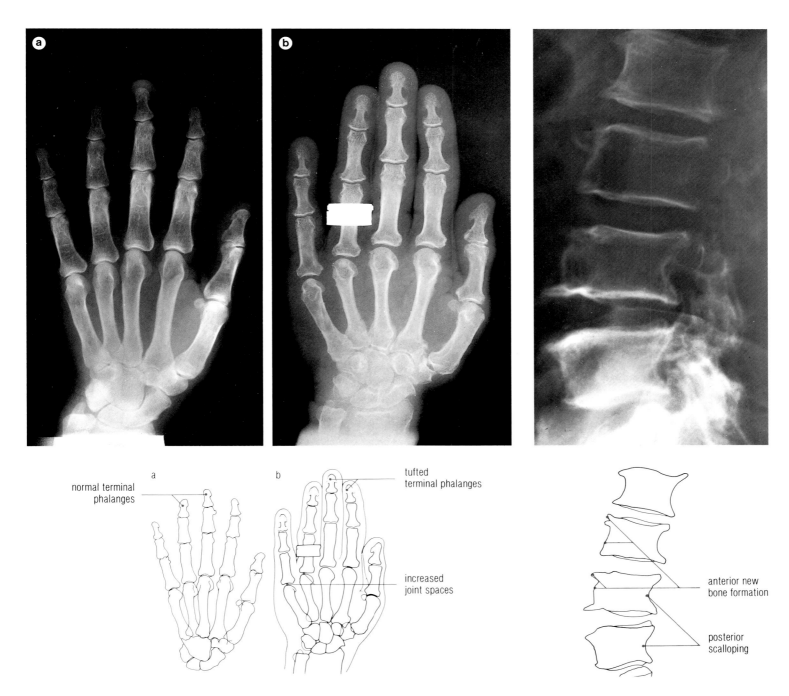

Fig. 3.8 Comparison of radiographs of (a) a normal and (b) an acromegalic hand. The characteristic tufting of the terminal phalanges in the acromegalic patient is shown together with an increase in joint space due to cartilaginous overgrowth.

Fig. 3.9 Radiographic appearance of the lumbar spine in acromegaly. Scalloping of the posterior margin of the vertebrae and anterior new bone formation are present.

3.5

Clinical Effects of Pituitary Tumours

Patients may present with headaches. The pituitary fossa is enlarged in the majority of cases (Fig. 3.10), the size of the pituitary fossa correlating with the circulating levels of GH.

Upward extension of the pituitary tumour, when present, may cause a characteristic bitemporal field defect best found with the Goldmann perimeter. The enlarged supraorbital ridges may produce technical problems with field plotting; this is therefore best performed by tilting the head backwards 20°. Lateral extension of the tumour may cause third, fourth and sixth cranial nerve palsies and, more rarely, temporal lobe epilepsy. Erosion into the sphenoid sinus may be associated with cerebrospinal fluid (CSF) rhinorrhoea.

Hyperprolactinaemia is common; females may therefore present with amenorrhoea and galactorrhoea or infertility, and males with low libido and impotence. Hypopituitarism also occurs and this most frequently affects gonadotrophin production. Later in the development of the disease, hypothyroidism and hypoadrenalism may occur due to decreased thyroid stimulating hormone (TSH) and adrenocorticotrophic hormone (ACTH) reserves. Hypopituitarism is often due to pressure on the stalk by the tumour. Diabetes insipidus, resulting from upward extension of the tumour into the hypothalamus is rare.

GROWTH HORMONE SECRETION IN ACROMEGALY

Basal GH levels are elevated but do not correlate with any clinical manifestation of the disease. This may be because of the variable secretion of immunoreactive but biologically non-active polymeric forms of GH. Somatomedin-C is invariably elevated. However, because of the pulsatile nature of GH secretion in normal subjects, it may not be possible to distinguish between normal and some acromegalic patients using basal GH concentrations; dynamic tests are therefore necessary.

A rise in circulating glucose normally causes a complete suppression of GH, but this is not the case in acromegaly (Fig. 3.11). Usually only a slight or no fall occurs in acromegaly and there may even be a paradoxical rise in GH. This phenomenon is not specific to acromegaly and may also occur in hepatic or renal disease, in anorexia nervosa and in patients on heroin or L-dopa. Dopamine and related drugs normally cause a rise in GH levels. L-dopa was first found, in 1972, to cause a paradoxical suppression of GH in acromegaly; bromocriptine, a long-acting dopamine agonist, also has this property (as do all dopamine agonists including lisuride and pergolide). These effects are antagonised by haloperidol, pimozide and metoclopramide which are specific dopamine antagonists. The cause of this paradoxical response to dopamine and its agonists is unclear.

Thyrotrophin releasing hormone (TRH) and gonadotrophin releasing hormone (GnRH) may also cause GH secretion in acromegaly but the reasons for this are also unclear.

PROGNOSIS AND TREATMENT

Mortality is approximately doubled in acromegaly compared with the normal population. The main reason for this is the presence of cardiovascular and cerebrovascular disease secondary to hypertension and diabetes mellitus. Respiratory disease also occurs with increased frequency. Early treatment is therefore recommended.

Aims of treatment should be the relief of symptoms, the reversal of the somatic changes occurring with acromegaly, together with reversal of the associated metabolic abnormalities. The ideal treatment should cause the minimum disturbance to the patient with no side-effects, particularly that of hypopituitarism. Early treatment avoids the subsequent complications of diabetes mellitus, enlargement of the tumour, hypopituitarism, osteoarthritis and cardiomyopathy. A summary of the possible treatment modalities in acromegaly is shown in Figure 3.12.

Regrettably, there is no agreed definition of cured acromegaly. GH is not detectable (< 1 mu/l or 0.5 ng/ml) in the circulation of normal subjects, except during stress or spontaneous brief pulses which occur five or six times during the day. In assessing activity, some authors use basal GH levels at 0900h, whilst others measure the mean GH concentration during a glucose tolerance test. It seems most logical to take several measurements during a normal day.

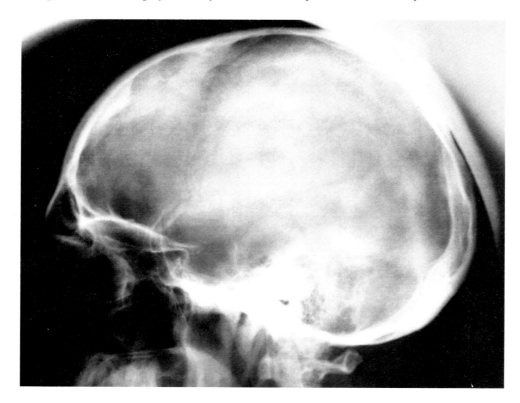

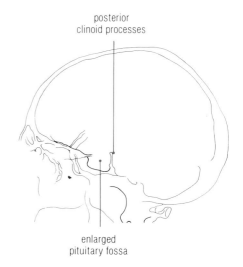

Fig. 3.10 The skull radiograph of an acromegalic patient with an enlarged pituitary fossa and thinning of the posterior clinoid processes. The expansion of the pituitary fossa occurs in over ninety-five per cent of patients with this disease and is best seen on the lateral view.

posterior
clinoid processes

enlarged
pituitary fossa

The treatments available fall into three groups: (i) surgery, via the trans-sphenoidal or transfrontal route; (ii) radiotherapy using a linear accelerator, a cobalt source, yttrium-90, or a proton beam, and (iii) medical therapy using a dopamine agonist (e.g. bromocriptine).

Surgery

Transfrontal surgery is recommended when there is a large suprasellar extension causing visual field defects. This rarely cures acromegaly and postoperative radiotherapy is usually necessary. Field defects improve, but not completely if they have been present for some time.

Trans-sphenoidal operations (Fig. 3.13) using either the transnasal or transethmoidal approach are best for small tumours associated with acromegaly; however, patients with small supra-sellar extensions may also be operated upon using this route. This is desirable because it has a lower morbidity than the transfrontal route, in which it is necessary to retract the frontal lobe and cut an olfactory nerve. Up to eighty per cent of patients may be 'cured' but the instance of hypopituitarism may be considerable (perhaps as much as twenty-five per cent), particularly in patients with larger tumours; however, there are insufficient data for calculating the frequency of recurrence. If acromegaly is not cured with a trans-sphenoidal operation, postoperative radiotherapy is necessary. Side-effects of surgery are most frequent with macro-adenomas. Intra-operative bleeding and postoperative pulmonary embolism may occur; this gives rise to a mortality rate for trans-sphenoidal operations of zero to three per cent. Transient third and fourth cranial nerve palsies may occur, as may CSF leakage.

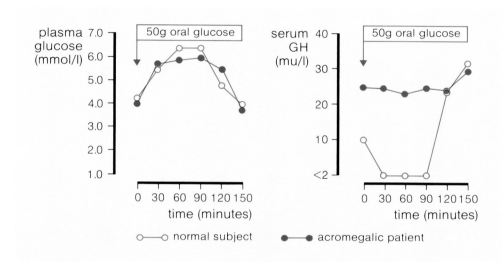

Fig. 3.11 **Graphs showing the effects of a 50g glucose load on blood glucose and GH levels in a normal subject and an acromegalic patient.** GH levels are acutely suppressed in normal subjects following a glucose load, whereas in acromegaly there is either no suppression or occasionally there is even a paradoxical rise. Carbohydrate tolerance is normal in both subjects shown.

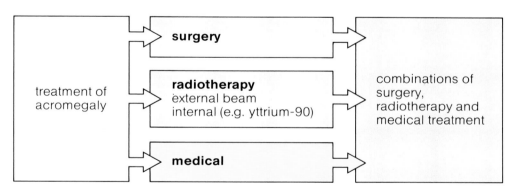

Fig. 3.12 **Table of the possible treatment modalities in acromegaly.**

Trans-Sphenoidal Surgery in Acromegaly

	number of patients	success rate (GH ⩽ 20 mu/l)	incidence of hypopituitarism
microadenomas	17	82%	0%
diffuse adenomas	38	68%	23%
invasive adenomas	25	54%	24%
total	80	66%	19%

Fig. 3.13 **Table showing the improvement of GH levels and the incidence of hypopituitarism following trans-sphenoidal surgery for acromegaly.** For all types of pituitary tumours, trans-sphenoidal surgery leads to an improvement in GH levels in sixty-six per cent of patients. The incidence of hypopituitarism following trans-sphenoidal surgery is lowest in microadenomas. Redrawn from Laws et al. (1979), by courtesy of the publishers, American Association of Neurological Surgeons.

Radiotherapy

Radiotherapy is an effective treatment for acromegaly but its effects are slow in onset and may take up to ten years to be fully developed. A great deal of skill and careful planning is necessary to ensure success. Best results occur using a linear accelerator and a three-field technique, which results in the largest dose of radiation being delivered safely to the tumour; this is not the case using the simpler two-field parallel opposed field technique. Pretreatment high resolution computed tomography (CT) (Fig. 3.14) is necessary to completely delineate the upper, lower and lateral margins of the tumour. A dose of 4,500 cGy should be delivered over twenty-six treatment days using five fractions per week, each fraction consisting of no more than 180 cGy. Using this technique no radiation-induced neurological damage has been recorded by the author. During treatment, an individual head mask is used to encompass and immobilise the whole of the patient's head; this improves accuracy and safety (Fig. 3.15).

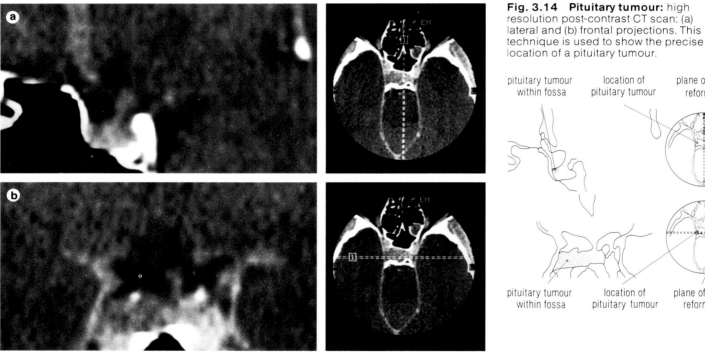

Fig. 3.14 Pituitary tumour: high resolution post-contrast CT scan: (a) lateral and (b) frontal projections. This technique is used to show the precise location of a pituitary tumour.

| pituitary tumour within fossa | location of pituitary tumour | plane of sagittal reformation |

| pituitary tumour within fossa | location of pituitary tumour | plane of coronal reformation |

Fig. 3.15 An individual head mask used to position the patient accurately during radiotherapy. Three fields are used and the daily dose of radiation should not exceed 180 cGy.

With external pituitary irradiation using a linear accelerator, a fall in GH levels of seventy-seven per cent after five years has been obtained (Fig. 3.16), and at the end of ten years eighty-one per cent of patients have serum GH concentrations of less than 20mu/1. Hypopituitarism occurs after external pituitary irradiation in approximately ten per cent of patients, and may develop gradually, becoming apparent some years after treatment.

Intrasellar implantation of radioactive yttrium-90 seeds results in an improvement in approximately fifty per cent of patients;

however, twenty-five per cent of these become hypopituitary (Fig. 3.17). Currently, complications resulting from this form of treatment are rare, but in inexperienced hands it may be associated with CSF rhinorrhoea, and later, meningitis, diabetes insipidus and impairment of visual fields. Proton beam irradiation is only available in a few centres and is associated with a higher incidence of hypopituitarism.

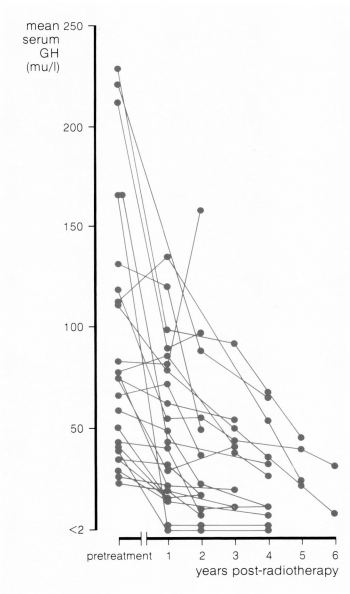

Fig. 3.16 Graph showing the fall in GH levels following external irradiation of the pituitary for the treatment of acromegaly. Data for twenty-two subjects are shown. Redrawn from Black et al. (1984), by courtesy of the publishers, Raven Press.

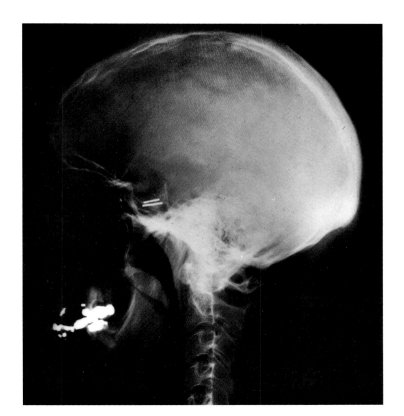

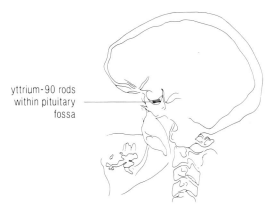

yttrium-90 rods within pituitary fossa

Fig. 3.17 Skull radiograph showing implanted radioactive yttrium-90. Intrasellar implantation of yttrium-90 improves the condition of approximately fifty per cent of the patients treated; however, twenty-five per cent of these become hypopituitary.

3.9

Medical Therapy

In normal subjects, dopamine and dopamine agonist drugs cause a rise in serum GH, but in acromegalic patients there is a paradoxical fall (Fig. 3.18).

Bromocriptine is a semi-synthetic ergot alkaloid which is a long-acting stimulator of dopamine receptors. The drug causes GH suppression in the majority of patients with acromegaly (Fig. 3.19) by acting on dopamine receptors of the somatotrophs. Although seventy per cent of patients respond to treatment with a reduction in GH, serum GH levels during treatment do not usually lie within normal limits, with only twenty per cent of patients having levels of 10mu/l or less (Fig. 3.20). The effects on GH secretion persist whilst the drug is taken, but GH levels rise when drug administration is stopped. It is best to withdraw the drug at yearly intervals to assess the effects of other ablative therapy such as external pituitary irradiation. However, it is impossible to predict whether a given acromegalic patient will respond to bromo-criptine using any pretreatment test.

Bromocriptine treatment should be started at night in a dose of 2.5mg. This is gradually increased to 20mg per day (5mg, six-hourly), all tablets being taken during meals; thereafter the dose should be increased further until maximum GH suppression is obtained.

Prolactin levels become undetectable in all patients and this may be associated with the resumption of normal periods in women and improved libido in men.

A reduction in pituitary tumour size during bromocriptine therapy has been reported in a number of patients. There may be an improvement of field defects to the normal state (Fig. 3.21), a decrease in pituitary fossa size, and serial CT scanning and contrast studies (Fig. 3.22) have indicated a disappearance of suprasellar extensions so that external pituitary irradiation may be carried out safely. Pituitary function may also improve if the tumour shrinks as pressure on the stalk is relieved, and patients with hypopituitarism may discontinue anterior pituitary replace-ment therapy after successful bromocriptine therapy.

Although only seventy per cent of patients on bromocriptine show GH suppression, there is an improvement of the clinical symptoms in over ninety per cent. This apparent discrepancy can be explained by the action of bromocriptine on monomeric GH in preference to oligomeric GH (Fig. 3.23). Oligomeric GH is much less biologically active than the monomeric form. For this reason, patients with clinically inactive acromegaly may have detectable GH in the circulation. There is a further group of patients in whom somatomedin-C levels fall, despite there being no change in circulating GH levels.

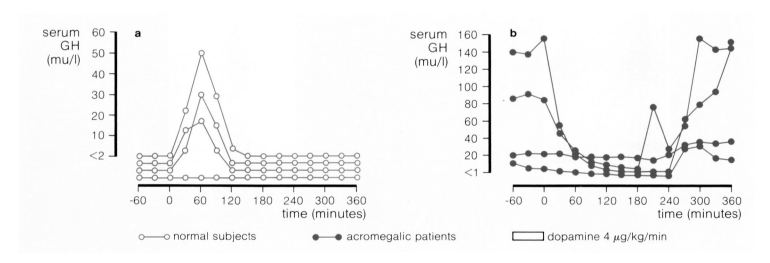

Fig. 3.18 The effects of intravenous dopamine on serum GH levels. The contrasting responses of (a) normal subjects and (b) acromegalic patients are shown.

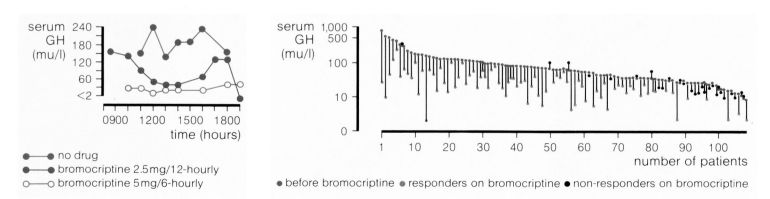

Fig. 3.19 The treatment of acromegaly using bromocriptine. Serum GH levels can be controlled in responsive patients when the drug is given six-hourly. Serum GH levels throughout the day for one acromegalic female are shown. Redrawn from Thorner et al. (1975), by courtesy of the publishers, The British Medical Journal.

Fig. 3.20 The change in mean serum GH concentration in 109 acromegalic patients treated with bromocriptine for up to five and one half years. There was a fall in GH levels in seventy per cent of patients in response to bromocriptine. However, GH levels were still not within normal limits; only twenty per cent of patients had levels of 10mu/l or less on treatment.

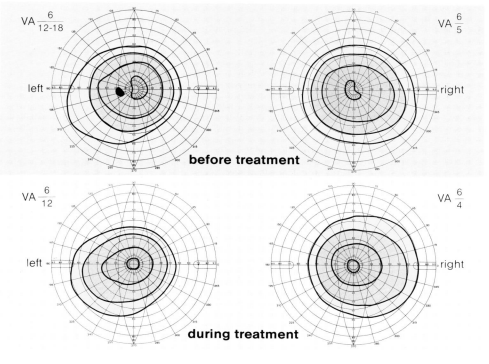

VA $\frac{6}{12-18}$ VA $\frac{6}{5}$

left   right

before treatment

VA $\frac{6}{12}$ VA $\frac{6}{4}$

left   right

during treatment

Fig. 3.21 Improvement in eyesight due to tumour reduction with bromocriptine therapy. Despite lack of improvement in visual acuity (VA), the field defects before treatment are no longer apparent following bromocriptine therapy. Redrawn from Belchetz (1984), by courtesy of the publishers, Chapman and Hall Ltd.

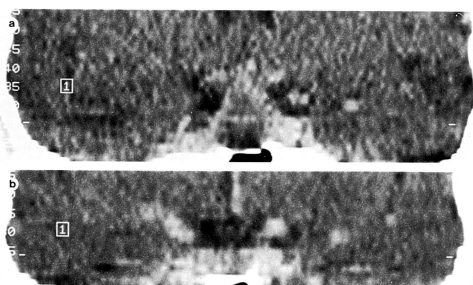

Fig. 3.22 Tumour size reduction with bromocriptine treatment: coronal CT scans, (a) before treatment and (b) after nine months of bromocriptine therapy. Tumour shrinkage can improve pituitary function and can obviate the need for anterior pituitary replacement therapy.

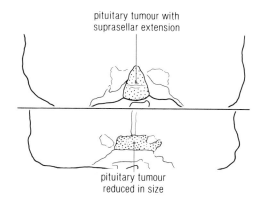

pituitary tumour with
suprasellar extension

pituitary tumour
reduced in size

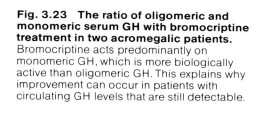

Fig. 3.23 The ratio of oligomeric and monomeric serum GH with bromocriptine treatment in two acromegalic patients. Bromocriptine acts predominantly on monomeric GH, which is more biologically active than oligomeric GH. This explains why improvement can occur in patients with circulating GH levels that are still detectable.

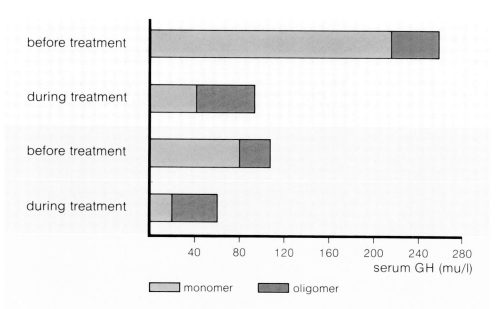

before treatment

during treatment

before treatment

during treatment

40   80   120   160   200   240   280
serum GH (mu/l)

□ monomer   ■ oligomer

The side-effects which occur with bromocriptine therapy do not cause serious problems (Fig. 3.24). Nausea and vomiting are largely obviated by starting bromocriptine gradually and increasing the dose slowly and, most important of all, by only taking the drug during meals. Constipation is the most frequent long-term side-effect and occurs in forty per cent of patients, although the taking of bulk fibre laxatives may alleviate this. A dry mouth, hyperkinesis and digital vasospasm have also been noted on rare occasions. None of these side-effects necessitate discontinuation of therapy.

Bromocriptine should be used as a sole treatment only in patients who are too old, unwell or unwilling to tolerate invasive investigations or radiotherapy. In general, it is used to complement unsuccessful surgery or external pituitary irradiation until the irradiation treatment is complete, a process which may take up to ten years. It has so far been used safely for over ten years. Alternative longer acting ergot alkaloids related to bromocriptine, which are also dopamine agonists, are being developed. Long-acting somatostatin analogues which may cause significant GH suppression may be an alternative to bromocriptine in the future.

CONCLUSIONS

Acromegaly is an insidious disease which requires a high degree of suspicion on the part of the clinician for early diagnosis to be made. This is important because of the greater mortality associated with this condition which is twice that of normal.

No treatment currently available satisfies all the requirements of an ideal therapy. Surgery, if successful, rapidly reduces GH levels to normal, but may not eradicate circulating GH and may cause hypopituitarism, particularly with large tumours. Radiotherapy is successful but takes time to act and causes hypopituitarism in a proportion of cases. Bromocriptine, which is only rarely used alone, improves symptoms but only occasionally reduces GH levels to normal. Its main use is as an adjunct to ablative treatment of the pituitary tumour. Occasionally, after careful judgement, all three types of treatment may be needed to reduce GH levels to normal.

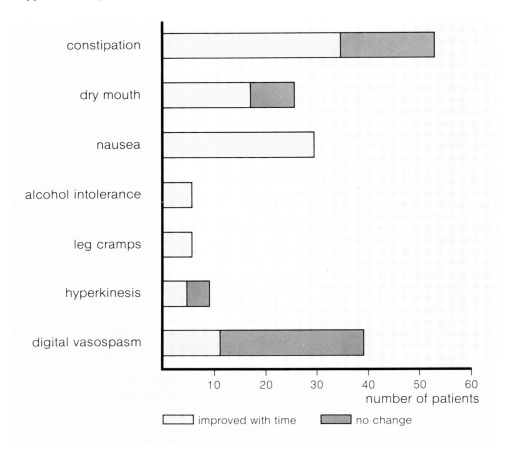

Fig. 3.24 Side-effects of bromocriptine treatment in 109 acromegalic patients. Dosages of between 10mg and 60mg can produce these symptoms. However, these side-effects do not warrant discontinuation of therapy.

4 Hyperprolactinaemia

Michael O Thorner, MB BS, FRCP

PROLACTIN SECRETION

Prolactin is secreted by the lactotroph cells of the anterior pituitary. The control of its secretion, like that of other anterior pituitary hormones, is regulated by the hypothalamus. Unlike the other anterior pituitary hormones, however, the hypothalamic influence is of tonic inhibition (Fig. 4.1).

The hypothalamus secretes two hypothalamic factors to control prolactin secretion: a prolactin releasing factor (PRF and a prolactin release inhibiting factor (PIF). The latter is almost certainly the catecholamine dopamine (DA) itself, although the possibility of the existence of non-catecholamine prolactin inhibiting factors cannot be excluded. Gamma-amino-butyric acid (GABA) may play a rôle as an inhibitor and there may well also be one or more PIF-peptides. The nature of PRF is unclear, although thyrotrophin releasing hormone can act in this way.

CAUSES OF HYPERPROLACTINAEMIA

The causes of hyperprolactinaemia may be considered, in a simplified fashion, as resulting from four basic abnormalities of prolactin secretion (Fig. 4.2).

Hypothalamic Dopamine Deficiency

Diseases of the hypothalamus, such as tumours, arteriovenous malformations, and inflammatory processes, might be expected to result in either diminished synthesis or release of dopamine. Furthermore, certain drugs (e.g. alpha methyldopa and reserpine) are capable of depleting the central dopamine stores.

Defective Transport Mechanisms

Section of the pituitary stalk results in deranged transport of dopamine from the hypothalamus to the lactotrophs; it is possible also to speculate that pituitary or stalk tumours with abnormal blood supplies, or their pressure effects, may interfere with the circulatory pathways to the normal lactotrophs or to those within the tumour.

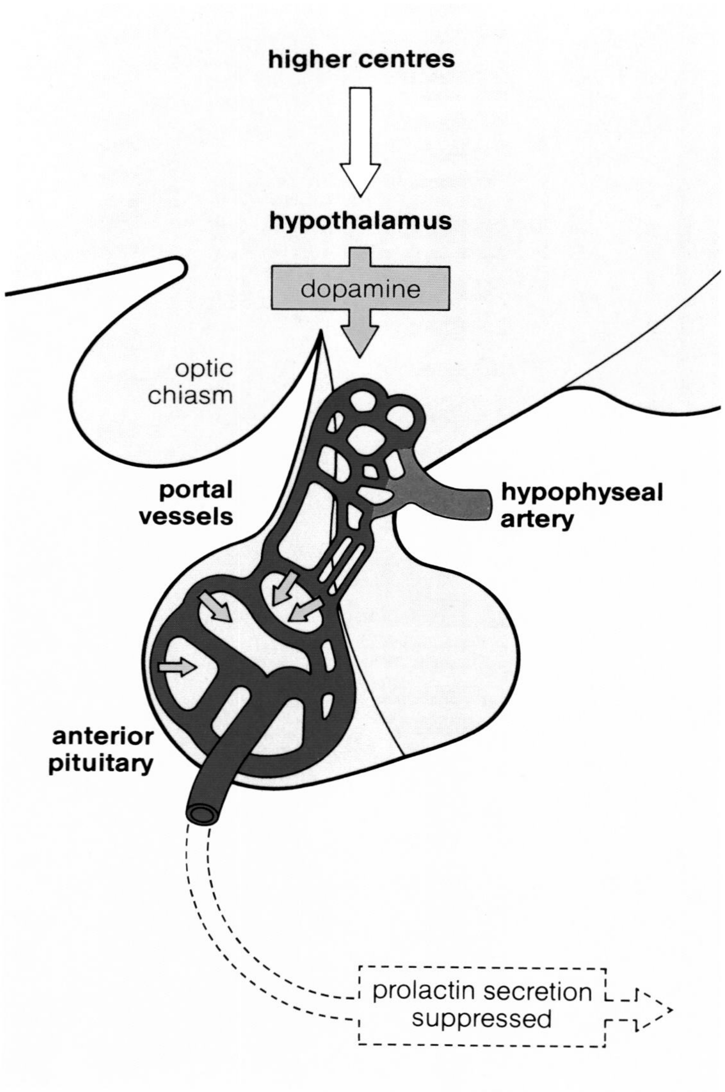

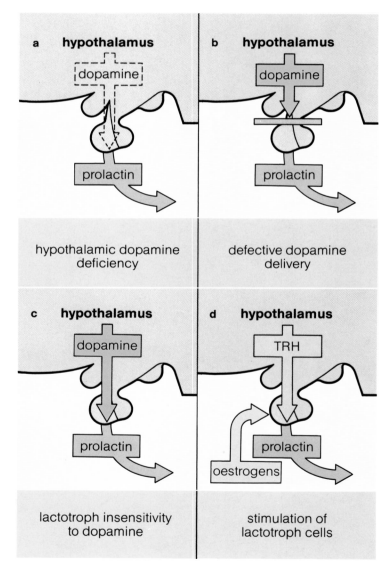

Fig. 4.1 Prolactin secretion. Dopamine is formed in the hypothalamus, and stored in the median eminence. It is secreted into the hypothalamo-hypophyseal portal capillaries to tonically inhibit prolactin release from pituitary lactotrophs. Any disruption of this pathway may therefore result in hyperprolactinaemia.

Fig. 4.2 Four basic mechanisms in hyperprolactinaemia. (a) Inadequate synthesis and/or secretion of dopamine from the hypothalamus. (b) Interruption of hypothalamo-hypophyseal portal circulation. (c) Decreased sensitivity of the dopamine receptors. (In all these cases, lactotrophs will be released from dopaminergic inhibition, thereby permitting the release of prolactin.) (d) Prolactin secretion may be stimulated by oestrogens, or by excess thyrotrophin releasing hormone in hypothyroidism.

Lactotroph Insensitivity to Dopamine

Although dopamine receptors have been found on human pituitary adenoma cells, it is not certain if they are functionally intact. Receptor sensitivity to dopamine may be diminished, which would explain the lack of response to increased endogenous dopamine stimulation; however, the receptors' obvious response to pharmacologic dopamine agonists makes this possibility less likely. Certain drugs act as dopamine receptor blocking agents, including phenothiazines (e.g. chlorpromazine), butyrophenones (haloperidol), and benzamides (metoclopramide, sulpiride and domperidone). These drugs block the effects of endogenous dopamine and thus release lactotrophs from their hypothalamic inhibition. This sequence of events results in hyperprolactinaemia.

Stimulation of Lactotrophs

Hypothyroidism may be associated with hyperprolactinaemia. If hypothyroidism results in increased thyrotrophin releasing hormone (TRH) production, then TRH (which can act as a PRF), could lead to hyperprolactinaemia. Oestrogens act directly at the pituitary level causing stimulation of lactotrophs and thus enhance prolactin secretion. Furthermore, oestrogens increase the mitotic activity of lactotrophs.

Chest wall injury can lead to hyperprolactinaemia. The mechanism is unclear but probably results from abnormal stimulation of the reflex associated with the rise in prolactin which is seen normally in lactating women during suckling. In some patients, it is not possible to elucidate the cause of hyperprolactinaemia.

CLINICAL MANIFESTATIONS OF HYPERPROLACTINAEMIA

The symptoms associated with hyperprolactinaemia may be due to several factors: either to the direct effects of excess prolactin, such as the induction of galactorrhoea or hypogonadism or to the effects of the structural lesion causing the disorder (i.e. the pituitary tumour) leading to, for example, headaches, visual field defects or external ophthalmoplegia, or associated dysfunction of secretion of other anterior pituitary hormones (Fig. 4.3).

The incidence of galactorrhoea in hyperprolactinaemic patients is between thirty and eighty per cent, depending on the care with which the physician looks for this sign. However, approximately fifty per cent of women with galactorrhoea have normal prolactin levels and, as mentioned below, it is particularly those patients with very high prolactin levels, i.e. greater than 100 ng/ml (2,000 mu/l), who often have no galactorrhoea. Thus galactorrhoea is a poor marker of hyperprolactinaemia.

Women with hyperprolactinaemia usually present with menstrual abnormalities; either amenorrhoea or oligomenorrhoea, or regular cycles with infertility. Occasionally patients may present with menorrhagia.

In contrast, men often present late in the course of their disease with symptoms of expansion of their pituitary tumour, i.e. headaches, visual defects and external ophthalmoplegia, or symptoms from secondary adrenal or thyroid failure. However, these men have usually been impotent for many years before their presentation. Occasionally the syndrome may occur in prepubertal or peripubertal children, when it may present with delayed or arrested puberty.

DIFFERENTIAL DIAGNOSIS

The theoretical causes of hyperprolactinaemia have already been discussed. However, in practice it is important to exclude two causes of hyperprolactinaemia: hypothyroidism, and the ingestion of drugs which either deplete central dopamine or block dopamine receptors.

Having excluded these two important causes, three diagnostic possibilities remain (Fig. 4.4): the patient may have a microadenoma, a macroadenoma, or no tumour at all. If the patient does not harbour an identifiable tumour he is described as having idiopathic hyperprolactinaemia. A microadenoma is described as having a maximum diameter of 10 mm and a macroadenoma as having a diameter in excess of 10 mm. The normal pituitary diameter does not exceed 10 mm.

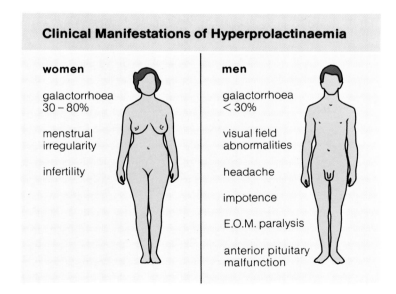

Clinical Manifestations of Hyperprolactinaemia

women	men
galactorrhoea 30–80%	galactorrhoea < 30%
menstrual irregularity	visual field abnormalities
infertility	headache
	impotence
	E.O.M. paralysis
	anterior pituitary malfunction

Fig. 4.3 Table of symptoms associated with hyperprolactinaemia. A variable incidence of galactorrhoea is reported in different studies.

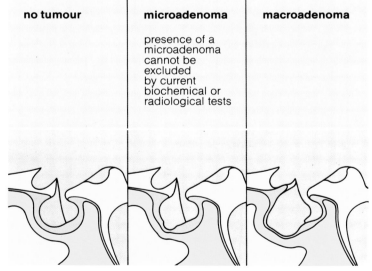

no tumour | microadenoma | macroadenoma

presence of a microadenoma cannot be excluded by current biochemical or radiological tests

Fig. 4.4 Table of differential diagnosis in hyperprolactinaemia.

Currently there are no tests which can exclude the possibility of a microadenoma. Its presence is suggested by radiological changes and usually the serum prolactin level is under 200 ng/ml (4,000mu/l). Prolactin levels may be much higher than this, however, and many microadenomas have been surgically removed when the prolactin level is higher than 200 ng/ml (4,000mu/l). As in Cushing's disease, the tumour may be too small to produce any change in the contour of the pituitary fossa on plain radiographs of the skull or tomograms of the sella turcica. The latest generation of computed tomographic (CT) scanners may help with this difficulty (Fig. 4.5). A macroadenoma can be diagnosed by the enlargement of the pituitary fossa, but as described below, care should be exercised to exclude the possibility of cisternal herniation (a partially empty fossa) as a cause for the enlargement. (CT scans are proving useful here, as is the use of limited metrizamide cisternography to delineate the chiasmatic cistern.)

CHANGES IN THE BREAST DUE TO PROLACTIN

The woman with amenorrhoea due to hyperprolactinaemia does not develop the breast atrophy of the postmenopausal woman, or that of the amenorrhoeic woman who is gonadotrophin deficient or has primary ovarian failure. On examination, the breast is well developed and the Montgomery tubercles are hyperplastic (Fig. 4.6). If the breast is correctly examined, first by expressing it from the periphery towards the areola to empty the milk ducts, followed by squeezing and lifting the areola (rather than the nipple itself) to empty the milk sinuses, galactorrhoea can usually be found.

In patients with extremely high prolactin levels galactorrhoea may not be found. In male patients with hyperprolactinaemia there is usually no gynaecomastia but milk may be expressed from an entirely normal-sized male breast. The incidence of galactorrhoea in men with hyperprolactinaemia is low, however, being less than thirty per cent (i.e. it is much less common than in women).

RADIOLOGY OF THE PITUITARY FOSSA

The radiologic evaluation of the pituitary fossa should include a lateral skull radiograph (Fig. 4.7) and a postero-anterior (PA) skull radiograph (Fig. 4.8) to demonstrate the floor of the pituitary fossa. (Fig. 4.9 is a normal lateral for comparison.) The routine use of tomography is now probably no longer necessary since many of the minor abnormalities that were detected probably represent normal variants rather than being the pathognomonic changes of small tumours. However, tomography of the sella may be necessary if there are difficulties in visualising the floor of the fossa, for instance due to overlying shadows or lack of pneumatisation of the sphenoid sinus, or if the patient is about to undergo trans-sphenoidal surgery. The patients who have macroadenomas usually have expanded pituitary fossae. One caveat is necessary however: the patient may have cisternal herniation (a partially empty fossa). The aetiology of this condition is unknown but it may be due to a defect in the diaphragma sellae, allowing the transmitted pressure changes of the cerebrospinal fluid to extend into the fossa, thereby expanding it. Another explanation may be that the fossa once contained a pituitary tumour which subsequently infarcted and therefore became smaller. The presence of cisternal herniation may be diagnosed either by means of contrast studies with tomography (e.g. metrizamide or air cisternography, Fig. 4.10) or CT scanning. Cisternal herniation may be diagnosed using new generation CT scanners, without any contrast injection.

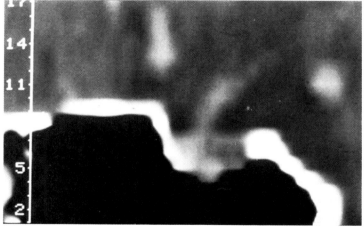

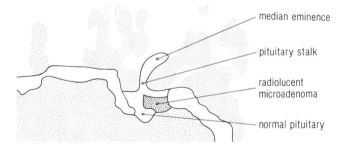

Fig. 4.5 CT scan of the pituitary fossa. This sagittal reconstruction was made using a GE 8800 scanner. The area of low attenuation within the pituitary indicates the presence of a prolactinoma. High dose intravenous contrast has been given to show up the most vascular structures such as the stalk and normal gland.

median eminence

pituitary stalk

radiolucent microadenoma

normal pituitary

Fig. 4.6 Changes in the breast due to prolactin secretion. Prominent Montgomery tubercles in the breast of a woman with hyperprolactinaemia.

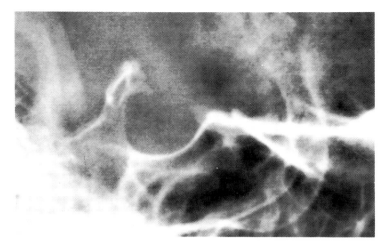

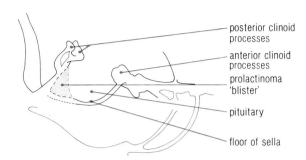

Fig. 4.7 Right lateral skull radiograph of the pituitary fossa. The postero-inferior blister is a prolactinoma.

posterior clinoid processes

anterior clinoid processes

prolactinoma 'blister'

pituitary

floor of sella

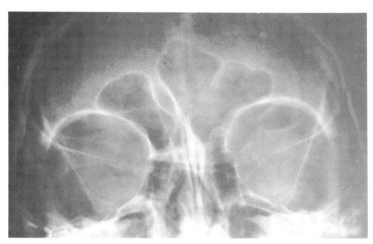

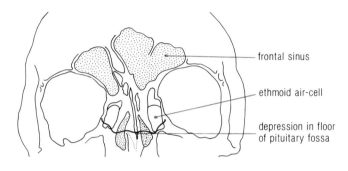

Fig. 4.8 PA skull radiograph. A prolactinoma has expanded the pituitary fossa. This distension is indicated here by the depression in the floor of the pituitary fossa.

frontal sinus

ethmoid air-cell

depression in floor of pituitary fossa

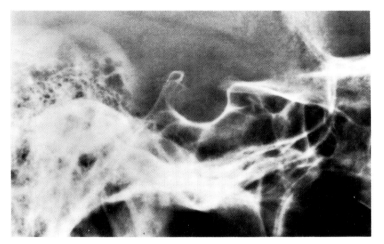

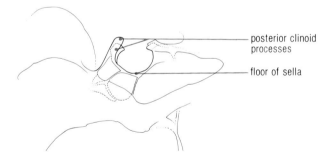

Fig. 4.9 Right lateral radiograph of a normal sella turcica. In this view of the normal sella the anterior cranial fossa appears as a 'single' floor. Note the apposition of the anterior and posterior clinoid processes.

posterior clinoid processes

floor of sella

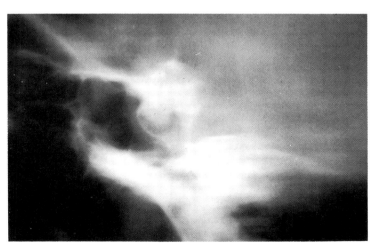

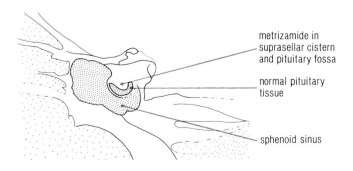

Fig. 4.10 Cisternal herniation. Metrizamide cisternogram showing a partially empty fossa.

metrizamide in suprasellar cistern and pituitary fossa

normal pituitary tissue

sphenoid sinus

4.5

TRANS-SPHENOIDAL SURGERY

Patients with hyperprolactinaemia and small pituitary tumours may be treated either by surgery, using the trans-sphenoidal approach, or medically, with dopamine agonist ergot drugs. For microadenomas the results, in the hands of most experienced surgeons, are similar. (In this discussion the relative advantages of medical therapy and surgery will not be dealt with; the emphasis, reflecting our expertise, will be on medical therapy.)

The trans-sphenoidal technique for approaching the pituitary gives the most satisfactory surgical results and often allows selective removal of the adenomas (Fig. 4.11). The operating microscope, image intensification (allowing video radiographic monitoring) and antibiotics (minimising post operative meningitis) are advances enabling this to be performed.

Trans-Sphenoidal Surgery – Microadenoma

Stages in the identification and removal of a prolactin microadenoma from the right of the gland are shown in Fig. 4.12. The first picture (a) shows the exposed but undisturbed gland, the second (b) shows the microadenoma being manipulated from the gland, and the third (c) shows the complete tumour just before excision from the lateral aspect of the gland. This patient was a 28 year-old woman with a two-year history of amenorrhoea and galactorrhoea. Serum prolactin pre-operatively was 159 ng/ml (3,180 mu/l).

Trans-Sphenoidal Surgery – Macroadenoma

A macroadenoma at surgery is shown in Fig. 4.13. The patient had a mass effect with bitemporal hemianopia. The first picture (a) shows the large tumour immediately upon opening the dura, before any of the tumour has been removed. The second picture (b) shows the tumour completely excised leaving the thin

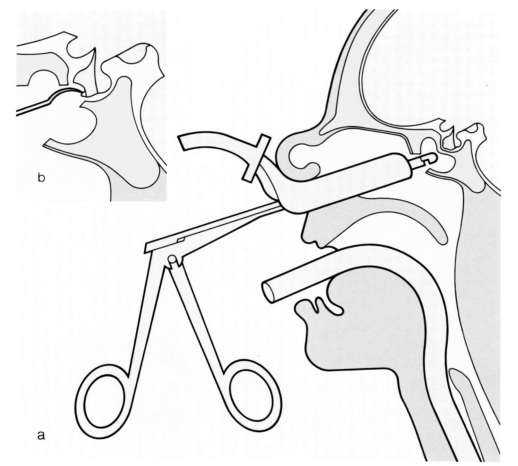

Fig. 4.11 Trans-sphenoidal surgery.
The sphenoidal sinus is reached by a transnasal route (a), and the floor of the sella and dura are opened, exposing the pituitary. This method allows the selective excision of adenomas (adenomectomy, b).

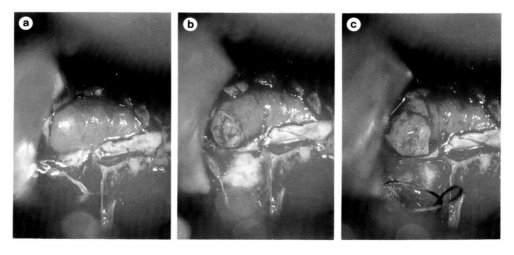

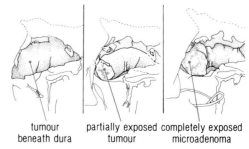

Fig. 4.12 Stages in the surgical removal of a microadenoma.
The exposed, undisturbed gland (a). The tumour being manipulated from the gland (b), and the completely exposed tumour just before excision, (c).

tumour beneath dura   partially exposed tumour   completely exposed microadenoma pituitary gland intact. The bluish structure, anterior to the gland, is the diaphragma sellae. In this case the removal of a moderately large adenoma was accomplished with preservation of the gland.

THE IN VITRO EFFECTS OF BROMOCRIPTINE
The first dopamine agonist ergot compound to be used in clinical practice was bromocriptine, a peptide ergot, having the advantage of a long duration of action, which can be demonstrated using an *in vitro* system. Anterior pituitary cells of a prolactinoma from a female patient were dispersed, placed in a perfusion apparatus, and perfused continuously. When the cells were exposed to dopamine, prolactin secretion was inhibited, but within ten minutes after the withdrawal of dopamine, prolactin secretion increased, becoming maximal after approximately fifteen minutes. Prolactin secretion was inhibited on exposure of the cells to bromocriptine. However, when the bromocriptine was withdrawn,

prolactin secretion remained suppressed for over three hours. On re-exposure to dopamine, prolactin secretion was once more inhibited, recovering again on withdrawal of dopamine. These results are summarised graphically in Fig. 4.14.

THE EFFECTS OF BROMOCRIPTINE IN VIVO
Bromocriptine acts like dopamine in stimulating dopamine receptors on the prolactin-secreting pituitary cells. Stimulation of this receptor leads to inhibition of both prolactin secretion and synthesis. After a single 2.5mg dose of bromocriptine administered at 0900h to women with hyperprolactinaemia, prolactin secretion was inhibited within two hours, and reached nadir at seven hours. When patients are treated chronically, on a 2.5mg dose three times daily, prolactin levels are maintained within the normal range, i.e. less than 20 ng/ml (400 mu/l), throughout a twenty-four hour period (Fig. 4.15).

Fig. 4.13 Stages in the surgical removal of a macroadenoma. The appearance of a macroadenoma after the dura has been opened (a), and the appearance of the pituitary gland after removal of the tumour (b). The bluish structure anterior to the gland is the diaphragma sellae.

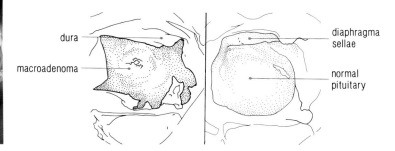

Fig. 4.14 The in vitro response of dispersed prolactinoma cells to dopamine and bromocriptine. Both suppressed prolactin secretion, but whereas prolactin secretion became maximal within fifteen minutes after withdrawal of dopamine, the effect of bromocriptine was longer-lasting, with prolactin levels remaining suppressed for three hours following withdrawal.

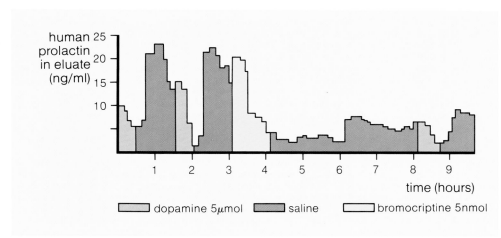

Fig. 4.15 The effects of bromocriptine in vivo. After a single 2.5mg dose of bromocriptine administered at 0900h, prolactin secretion was inhibited within two hours, and reached nadir at seven hours. With chronic treatment (2.5mg three times daily) at both three and six months, prolactin levels were maintained within the normal range throughout a twenty-four hour period.

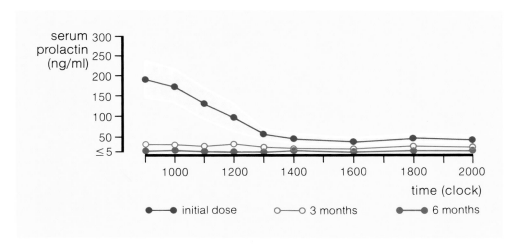

EFFECTS OF BROMOCRIPTINE IN MEN

The first male patient started bromocriptine treatment at St. Bartholomew's Hospital, London, in 1971 and his case illustrates a number of important points (Fig. 4.16). Initially, his prolactin levels were extremely elevated, but the administration of bromocriptine lowered them into the normal range (undetectable by bioassay) and this was associated with cessation of his galactorrhoea. Bromocriptine therapy normalised his prolactin levels and his gonadal function, restoring his potency. Following withdrawal of bromocriptine, hyperprolactinaemia recurred, with associated galactorrhoea and impotence. After restoration of bromocriptine, prolactin levels rapidly returned to normal, galactorrhoea ceased, and potency was restored.

EFFECTS OF BROMOCRIPTINE IN WOMEN

The second patient to be treated was a woman with a large pituitary tumour and extremely high prolactin levels. Bromocriptine lowered her prolactin levels into the normal range, her galactorrhoea ceased, and menstruation returned within one month of starting therapy, even though she had been amenorrhoeic for several years.

The third patient had post-oral contraceptive amenorrhoea and galactorrhoea associated with hyperprolactinaemia. Bromocriptine therapy lowered the prolactin levels to normal, led to cessation of her galactorrhoea, and to normal menstruation (Fig. 4.17).

BROMOCRIPTINE IN AMENORRHOEA

In our experience of treating a large number of amenorrhoeic hyperprolactinaemic women, the results of treating the first fifty-eight appear to be representative (Fig. 4.18). Within one month of starting therapy about twenty-five per cent of patients have a return of regular menstrual cycles. Within two months the number rises to over sixty per cent and within ten months approximately eighty per cent have menstrual cycles. Those who do not are, with only one or two exceptions, patients who have previously undergone pituitary surgery and irradiation and are gonadotrophin deficient. Thus, if hyperprolactinaemia is the cause

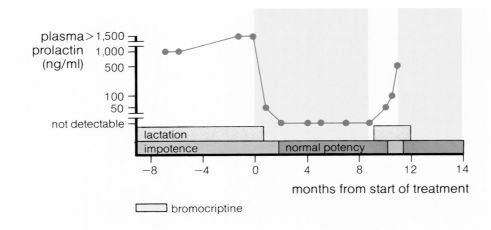

Fig. 4.16 The effects of bromocriptine in a male prolactinoma. Normalisation of serum prolactin by bromocriptine was associated with cessation of galactorrhoea, and with restoration of potency. On stopping the drug, however, both galactorrhoea and impotence returned, only to disappear after reinstitution of bromocriptine therapy.

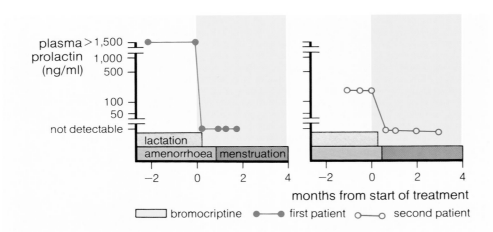

Fig. 4.17 Effects of bromocriptine in a female patient. The first female patient treated had hyperprolactinaemia associated with a large pituitary tumour, and the second had post oral-contraceptive amenorrhoea and galactorrhoea with hyperprolactinaemia. In both cases bromocriptine therapy led to cessation of galactorrhoea and the return of normal menstrual cycling.

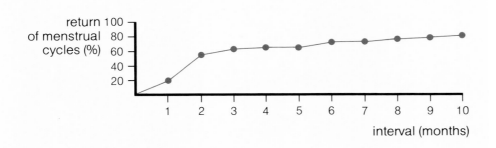

Fig. 4.18 The success rate of bromocriptine in amenorrhoea. If hyperprolactinaemia is the cause of a patient's amenorrhoea, the chances of restoring normal gonadal function with bromocriptine are very good. After one month of treatment, one woman in four will return to normal menstrual cycling; within two months this number will increase to six out of ten, and after ten months, eight out of ten women will be menstruating normally. (Most of the remaining twenty per cent have had pituitary surgery and irradiation therapy and are gonadotrophin deficient.)

of the patient's amenorrhoea, the chances of restoring normal gonadal function by medical therapy alone are extremely good.

LONG-TERM EFFECTS OF BROMOCRIPTINE

To study the long-term effects of bromocriptine on prolactin secretion we carefully evaluated a group of patients (Fig. 4.19). Ten blood samples were taken from each patient before treatment, at three, six and twelve months on therapy, and two months following drug withdrawal. All patients were treated with the same dose of bromocriptine (2.5 mg three times a day). In all cases bromocriptine lowered prolactin levels and in nine of the twelve patients prolactin secretion was suppressed throughout the year. After withdrawal of bromocriptine, prolactin levels rose in all patients to levels similar to those seen prior to therapy. The three patients in whom the prolactin levels were not lowered into the normal range nevertheless regained normal gonadal function.

HYPERPROLACTINAEMIA AND OVULATION

Ovulation is normally associated with a dip in basal body temperature, and normal luteal function with a temperature rise. Basal body temperature is therefore useful as a means of documenting ovulation. When hyperprolactinaemic patients have had prolactin levels and periods restored to normal by bromocriptine, they usually demonstrate a biphasic temperature pattern. One patient had had polymenorrhoea for many years and was found to be hyperprolactinaemic. Bromocriptine normalised her periods and after one year therapy was withdrawn. During therapy her basal body temperature chart (Fig. 4.20) showed a normal biphasic pattern, but following withdrawal of bromocriptine, prolactin levels rose to more than 100 ng/ml (2,000 mu/l), her galactorrhoea returned, and her temperature pattern immediately became monophasic. She did not become amenorrhoeic but developed irregular (presumably anovulatory) periods. Following reinstitution of therapy, circulating prolactin levels normalised, galactorrhoea ceased, and within two weeks she ovulated, demonstrating a post-ovulatory temperature rise. She has subsequently had regular cycles and three successful pregnancies, each with the help of bromocriptine.

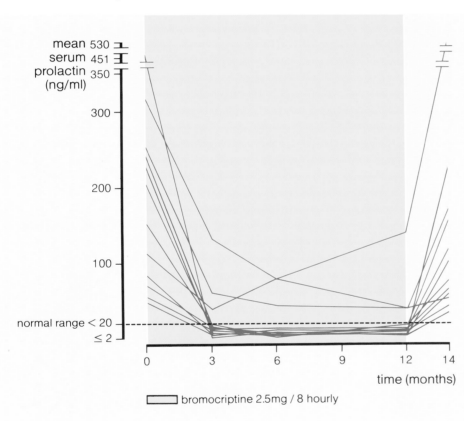

bromocriptine 2.5mg / 8 hourly

Fig. 4.19 The long-term effects of bromocriptine therapy. Prolactin levels in a group of patients on long-term bromocriptine therapy were tested before therapy, after three months, six months, and one year of treatment, (during which all patients received bromocriptine 2.5mg *t.d.s.*), and two months after cessation of treatment. In all cases, prolactin remained suppressed throughout the year, and in most cases, prolactin levels were held within the normal range. Gonadal function was restored even in those patients whose prolactin levels did not return to normal.

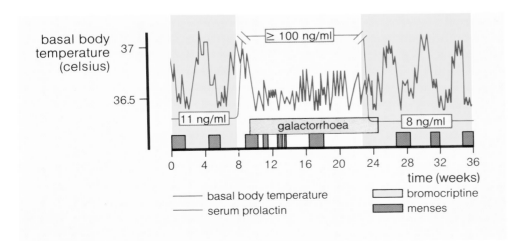

basal body temperature
serum prolactin
bromocriptine
menses

Fig. 4.20 Hyperprolactinaemia and ovulation. Normal ovulation and luteal function are associated with a biphasic basal body temperature. When patients have prolactin levels and periods restored to normal with bromocriptine, their temperature charts demonstrate the normal biphasic pattern. When therapy is withdrawn, the temperature chart shows a monophasic pattern, becoming biphasic again on reinstitution of bromocriptine.

HYPERPROLACTINAEMIC HYPOGONADISM

The pathogenesis of the hypogonadal state in hyperprolactinaemia is poorly understood. In men, testosterone levels may be normal or low, while in women a hypo-oestrogenic state may occur, with loss of ovulation. However, the clinical features in hyperprolactinaemic women differ from those in the postmenopausal state since breast atrophy is absent and gonadotrophin levels are not elevated.

Proposed explanations for the suppression of gonadal function in hyperprolactinaemia include: (i) suppression of gonadotrophin secretion, (ii) inhibition of positive oestrogen feedback on LH secretion in women, (iii) increase in adrenal androgen secretion, and (iv) blockade of the effects of gonadotrophins at the gonadal level (Fig. 4.21). It is probable that an important mechanism is prolactin feedback at the hypothalamus, which alters secretion of gonadotrophin releasing hormone (GnRH), causing LH and FSH secretion to become inappropriately low relative to gonadal steroid levels. Abnormalities in LH pulsatility also occur. Prolactin may interfere with LH and FSH action at the gonad, blocking progesterone synthesis, and may stimulate adrenal androgen secretion.

SIZE REDUCTION OF PROLACTINOMAS

Dopamine agonist therapy for hyperprolactinaemia has usually been reserved for patients with idiopathic hyperprolactinaemia, or small pituitary tumours. However, since surgical therapy of large prolactin-secreting pituitary tumours normalises serum prolactin or gonadal function in less than twenty per cent of patients, particularly those with high prolactin levels, there is a need for a new approach to the problem. Three major pieces of

evidence suggest that medical therapy may help in the treatment of these large tumours:

(i) visual field defects, due to prolactinomas pressing on the optic chiasm, have improved with bromocriptine therapy alone.

(ii) dopamine agonist therapy (with bromocriptine and lisuride) has been shown by neuroradiologic evaluations, to reduce the size of prolactinomas.

(iii) bromocriptine reduces DNA turnover, and the mitotic index, in the *in situ* pituitary of the rat.

These observations have led several groups to evaluate the rôle of bromocriptine as primary therapy for large prolactinomas. Others are assessing bromocriptine as preparation for surgery in the hope of improving surgical results.

Bromocriptine appears to reduce pituitary tumour size in seventy-five to eighty per cent of patients with large prolactin-secreting tumours even with gross extrasellar extension. The type of results that can be expected are illustrated by a patient with a large prolactin-secreting tumour, treated with bromocriptine alone. The patient had a suprasellar extension and visual field defects. Fig. 4.22 represents visual field plots from this patient before and during treatment as well as after withdrawal and reinstitution of bromocriptine. Before therapy (baseline) the patient had a bitemporal hemianopia, complete in the left eye and incomplete in the right eye. The visual fields were greatly improved after ten days, and only an equivocal superior bitemporal quadrantic defect to the low intensity object was present after nearly one year. Thirteen days after withdrawal of medical therapy the tumour had enlarged again and the field defects recurred as an almost complete temporal hemianopia in the left eye and a partial temporal hemianopia in the right. Progressive

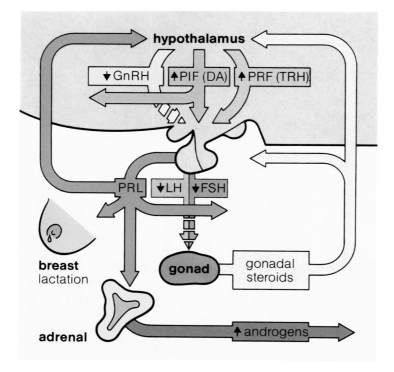

Fig. 4.21 Mechanisms of hyperprolactinaemic hypogonadism. Hyperprolactinaemia causes hypogonadism by several mechanisms: (i) High prolactin (PRL) levels lead to partial suppression of GnRH release, as well as loss of its pulsatility, and (ii) prolactin also interferes with the action of LH and FSH on the gonad. (iii) Prolactin causes an increase in adrenal androgen secretion, and (iv) leads to inhibition of positive oestrogen feedback on GnRH and LH secretion in women.

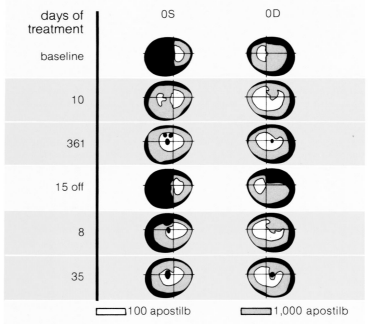

Fig. 4.22 Visual field plots of a patient with hyperprolactinaemia. The visual fields shown here were plotted using a Goldmann perimeter under identical conditions with a 0.25mm² object at two different light intensities: 1,000 apostilb (I_4) and 100 apostilb (I_2). The black periphery indicates a normal visual field for comparison. An almost complete bitemporal hemianopia (pre-therapy) which had nearly gone after a year of treatment with bromocriptine, returned on cessation of therapy and began to subside after reinstitution of bromocriptine.

improvement in visual fields was again observed over the subsequent six months after reintroduction of therapy.

Changes in Pituitary Volume During Bromocriptine Therapy

Fig. 4.23 shows coronal CT head scans (post–enhancement) from the patient whose visual fields are shown in Fig. 4.22. The left panel CT scan performed on a Delta 25 scanner illustrates the situation before therapy, the right panel performed on a GE 8800 scanner two weeks after starting bromocriptine therapy, 2.5 mg three times a day. Before therapy (left panel) the scan shows an enlargement of the pituitary fossa and an enhancing mass extending inferiorly into the sphenoid sinus, superiorly into the chiasmatic cistern and abutting on the third ventricle. Two weeks after starting bromocriptine therapy (right panel) the scan shows marked reduction in tumour size, with regression of the suprasellar extension. The chiasmatic cistern is now largely free of tumour, apart from a finger-like process to the left of the midline. The intrasellar high density is present in the pre-enhancement scan and represents calcification within the tumour. Within the short space of two weeks, therefore, there was marked reduction in the size of the pituitary and a consequent decompression of the optic chiasm which explains the rapid improvement in visual fields observed in this patient. From our experience of sixteen patients with large prolactin-secreting tumours, thirteen showed similar changes. The three patients in whom these changes were not observed consisted of:

(i) a patient with a pituitary cyst which was associated with a small prolactinoma, but in whom the majority of the pituitary mass was the cyst,

(ii) a patient with an extremely large tumour which was reduced in size but still remained large. (His serum prolactin level fell by ninety per cent but still remained elevated at 328 ng/ml at the end of nine months of therapy) and,

(iii) a patient who had only been treated for six weeks and in whom there was as yet only equivocal evidence of reduction in size of the tumour.

Other groups have had similar results. It seems that about sixty-five per cent of macroadenomas with large extrasellar extensions may be treated with bromocriptine alone to shrink the tumours and relieve both the mass effects and the hormonal excess.

CHANGES IN SERUM PROLACTIN LEVELS

In patients with macroadenomas the serum prolactin levels can be readily suppressed with bromocriptine therapy. Fig. 4.24 shows serum prolactin levels throughout the day after the initial 2.5 mg oral dose of bromocriptine administered at 0900h to the patient whose visual field plots and CT scans are shown in Figure 4.22 and 4.23, as well as those from a patient with a similar problem. After a single dose of bromocriptine the prolactin levels fell by approximately ninety per cent. In the box are the mean and absolute range of prolactin levels in samples taken at the same time intervals before therapy (baseline) and during bromocriptine therapy, 7.5 mg/day. In the first patient the prolactin levels were suppressed into the normal range (less than 20 ng/ml) and in the second patient prolactin levels, although lowered, did not come down to normal. However, with treatment over one year the levels continued to fall to 78 ng/ml. In these patients, as with the patients with microadenomas, gonadal function is usually restored to normal. As previously noted, when therapy was withdrawn at one year, visual field defects recurred in the first patient and this was associated with prolactin levels rising again to 2,580 ng/ml at

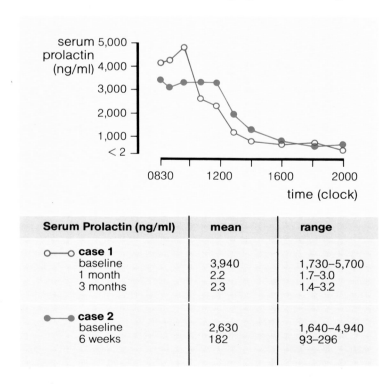

Serum Prolactin (ng/ml)	mean	range
○——○ **case 1**		
baseline	3,940	1,730–5,700
1 month	2.2	1.7–3.0
3 months	2.3	1.4–3.2
●——● **case 2**		
baseline	2,630	1,640–4,940
6 weeks	182	93–296

Labels on Fig. 4.23 diagram (left): 3rd ventricle; suprasellar extension of tumour; calcification within tumour; tumour in sphenoid sinus.
Labels (right): falx cerebri; 3rd ventricle; regressed tumour; sphenoid sinus.

Fig. 4.23 Coronal CT head scans before and during treatment with bromocriptine. The left scan (before therapy) shows enlargement of the pituitary fossa and an enhancing mass extending inferiorly into the sphenoid sinus, superiorly into the chiasmatic cistern, and abutting on the third ventricle. The right scan (taken after two weeks of therapy) shows a marked reduction in tumour size, with regression of the suprasellar extension.

Fig. 4.24 Changes in serum prolactin levels. The effect on serum prolactin levels throughout the day of a single 2.5mg oral dose of bromocriptine at 0900h. Case one is the patient whose visual field chart and CT scans are shown in Figs. 4.22 and 4.23. Case two is a patient with a similar problem. In patients like these, even when prolactin levels do not come down to the normal range, gonadal function is usually restored.

thirteen days in comparison to the pre-treatment level (3,940 ng/ml). It should be noted, however, that in male patients on bromocriptine prolactin levels usually fall rapidly and easily into the normal range. If this does not occur gonadal function may not return to normal.

SIDE EFFECTS
These occur only at the start of treatment and disappear with continued therapy. There are no long-term problems associated with chronic treatment at the doses used for hyperprolactinaemia, usually 7.5mg/day, rarely more than 15mg/day.

Initiating Side Effects
If treatment is started with full doses or increased too quickly, dizziness, nausea and postural hypotension may occur. To avoid these, bromocriptine must always be taken during a meal. It should be started at night on retiring with a sandwich and glass of milk. After taking half a tablet (1.25 mg) for three nights, one tablet may be taken. After taking this dose for three further nights this dose may be taken instead during the evening meal. At intervals of three days additional half tablets (1.25mg increments) may be progressively added until achievement of the usual dose of one tablet (2.5 mg) taken three times daily, in the middle of breakfast, lunch and the evening meal. If side effects still occur longer intervals and smaller increments should be used.

The only group of patients not suffering these side effects if given the full dose immediately is puerperal women. They may be given bromocriptine 2.5 mg two or three times daily to suppress puerperal lactation, without side effects, if treatment is started within twenty-four hours of delivery. The reasons for this difference are unknown.

PREGNANCY AND BROMOCRIPTINE
Many hyperprolactinaemic women desire pregnancy. The administration of bromocriptine lowers the prolactin levels and restores gonadal function, therefore conception presents little difficulty. There are, however, several important considerations that must be recognised by both physician and patient. The possible teratogenic sequelae of foetal exposure to bromocriptine merit consideration. There is no evidence for teratogenicity in animal studies, and in 1,400 pregnancies in women who were taking bromocriptine when they conceived there is no evidence of increased incidence of abortion, multiple pregnancy, or fetal abnormalities. However, until these babies have lived their own complete life cycles, the possibility of unexpected late effects cannot be excluded. In order to minimise fetal exposure to bromocriptine, it is suggested that the patient should use mechanical contraception. Once three regular menstrual cycles have occurred, contraceptive precautions are discontinued. In this way pregnancy can be suspected as soon as a menstrual period is forty-eight hours overdue. At that time a serum beta HCG assay should be performed to confirm the pregnancy and the patient should discontinue bromocriptine. In this way the fetus is exposed to bromocriptine for a theoretical maximum of sixteen days.

There is little doubt that patients with pituitary tumours run a small but significant risk of expansion of the tumour during pregnancy. It is very difficult to assess the absolute risk. With microadenomas the incidence seems to be less than one per cent and probably less than 0.5 per cent. In patients with macro-adenomas the incidence is probably higher, perhaps between five and twenty per cent. This risk is unrelated to bromocriptine therapy prior to pregnancy but may occur when fertility is induced with other drugs, including exogenous gonadotrophins and clomiphene, and even when no drug therapy has been employed in patients with pre-existing pituitary adenomas.

In practice the problem of pregnancy is not great since the vast majority of women who present with hyperprolactinaemia have only microadenomas. To avoid major problems it is extremely important that the patients undergo careful endocrine, neuro-radiological, and neuro-ophthalmological evaluation prior to treatment. If there is no suprasellar extension and if the patient harbours only a microadenoma then the risk of swelling of the pituitary is extremely small; it is therefore suggested that the patient be evaluated clinically at bi-monthly intervals throughout pregnancy. If the patient has a macroadenoma and suprasellar extension, a strong case can be made for decompression of the tumour prior to pregnancy or, alternatively, for the patient to be treated with external pituitary irradiation. However, it is possible even for these patients to go through pregnancy without developing visual disturbances and, furthermore, even if visual disturbances occur in one pregnancy, the problem may not recur in subsequent pregnancies.

Thus the approach to the patient with the prolactin-secreting macroadenoma who desires pregnancy can be either expectant or prophylactic. I believe that as the risk of swelling of the adenoma is less than twenty per cent, it is reasonable to adopt an expectant policy. Others suggest that pituitary decompression should be performed surgically and still others recommend that external pituitary irradiation be given. It is not clear whether external pituitary irradiation or decompression of the pituitary by surgery, or both, completely prevents symptom-generating pituitary enlargement. It should be stressed that so far no patient has become permanently blind following expansion of the tumour during pregnancy.

If visual field defects or headaches from tumour expansion do occur during pregnancy a number of therapeutic options are available. Following termination of the pregnancy, either by abortion or delivery of the baby, tumours have become smaller and visual symptoms and headaches have resolved in all cases. Thus, if such symptoms occur early in pregnancy, abortion may be indicated. If they occur in the eighth month of pregnancy, premature delivery of the baby may be decided upon although if field defects and symptoms are minor careful observation may be all that is required. The most problematic situation arises when symptoms occur in the middle trimester. At that time it is suggested that bromocriptine therapy be restarted in the hope of reducing the tumour size or at least preventing further swelling. If this is unsuccessful high dose dexamethasone can be used to achieve the same ends. Dexamethasone also reduces the chances of fetal respiratory distress should premature delivery be needed. As a last resort trans-sphenoidal surgery during pregnancy can and has been used to decompress the tumour. As such complications are extremely rare, no one has accumulated any large experience of them.

CONCLUSION
Dopamine agonist therapy such as with bromocriptine for hyperprolactinaemia leads to a reversal of the hyperprolactinaemic-hypogonadal state without risk of the development of pituitary insufficiency. Dopamine agonist therapy is effective not only in patients with microadenomas, but also in the majority of patients with large prolactin-secreting tumours in reducing tumour size; however, the tumour size will increase (as will prolactin levels) after withdrawal of therapy. This may give rise to problems from compression of vital structures by the tumour.

5 The Posterior Pituitary

Peter H Baylis, BSc, MD, FRCP

ANATOMICAL RELATIONSHIP OF THE POSTERIOR PITUITARY TO SURROUNDING STRUCTURES

The pituitary is a composite gland, the anterior lobe being derived from an evagination of the stomodeal ectoderm called 'Rathke's pouch', while the posterior lobe is an extension of the forebrain. The weight of the adult human gland is approximately 620 mg; in females twenty per cent and in males twenty-five per cent of this gland is posterior pituitary. Nervous tissue is the principal component of the posterior pituitary.

The immediate anatomical relationships of the pituitary gland are seen in Figure 5.1, which represents a sagittal section through the pituitary and hypothalamus. The gland lies in a bony fossa, and its stalk pierces the fibrous diaphragma sellae. The lateral wall of the fossa is made up of the cavernous sinus in which lie the carotid syphon and the cranial nerves III, V and VI. The optic chiasm is situated immediately above the pituitary fossa, anterior to the pituitary stalk. The hypothalamus lies above the pituitary stalk and extends to the lateral walls of the third ventricle. Bounded anteriorly by the anterior commissure and posteriorly by the mammillary body, it is composed of many sets of nuclei and neuronal tracts many of which terminate in the median eminence.

Neuronal Tracts from the Paraventricular and Supraoptic Nuclei

Two major nuclei in the hypothalamus synthesise both the peptides antidiuretic hormone (ADH or vasopressin) and oxytocin, the supraoptic and paraventricular (Fig. 5.2). (Smaller groups of neurons synthesising these neurohypophyseal hormones are clustered in the suprachiasmatic region in some, but not all, mammals.) Each neuron in these nuclei synthesises either oxytocin or ADH as part of a larger precursor molecule. In the rostral part of the supraoptic nucleus, oxytocin and ADH neurons are equally distributed, but in the caudal part only oxytocin neurons are found. Similarly, both hormones are present in the rostral paraventricular nucleus, the neurons close to the third ventricle contain oxytocin while those more laterally situated contain ADH. At least four neuronal tracts arise from the supraoptic and paraventricular nuclei. The main pathway terminates in the posterior pituitary to release its peptides into the systemic circulation. Both ADH and oxytocin are found in the zona externa of the median eminence, and the majority of fibres to this region arise from the paraventricular nucleus. From the median eminence, the peptides are secreted into the hypothalamo-pituitary-portal circulation. A third tract passes to the floor of the

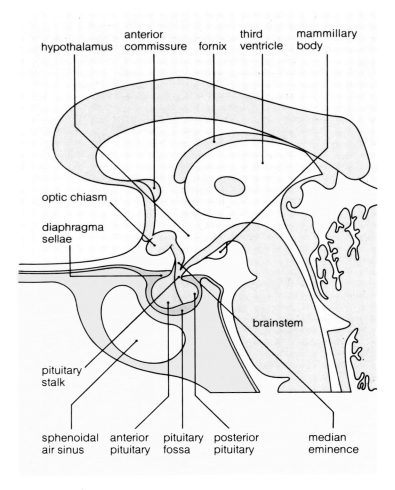

Fig. 5.1 Diagram of the anatomical relationships of the posterior pituitary and hypothalamus to surrounding structures. The diagram represents a sagittal section through the pituitary and hypothalamus.

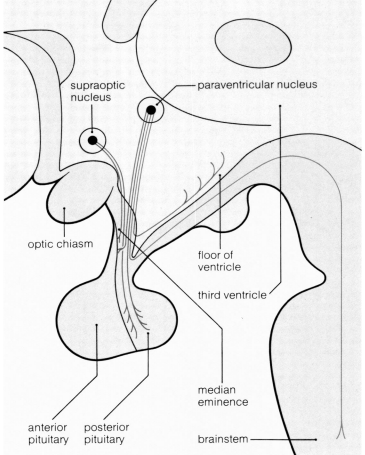

Fig. 5.2 Schematic representation of the neuronal pathways from the paraventricular and supraoptic nuclei. Neuronal tracts from the paraventricular and supraoptic nuclei connect with the posterior pituitary, the median eminence, the floor of the third ventricle, and the brainstem.

third ventricle. Whether the peptide hormones are actively secreted via this tract into the cerebrospinal fluid is unknown, but they are undoubtedly present. The final neuronal pathway terminates in the brainstem in close proximity to the vasomotor centre.

Sensory Tracts to the Paraventricular and Supraoptic Nuclei

Changes in the plasma tonicity are recognised by a putative osmoreceptor which is believed to be situated in the anterior hypothalamus. In man, it appears to be distinct from the paraventricular and supraoptic nuclei and from the thirst centre. It is presumed that afferent fibres from the osmoreceptor go to both ADH and oxytocin synthesising neurons (Fig. 5.3). Baroregulatory afferent fibres arise in low pressure receptors sited in the atria of the heart and the great veins of the chest, and high pressure receptors in the carotid body and arch of the aorta. They terminate in a group of nuclei within the brainstem. Fibres then relay in the posteromedial nucleus of the hypothalamus before ending in the paraventricular and supraoptic nuclei.

The potent stimulatory effect that vomiting has on ADH release is probably mediated by the vagus nerve. It remains unclear whether the effects of hypoglycaemia are monitored by a glucostat and whether an angiotensin sensor exists to appreciate changes in plasma angiotensin concentration. The release of oxytocin by suckling is a neurohormonal reflex, the afferent fibres being carried by the vagus nerve.

Arterial Supply to the Hypothalamus and Pituitary Gland

The majority of the arterial blood supply to the hypothalamus and pituitary gland arises from the internal carotid artery or its branches (Fig. 5.4). The posterior lobe is supplied by the inferior hypophyseal artery and the artery of the trabecula, which is a branch of the superior hypophyseal artery. There is no direct arterial supply to the anterior pituitary, and all its blood comes from the long and short hypophyseal portal vessels which drain the median eminence. Branches from the circle of Willis supply the hypothalamus which is extremely well-perfused. The paraventricular and supraoptic nuclei receive blood from branches of the suprahypophyseal, anterior communicating, anterior cerebral, posterior communicating and posterior cerebral arteries. Venous blood draining from both anterior and posterior lobes of the pituitary enters the dural sinus.

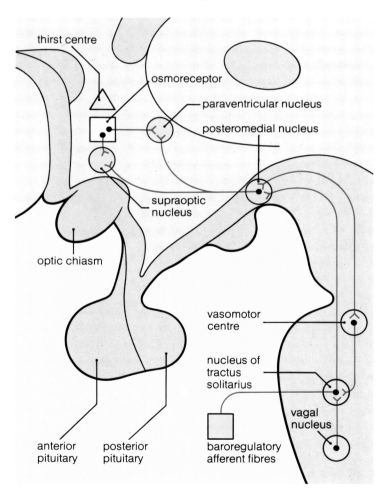

Fig. 5.3 Diagram of the sensory pathways to the paraventricular and supraoptic nuclei. It is believed that changes in plasma tonicity are recognised by an osmoreceptor situated in the anterior hypothalamus. Presumably, afferent fibres connect this osmoreceptor with the neurons synthesising ADH and oxytocin. Baroregulatory information from afferent fibres terminating in brainstem nuclei is relayed to the paraventricular and supraoptic nuclei via the posteromedial nucleus of the hypothalamus.

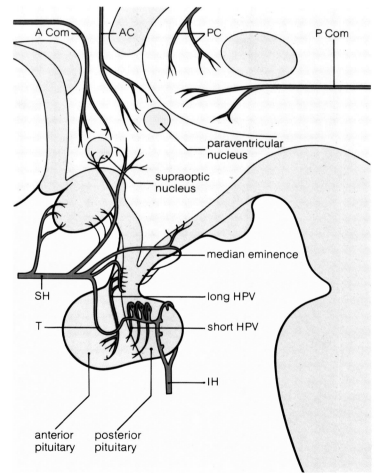

Fig. 5.4 Diagram of the arterial blood supply to the hypothalamus and pituitary gland. Most of the blood supply to the hypothalamus and pituitary arises from the internal carotid artery or its branches. The posterior lobe of the pituitary is supplied by the inferior hypophyseal artery (IH) and the artery of the trabecula (T), while the anterior lobe is supplied indirectly via the hypophyseal portal vessels (HPV). Branches from the circle of Willis supply the hypothalamus, and the paraventricular and supraoptic nuclei in particular are served by branches from the suprahypophyseal (SH), the anterior communicating (ACom), the anterior cerebral (AC), the posterior communicating (PCom) and posterior cerebral (PC) arteries.

CHEMISTRY OF ADH AND OXYTOCIN

The structure of the neurohypophyseal hormones, ADH and oxytocin (Fig. 5.5), was elucidated and their synthesis completed by 1954. Arginine ADH is the antidiuretic hormone of most mammals, except the pig family in which it is lysine ADH. Both are basic molecules with isoelectric points in the region of pH9–10 while oxytocin is more neutral. The ring is essential for biological activity. Position 8 plays a key role in determining oxytocic or vasopressor characteristics. The more basic the amino acid in this position the more vasopressor activity the molecule possesses.

Structure-activity data on a large number of analogues have facilitated the design of analogues possessing desired biological properties. An example is the synthesis of a long-acting antidiuretic molecule (1-deamino, 8-D-arginine vasopressin, desmopressin) which has little pressor activity and is ideal for the treatment of ADH deficiency. Other modifications should lead to ADH antagonists suitable for the treatment of disorders associated with ADH excess.

After secretion by exocytosis from the neurohypophysis, the native nonapeptides circulate unbound to plasma proteins. Their plasma half-life is extremely short (Fig. 5.5) due to efficient clearance by the kidney and liver (ADH) and uterus, kidney and liver (oxytocin). This clearance is so rapid that changes in plasma concentration are usually a reflection of changes in secretion rate rather than clearance rate. In pregnancy, the plasma enzyme oxytocinase degrades both oxytocin and ADH rapidly.

Neurosecretion of Neurohypophyseal Hormones

The principal sites of biosynthesis of ADH and oxytocin are the magnocellular neurons of the supraoptic and paraventricular nuclei (Fig. 5.6). Each neuron synthesises either oxytocin or ADH. They arise as part of larger precursor molecules, pro-oxyphysin and pro-pressophysin respectively. The neurophysin-nonapeptide complex migrates, as neurosecretory granules, along the axons of the neurons from each nucleus at a rate of one to three millimetres per hour. The complex is then stored as granules at the end of the neuronal tracts to be released under the influence of specific stimuli. The common final pathway of these stimuli is phasic electrochemical 'firing' of the neurons themselves. The

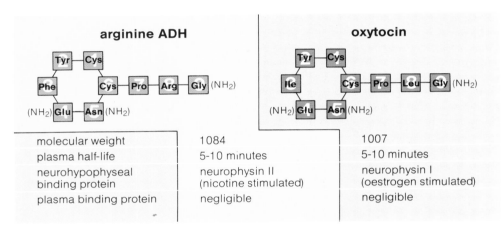

	arginine ADH	oxytocin
molecular weight	1084	1007
plasma half-life	5-10 minutes	5-10 minutes
neurohypophyseal binding protein	neurophysin II (nicotine stimulated)	neurophysin I (oestrogen stimulated)
plasma binding protein	negligible	negligible

Fig. 5.5 Diagram comparing the chemical characteristics of arginine ADH and oxytocin. Arginine ADH is the antidiuretic hormone of most mammals. ADH's are basic molecules (pH 9–10) while oxytocins are more neutral. The more basic the amino acid in position 8, the more vasopressor activity the molecule possesses.

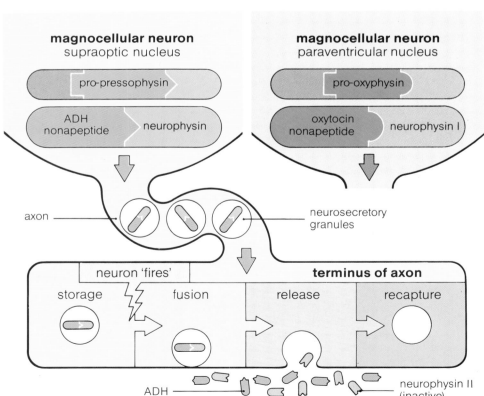

Fig. 5.6 Diagram representing synthesis and release of ADH and oxytocin. ADH and oxytocin are synthesised in the magnocellular neurons of the supraoptic and paraventricular nuclei. Each neuron synthesises either oxytocin or ADH which arise from precursor molecules, pro-oxyphysin and pro-pressophysin respectively. The neurophysin-nonapeptide groups migrate, in the form of neurosecretory granules, along the axons of the magnocellular neurons to be stored at the ends of the neuronal tracts. When the neurons 'fire', the granules fuse with the axonal plasmalemma, and then each nonapeptide and its specific neurophysin are released separately. Once released the neurophysin has no apparent physiological function.

neurosecretory granules then fuse with the plasmalemma of the axon, and the nonapeptide and its specific neurophysin are released separately by exocytosis. The membrane of the granule is then recaptured by micropinocytosis. Once released into the circulation, the neurophysin no longer appears to have any physiological function. Figure 5.7 shows the distribution of ADH in neurosecretory granules within a rat neurohypophysis, demonstrated by immunocytochemical reactions specific for arginine ADH.

FUNCTIONS OF ADH AND OXYTOCIN

The functions of ADH and oxytocin are shown diagrammatically in Figure 5.8. The main physiological rôle of ADH is reduction of free water clearance by the kidney to produce concentrated urine. ADH acts on the distal nephron to increase water permeability of the tubular cell so that solute-free water may pass along the osmotic gradient from the lumen of the nephron to the renal interstitial medulla. At supraphysiological plasma concentrations, ADH contracts smooth muscle, resulting in pressor activity.

Again at high concentrations, it activates liver glycogen phosphorylase to convert glycogen to glucose. Lipolysis is also increased. The secretion of ADH from the median eminence into the portal circulation of the hypothalamo-pituitary region may modulate the release of adrenocorticotrophin (ACTH) from the anterior pituitary gland. Recent studies suggest that intracerebral ADH may modify behaviour and improve memory in animals.

Oxytocin has no definitely known rôle in the male, although it may aid contraction of the seminal vesicles of the testis. In the female, it contracts the pregnant uterus, although it is not the sole initiator of parturition. During lactation, oxytocin promotes milk ejection by contraction of smooth muscle in the breast ducts; an effect that is mediated by a neurohormonal reflex. Like ADH, oxytocin is released from the median eminence and may affect the anterior pituitary. The response of gonadotrophins to the gonadotrophin releasing hormone appears to be modified by oxytocin. There is tentative evidence that oxytocin increases lipolysis in the adipocyte.

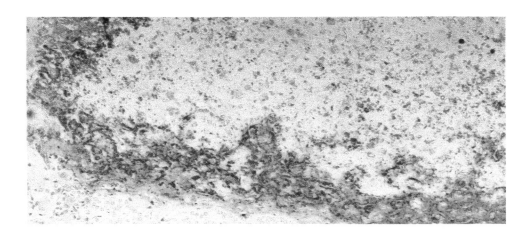

Fig. 5.7   Histological section of a rat neurohypophysis. The distribution of ADH in the form of neurosecretory granules is demonstrated by immunocytochemical reactions specific for arginine ADH.

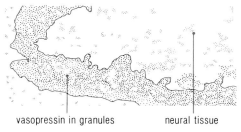

vasopressin in granules   neural tissue

Fig. 5.8   Diagram showing the functions of ADH and oxytocin. The most important function of ADH is the reduction of free water clearance by the kidney. At high concentrations it contracts smooth muscle, and initiates the conversion of glycogen to glucose in the liver. Secretion of ADH into the hypothalamo-pituitary circulation modulates the release of ACTH from the anterior pituitary. Oxytocin aids contraction of the pregnant uterus and assists milk ejection during lactation. There is evidence that oxytocin may aid contraction of the seminal vesicles of the testis, may have some effect in the anterior pituitary on the response of gonadotrophins to gonadotrophin releasing hormone and may also increase lipolysis in the adipocyte.

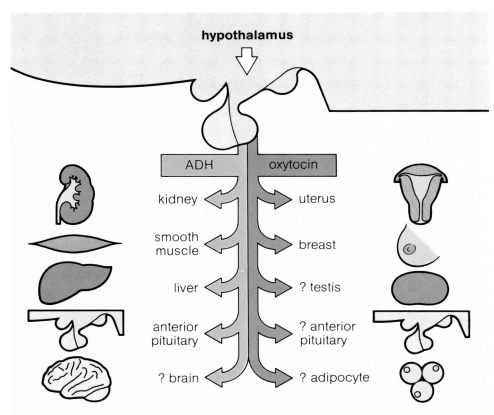

hypothalamus

| ADH | oxytocin |

kidney ← → uterus

smooth muscle ← → breast

liver ← → ? testis

anterior pituitary ← → ? anterior pituitary

? brain ← → ? adipocyte

Regulation of ADH Secretion

The factors that regulate ADH secretion have been clearly defined (Fig. 5.9), the major determinant being plasma osmolality. However, different solutes have varying abilities to stimulate ADH release. Sodium and mannitol appear to be the most potent, while glucose has little or no effect on ADH secretion. Large quantities of ADH are released after marked hypotension, hypovolaemia and vomiting. Angiotensin II and hypoglycaemia both appear to be specific stimuli of ADH secretion. Although many other factors have been reported to stimulate ADH release (e.g. pain, stress, emotion), these observations have not been confirmed using direct methods to measure plasma ADH.

Factors Regulating Oxytocin Secretion

The factors that control oxytocin secretion in the male and in the non-pregnant, non-suckling female are unclear (Fig. 5.10). Recent studies in animals show that osmotic stimulation releases oxytocin in similar quantities to ADH but that the quantity of oxytocin released after haemorrhage is considerably smaller than the quantity of ADH released. Oxytocin secretion appears to increase with the duration of pregnancy but the regulating factors are unknown. Suckling is a specific stimulus for oxytocin release. At the time of parturition, plasma oxytocin concentrations are very high, although the mechanism controlling its release is not fully understood.

Osmoregulation of ADH Secretion

Slow infusion of hypertonic saline (5% NaCl, 0.06 ml/kg/min) into normal healthy individuals causes a linear increase in plasma osmolality (Fig. 5.11). Plasma ADH concentration rises in response to plasma hypertonicity. Conversely, a fall in plasma osmolality induced by a standard oral water load (20 ml/kg) suppresses ADH secretion so that plasma ADH becomes undetectable. As plasma osmolality rises to values of 298 mmol/kg and above, thirst is experienced. Under normal circumstances, healthy individuals maintain their plasma osmolality within the range 282 to 295 mmol/kg, with plasma ADH concentration varying from 0.5 to 6.0 pg/ml which allows the formation of maximally dilute and concentrated urine, respectively.

The relationship between plasma ADH (pADH) and osmolality (pOS) appears to be linear, and may be defined by the function pADH = 0.6 (pOS-284), r = + 0.80, p<0.001. The slope of the regression line is a measure of the sensitivity of the osmotic-sensor and ADH-releasing unit. Thus, in this instance, there is a rise in plasma ADH of 0.6 pg/ml for every unit rise in plasma osmolality. The abscissal intercept defines the theoretical threshold for ADH release, and is approximately 284 mmol/kg. At plasma osmolalities below this value, plasma ADH remains undetectable, while those above cause a linear increase in plasma ADH concentration.

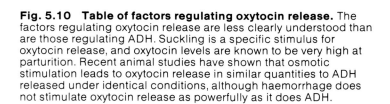

Factors Regulating ADH Release

osmotic regulation	non-osmotic regulation
	haemodynamic:
stimulatory solutes:	hypotension, hypovolaemia
sodium, mannitol, urea	nausea and/or vomiting
	hypoglycaemia
non-stimulatory solutes:	renin-angiotensin
glucose	pain, stress, emotion?

Fig. 5.9   Table of factors regulating ADH release. ADH secretion is mainly determined by plasma osmolality, with sodium and mannitol being the most potent stimulatory solutes. The main non-osmotic factors regulating ADH release are hypotension, hypovolaemia and vomiting. Angiotensin II and hypoglycaemia also stimulate ADH release. It has been suggested that pain, stress and profound emotion may also be ADH stimuli, although definite evidence is so far unavailable.

Factors Regulating Oxytocin Release

physiological regulation largely unknown
suckling
pregnancy and parturition
osmotic and haemodynamic factors?

Fig. 5.10   Table of factors regulating oxytocin release. The factors regulating oxytocin release are less clearly understood than are those regulating ADH. Suckling is a specific stimulus for oxytocin release, and oxytocin levels are known to be very high at parturition. Recent animal studies have shown that osmotic stimulation leads to oxytocin release in similar quantities to ADH released under identical conditions, although haemorrhage does not stimulate oxytocin release as powerfully as it does ADH.

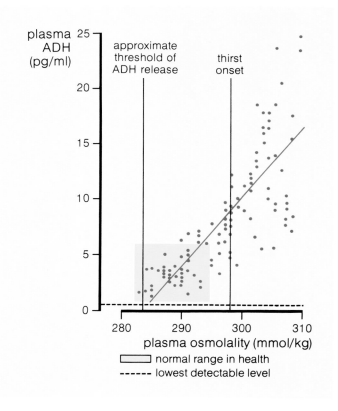

Fig. 5.11   Graph delineating the relationship of plasma osmolality to ADH secretion. Plasma ADH concentration rises in response to plasma hypertonicity, and falls to undetectable levels in response to a standard oral water load of 20ml/kg. Thirst is normally experienced when plasma osmolality reaches 298 mmol/kg or more. Healthy individuals maintain their plasma osmolality within the range 282 to 295 mmol/kg, with plasma ADH concentration varying between 0.5 to 6.0 pg/ml. From this graph, it can be seen that there is a rise in plasma ADH of 0.6 pg/ml for every unit rise in plasma osmolality. The abscissal intercept defines the theoretical threshold for ADH release, at approximately 284 mmol/kg.

This functional analysis of osmotically-mediated ADH release is helpful in defining disorders of ADH secretion. Abnormalities in the sensitivity of the ADH-releasing unit and in the threshold of ADH secretion have been defined.

Baroregulation of ADH Secretion

An acute fall in blood pressure or blood volume causes release of ADH. Whether hypertension or hypervolaemia affect ADH secretion is not known. Figure 5.12 shows the exponential rise in plasma ADH concentrations in response to progressive hypotension induced in healthy normal subjects by infusion of the ganglion-blocking drug trimetaphan over periods of fifteen to thirty minutes. Similar large increases in plasma ADH have been demonstrated in normal humans rendered hypotensive after tilting or hypovolaemic after phlebotomy. The relationship between the rate of fall of blood pressure to the ADH response is not known.

Minor fluctuations in blood pressure appear to have very little effect on plasma ADH concentration. A fall in blood pressure of ten per cent or more must be attained before a significant rise in ADH is achieved. However, a forty per cent reduction in pressure produces plasma ADH levels approximately one hundred times greater than the normal basal concentrations.

Inter-Relationship between Osmoregulation and Baroregulation of ADH Secretion

The two main systems controlling ADH secretion do not appear to operate independently. Osmotic stimulation by hypertonic saline infusion of rats rendered hypotensive or hypovolaemic shows a subtle but definite change in osmoregulation of ADH secretion. This is demonstrated schematically in Figure 5.13. The regression line labelled N represents normotensive/normovolaemic osmoregulation of ADH. As either blood pressure or blood volume is reduced, the line moves to the left of N and its slope becomes steeper. Thus, with these moderate degrees of hypotension/hypovolaemia, the sensitivity of ADH release is increased and the osmotic threshold for its release is lowered.

The pathophysiological consequence of these alterations is the preservation of osmoregulation despite moderate degrees of hypotension or hypovolaemia. Baroregulation of ADH does not over-ride osmoregulation, and animals can continue to excrete free water, or concentrate urine, but at a lower plasma osmolality 'set-point'.

Because there is an inter-relationship between these two ADH regulating mechanisms there must be some form of integration of the sensory information which is fed to the neurons synthesising and releasing ADH in the hypothalamus.

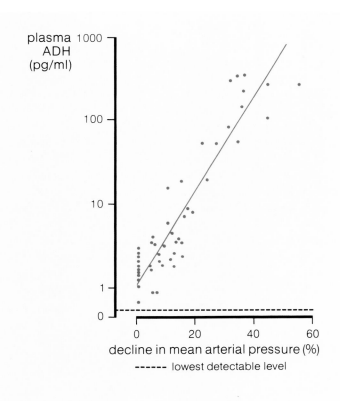

Fig. 5.12 Graph delineating the relationship between mean arterial pressure and ADH release. An acute fall in blood pressure or volume causes release of ADH. The graph shows the exponential rise in ADH in response to progressive hypotension induced in normal subjects by infusion of trimetaphan over periods ranging from fifteen to thirty minutes. Blood pressure must be reduced by at least ten per cent before any significant rise in ADH secretion occurs, although a forty per cent reduction in blood pressure leads to plasma ADH concentrations about one hundred times the normal basal level.

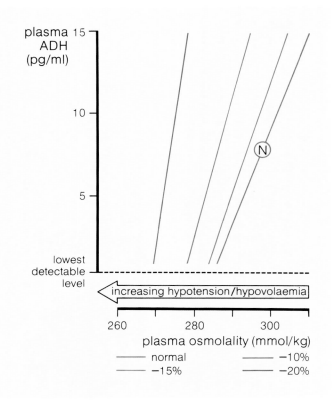

Fig. 5.13 Diagram of the relationship between osmoregulation and baroregulation of ADH secretion. Osmotic stimulation of hypotensive or hypovolaemic rats induces a definite change in osmoregulation of ADH secretion. The regression line (N) represents normotensive/normovolaemic osmoregulation of ADH. With moderate reductions in blood volume or pressure, the line moves to the left and becomes steeper, demonstrating an increase in sensitivity of ADH releasing mechanisms and a lowering of the osmotic threshold for its secretion.

CAUSES OF POLYURIA AND POLYDIPSIA

Figure 5.14 delineates the only three basic disorders which can account for polyuria (arbitrarily defined as a persistent twenty-four hour urine volume greater than 2.5 litres) and polydipsia (excessive thirst). These disorders are: (i) primary polydipsia; (ii) cranial diabetes insipidus; (iii) nephrogenic diabetes insipidus.

Primary polydipsia may occur for no apparent reason, but more often is related to some form of psychiatric illness. Mouth dryness caused by drugs (e.g. mono-amine oxidase inhibitors) or mouth-breathing must be distinguished from true polydipsia. ADH secretion is normally suppressed by the low plasma osmolality in primary polydipsia but its renal action may also be impaired if excessive fluid intake is prolonged, because the solute concentration within the renal interstitial medulla is reduced by a 'wash-out' effect. This leads to a reduction in the osmotic gradient across the renal tubular cell. Thus, even when there is maximum tubular permeability under the action of ADH, free water is unable to flow from the lumen to the medulla and consequently urinary concentrating ability is impaired.

Cranial diabetes insipidus is due to an absolute or more often a relative lack of ADH. (The causes are listed in Fig. 5.15.) The majority of patients have measurable plasma ADH, but its concentration is inappropriately low for the concomitant plasma osmolality.

Acquired nephrogenic diabetes insipidus is probably the commonest cause of polyuria, particularly in association with the osmotic diuresis of diabetes mellitus. The hereditary, sex-linked form of nephrogenic diabetes insipidus is extremely rare.

In all instances, there is resistance to the renal action of ADH and consequently plasma ADH is inappropriately high with respect to urine osmolality. Renal infection, post-obstructive uropathy, vascular lesions, electrolyte disturbances (hypokalaemia and hypercalcaemia), amyloid and sickle-cell anaemia are among the commonest causes of nephrogenic diabetes insipidus.

Causes of Cranial Diabetes Insipidus

Cranial diabetes insipidus is an uncommon condition characterised by an absolute or relative lack of ADH (see Fig. 5.15). The familial forms of the disorder are very rare. It may be inherited as a dominant or recessive trait in patients with the isolated ADH deficiency. These patients become obviously polyuric in the first year or two of life. Plasma ADH is undetectable under basal conditions, but it may be released following profound stimulation.

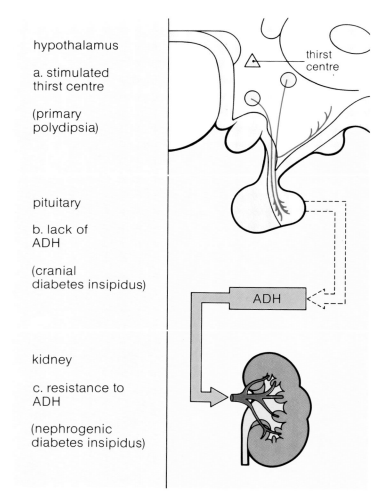

hypothalamus

a. stimulated thirst centre

(primary polydipsia)

pituitary

b. lack of ADH

(cranial diabetes insipidus)

kidney

c. resistance to ADH

(nephrogenic diabetes insipidus)

Causes of Cranial Diabetes Insipidus

familial

as isolated defect

or in association with diabetes mellitus, optic atrophy, nerve deafness, bladder and ureter atonia (DIDMOAD syndrome)

acquired

idiopathic (approx. 50% of patients)

trauma (head injury, surgery to hypothalamo-pituitary region)

rare

tumour (pituitary macroadenoma, craniopharyngioma, metastatic carcinoma)

granulomata (sarcoid, eosinophilic granuloma)

infection (pyogenic or tuberculous basal meningitis, encephalitis)

vascular (peripartum hypotension, aneurysm)

external irradiation

Fig. 5.14   Diagram of the causes of polyuria and polydipsia.
Primary polydipsia (a) is usually related to psychiatric illness. ADH secretion is suppressed by low plasma osmolality induced by the excessive water intake which, if prolonged, may also affect the kidney. Cranial diabetes insipidus (b) is due to a shortage or absence of ADH. In nephrogenic diabetes insipidus (c), there is resistance to the renal action of ADH, with a consequent raising of plasma ADH concentration to a level inappropriately high relative to urine osmolality.

Fig. 5.15   Table of the causes of cranial diabetes insipidus.
All patients have low or undetectable plasma ADH levels relative to their plasma osmolality. There is evidence that two types of functional defect may occur; one in the osmotic-sensing unit and the other in the neurons which should synthesise and release the ADH.

The polyuria in patients with the DIDMOAD syndrome (see Fig. 5.15) is less profound than in those with the isolated defect. No specific cause can be found for about fifty per cent of patients with acquired cranial diabetes insipidus.

Surgery to a pituitary tumour or the tumour itself may cause cranial diabetes insipidus, if there is injury to the hypothalamus or the upper part of the pituitary stalk, and this accounts for a large proportion of cases. The other causes of cranial diabetes insipidus are rare.

All patients have low or undetectable plasma ADH concentration in relation to their plasma osmolality. Investigation of the pattern of ADH secretion in response to osmotic and non-osmotic stimulation suggests that two types of functional defect may occur; one defect appears to be in the osmotic-sensing unit and the other in the neurons that synthesise and release the hormone.

WATER DEPRIVATION TEST

Some form of water deprivation test has long been the 'cornerstone' for differentiating the causes of polyuria. The protocol for a modified Dashe dehydration test combined with an assessment of response to exogenous ADH is given in Figures 5.16 – 5.18. Patients with moderate or severe cranial diabetes insipidus will be clearly distinguished from others by the observation of consistently hypotonic urine during fluid restriction, together with concentrated urine after exogenous ADH. Hypotonic urine following exogenous ADH strongly suggests nephrogenic diabetes insipidus.

Difficulty is often experienced differentiating primary polydipsia from mild cranial and nephrogenic diabetes insipidus. This is due to the fact that many polydipsic patients have a minor concentrating defect secondary to the solute loss from the renal interstitial medulla. Measurement of plasma ADH in response to osmotic stimulation and the relationship of endogenous plasma ADH to urine osmolality after overnight dehydration will aid the differentiation of these disorders.

The water deprivation test is difficult to perform correctly, unpleasant for the patient (who may also drink surreptitiously during the test) and relies heavily on the patient's ability to empty the bladder completely. For these reasons it is far from ideal. Furthermore, the stimulus to ADH secretion is a combination of hypertonicity and hypovolaemia, especially towards the end of the period of dehydration. Although the test mimics the physiological situation, it fails to provide a pure osmotic or haemodynamic stimulus.

Water Deprivation Test

preparation of patient

fluid intake encouraged during night before test

light breakfast, no tea, coffee, alcohol or smoking for 12 hours before test

patient to be supervised throughout test

Fig. 5.16 Table of preparatory procedures for a water deprivation test. This should be performed during the working day rather than overnight, so that the patient may be adequately supervised and severe dehydration avoided.

Water Deprivation Test

dehydration test

no fluids for 8 hours: allow only dry snacks

weigh patient hourly: consider stopping test if there is more than 3% loss of initial body weight

take urine sample every hour to measure volume and osmolality

draw blood every hour to measure plasma osmolality and ADH if possible.

patient to be supervised throughout test

Fig. 5.17 Table of procedures comprising a water deprivation test.

Water Deprivation Test

response to ADH

after 8 hours dehydration, administer desmopressin 40 μg intranasally or 2 μg intramuscularly, patient allowed to eat and drink

collect urine at 3 and 5 hours after desmopressin to measure volume and osmolality

draw blood at 5 hours to measure plasma osmolality

patient to be supervised throughout test

Fig. 5.18 Table of procedures for testing response to an exogenous ADH analogue after a water deprivation test.

Differentiation of the Causes of Polyuria

The most precise way to diagnose the three basic causes of polyuria rests on the measurement of plasma ADH, plasma osmolality and urine osmolality after osmotic stimulation or dehydration or both. Figure 5.19a shows that, after five per cent hypertonic saline infusion, patients with cranial diabetes insipidus (CDI) have values that fall to the right of the normal range, while those with primary polydipsia or nephrogenic diabetes insipidus remain in the normal range.

Nephrogenic diabetes insipidus (NDI – Fig. 5.19b) can be readily distinguished by the inappropriately high plasma ADH in relation to the low urine osmolality attained after dehydration.

Occasionally polydipsic patients fall into the NDI area, but a week of treatment with desmopressin will restore the responsiveness of the renal tubule to endogenous ADH. Indeed, these patients may even develop hyponatraemia because of persistent inappropriate drinking in the presence of exogenous ADH. This observation has been recommended as the basis of a specific test for primary polydipsia.

Treatment of Cranial Diabetes Insipidus

Many patients with mild cranial diabetes insipidus, i.e. twenty-four hour urine volume up to four litres, may elect to have no therapy, and appear to remain well. These patients rely on their thirst mechanism to maintain water homeostasis. If an untreated patient is unable to obtain fluid or loses thirst awareness (e.g.

coma), the condition can be life-threatening. Furthermore, long-standing cranial diabetes insipidus can lead to hydroureter and hydronephrosis, and possibly a degree of nephrogenic diabetes insipidus due to solute 'wash-out' from the kidney. Therefore there are arguments for treating all patients.

Non-hormonal drugs (Fig. 5.20) have been strongly advocated in the past when ADH preparations were hazardous to administer. Chlorpropamide and clofibrate appear to act by increasing the renal tubular sensitivity to circulating endogenous ADH, while carbamazepine probably increases ADH secretion. These drugs are only appropriate for patients with mild or moderate diabetes insipidus who have detectable basal plasma ADH. The precise mechanism of action of thiazide drugs is unknown, but it is probably related to the reduction in total body sodium and reduced glomerular filtration. All these oral preparations may reduce the polyuria by twenty-five to fifty per cent.

Desmopressin is a long-acting ADH analogue with potent antidiuretic and minimal pressor characteristics, administered intranasally or parenterally. Care must be taken to avoid overdosage. Persistent antidiuresis even with only moderate drinking will eventually lead to severe hyponatraemia. It is therefore wise to allow the patient to develop polyuria for a short period each week. Lysine ADH is a poor substitute for desmopressin because its therapeutic action lasts for only one to three hours and it retains pressor activity.

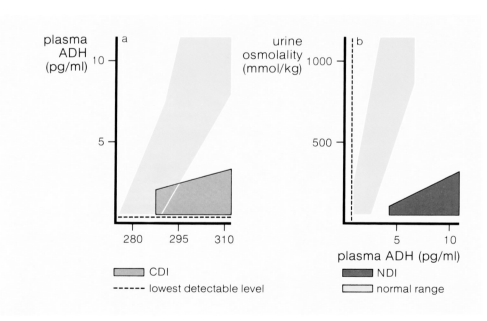

CDI
------ lowest detectable level
NDI
normal range

Fig. 5.19 Diagram of measurements used to differentiate the causes of polyuria. After osmotic stimulation with 5% hypertonic saline (a), patients with cranial diabetes insipidus (CDI) exhibit values to the right of the normal range, while those with nephrogenic diabetes insipidus (NDI) and primary polydipsia will show values within the normal limits. After overnight dehydration (b) nephrogenic diabetes insipidus is usually distinguishable from primary polydipsia by the inappropriately high levels of plasma ADH relative to urine osmolality. If a polydipsic patient has ADH levels in the NDI area (because of kidney 'wash-out') a week of treatment with an exogenous ADH will restore the responsiveness of the renal tubule to endogenous ADH.

Fig. 5.20 Table of drugs used in the treatment of cranial diabetes insipidus.

Treatment of Cranial Diabetes Insipidus

non-hormonal oral drugs	ADH analogues
thiazide diuretic (e.g. bendrofluazide 5mg daily)	desmopressin intranasal 10-40µg daily intramuscular 1-4µg daily
chlorpropamide 250-500mg daily	
clofibrate 1–2g daily	lysine ADH intranasal 5-20 units daily
carbamazepine 200-400mg daily	

CARDINAL FEATURES OF THE SYNDROME OF INAPPROPRIATE ANTIDIURETIC HORMONE

Although many separate descriptions of the electrolyte disorders that occur in this syndrome were recorded in the first half of this century, the true pathogenesis of the syndrome was not deduced until 1957 by Schwartz and co-workers who set out fundamental criteria (Fig. 5.21). Circulating levels of ADH often tend to be in the same range as the normally hydrated adult, and they are only recognised as abnormal in relation to the concurrent overhydration and plasma hypotonicity. An unambiguous diagnosis of the syndrome of inappropriate antidiuretic hormone (SIADH) can be made by measuring plasma ADH when the patient is hyponatraemic and hypotonic.

Causes of the Syndrome of Inappropriate Antidiuretic Hormone

Many conditions have been described in association with the cardinal manifestations of SIADH (Figs. 5.22 and 5.23). In the majority, ADH measurements have not been made, so doubt must remain about some of the causes. Four main groups of disorders emerge: neoplastic, central nervous, respiratory and drug-related.

Features of the Syndrome of Inappropriate Antidiuretic Hormone

hyponatraemia and hypotonicity of plasma

less than maximal urinary dilution in the presence of plasma hypotonicity

excessive renal excretion of sodium

absence of volume depletion or oedema-forming states

normal renal and adrenal function

Fig. 5.21 Table of the criteria for diagnosis of the syndrome of inappropriate antidiuretic hormone (SIADH).

Causes of the Syndrome of Inappropriate Antidiuretic Hormone

tumours	central nervous system disorders	respiratory disorders
carcinoma	meningitis, encephalitis	pneumonia
thymoma	head injury	tuberculosis
lymphoma	brain abscess and tumour	empyema
leukaemia	subarachnoid haemorrhage, cerebral thrombosis	pneumothorax
sarcoma	Guillain-Barré syndrome	asthma
mesothelioma	acute intermittent porphyria	positive-pressure ventilation

Fig. 5.22 Table of neoplastic central nervous system and respiratory disorders associated with SIADH.

Causes of the Syndrome of Inappropriate Antidiuretic Hormone

drugs		miscellaneous
ADH, oxytocin	clofibrate	acute psychosis
	thiazide diuretic	hypothyroidism
vincristine, vinblastine, cyclophosphamide	mono-amine oxidase inhibitors	glucocorticoid deficiency
chlorpropamide	phenothiazines	postoperative period
carbamazepine	nicotine	'idiopathic'

Fig. 5.23 Table of drugs and miscellaneous disorders associated with SIADH.

5.11

Types of the Syndrome of Inappropriate Antidiuretic Hormone

Following extensive osmoregulatory studies of ADH secretion in hyponatraemic patients who all fulfilled the criteria for SIADH, four patterns of ADH secretion emerged (Fig. 5.24).

The first and most common pattern (Type I), accounting for approximately forty per cent of patients with SIADH is characterised by excessive and erratic ADH secretion which is totally unaffected by changes in plasma osmolality. Although neoplastic conditions often demonstrate this pattern, many other causes of SIADH show the same abnormality. The pathogenesis of this type of defect is unknown, but several different mechanisms are possible. Ectopic production of ADH by neoplasms might be expected to cause random release. Rapidly fluctuating non-osmotic stimuli (e.g. hypotension) might also be responsible. Electrical instability of the neurogenic pathways controlling ADH or the neurohypophysis itself is a further possible mechanism.

Type II is the second most common osmoregulatory defect and has been termed the 'reset osmostat'. These patients continue to regulate water excretion about a lowered plasma osmolality. This pattern of ADH secretion is observed in patients with neoplasms, chest disease and nervous disorders. The pathogenesis of the pattern remains unknown, but interruption of the afferent limb of the baroregulatory reflex arc which normally inhibits ADH secretion is one possible mechanism.

The third type of defect is characterised by normal and appropriate osmoregulation of the hormone except under conditions of plasma hypotonicity when there is constant non-suppressible ADH secretion. It is rarely seen in malignant disease.

The abnormality may be due to a persistent 'leak' of ADH due to neurohypophyseal damage, loss of inhibitory osmoregulator neurons, or persistent non-osmotic stimulation.

The fourth type is uncommon, accounting for less than ten per cent of all cases. Osmoregulated ADH is entirely normal, yet the patients still fulfil the criteria of SIADH. Antidiuretic hormones other than ADH, for example vasotocin, may be responsible or the defect may lie within the kidney.

Treatment of the Syndrome of Inappropriate Antidiuretic Hormone

When the underlying cause of SIADH cannot be treated sufficiently well to correct the hyponatraemia, alternative management may be required (Fig. 5.25). Therapy has traditionally been based on free water restriction. Since in the long-term, management of SIADH fluid restriction may be inconvenient and unpleasant for the patient, drugs to inhibit the renal action of ADH have been prescribed. Lithium provides a less consistent response than demeclocycline and is associated with some toxicity. No ADH analogue which inhibits its renal action is yet available commercially. Phenytoin suppresses ADH release when administered intravenously and orally. The opiate agonist, oxilorphan, also suppresses the central release of the hormone.

Hypertonic saline infusion should only be considered in severely hyponatraemic patients who are at risk from cerebral thrombosis or are close to death, since this treatment is dangerous. Hypertonic saline should be infused slowly, and should replace only about half the apparent sodium deficit. Oral salt and salt-retaining drugs have no place in the long-term treatment of SIADH.

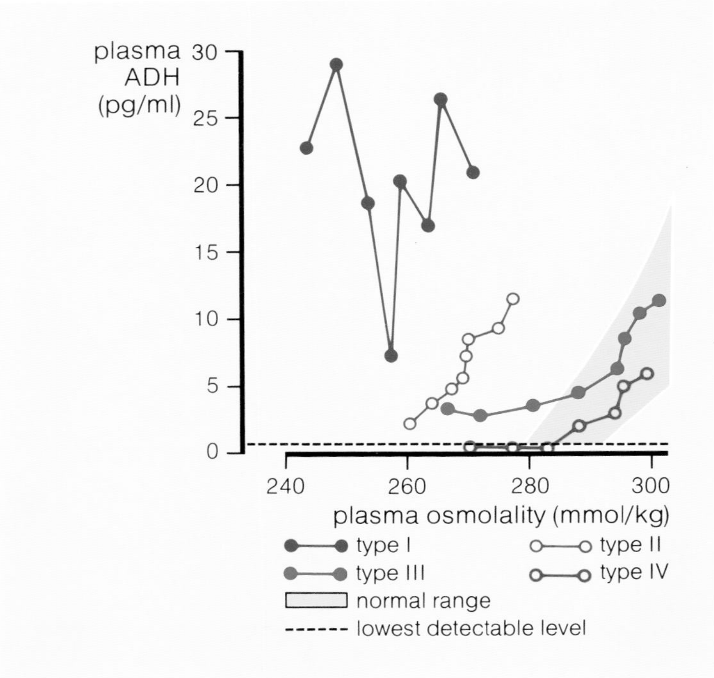

Fig. 5.24 Diagram of ADH measurements found in the four types of SIADH. Type I SIADH accounts for about 40% of cases, and is characterised by excessive and erratic ADH secretion unrelated to changes in plasma osmolality. Type II SIADH ('reset osmostat') is the second most common variant. Patients continue to regulate water excretion about a lowered plasma osmolality. Type III SIADH is characterised by normal osmoregulation of ADH except when the plasma is hypotonic, when there is constant and non-suppressible ADH secretion. Type IV SIADH accounts for less than 10% of cases. Osmoregulation of ADH secretion is entirely normal, and yet patients fulfil the criteria for SIADH.

Treatment of the Syndrome of Inappropriate Antidiuretic Hormone

fluid restriction

500ml/24hr or less (as long as plasma remains dilute)

drugs

induction of partial nephrogenic diabetes insipidus (demeclocycline, lithium)

inhibition of ADH release (phenytoin, oxilorphan)

induction of osmotic diuresis (oral urea)

hypertonic saline infusion

to be used only in the emergency situation replace half the apparent sodium deficit by infusion of 5% saline over 12 hours

Fig. 5.25 Forms of management of SIADH. Long-term fluid restriction may be inconvenient and unpleasant for the patient, therefore drug therapy may be a more useful solution. Hypertonic saline infusion should be used only in emergencies.

6 Adrenal Cortex Physiology

Vivian H T James, PhD, DSc, FRCPath

The human adrenal glands are paired structures, situated at the upper pole of each kidney; each is shaped roughly like a cocked hat. Each gland is highly vascularised, and weighs approximately 4–5g in the normal healthy adult. The outer cortex, comprising ninety per cent of the gland, surrounds the central medulla. The cortex is a zonated structure (Fig. 6.1) and is covered by a thin capsule below which are isolated groups of glomerulosa cells. Most of the cortex is made up of the zona fasciculata and the zona reticularis, the latter adjoining the medulla. The blood supply is derived from the inferior phrenic artery, the aorta and the renal arteries, and is largely subcapsular. The venous circulation within the gland is complex and is thought to play an important role in regulating steroid synthesis. The central vein from the right adrenal is short and enters the inferior vena cava directly, whereas that from the left adrenal drains into the left renal vein.

HORMONE PRODUCTION IN THE GLOMERULOSA CELLS

The adrenal cortex produces three major types of steroid hormones – mineralocorticoids, glucocorticoids and androgens.

The source of the mineralocorticoids, aldosterone and in part, deoxycorticosterone, is the glomerulosa cells. The major factor controlling aldosterone secretion is angiotensin, but increased plasma potassium concentration is also an efficient aldosterone stimulating agent (Fig. 6.2). The role of corticotrophin (ACTH) is less clear. It is more effective in salt-depleted subjects than in those with normal salt balance and is probably relatively unimportant in the normal situation. There is evidence of the existence of other, as yet unknown, factors. Angiotensin I is formed from angiotensinogen substrate by the action of renin. Renin synthesis occurs in the juxtaglomerular cells of the kidney and is released in response to changes in tubular sodium concentration, renal arteriolar blood pressure, and stimulation via sympathetic nerves. The decapeptide angiotensin I is converted into the octapeptide angiotensin II by a converting enzyme (ACE); this conversion takes place primarily, but not exclusively, in the lung. The heptapeptide angiotensin III is also formed and this can stimulate aldosterone secretion, but a physiological role for it is not yet established.

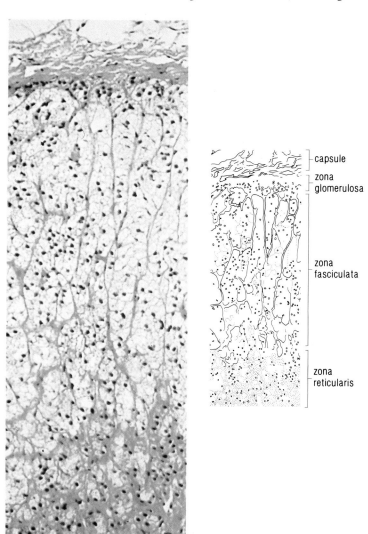

Fig.6.1 Histological section of an adrenal gland. The medulla represents 10% of the gland, whilst the remaining 90% is made up of cortical tissue – the zonae glomerulosa, fasciculata and reticularis. The whole gland is surrounded by a fibrous capsule below which the zona glomerulosa cells appear only focally. Haematoxylin and eosin stain, magnification x250.

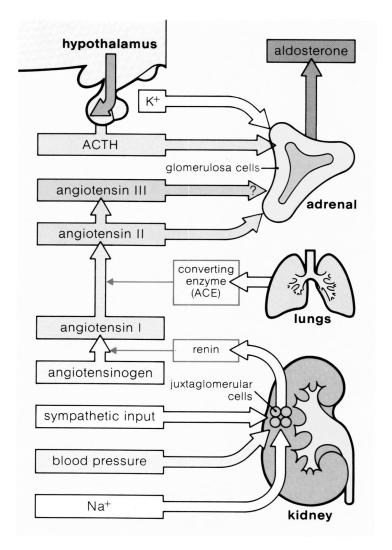

Fig.6.2 Physiological mechanisms governing the production and secretion of aldosterone. The major factor influencing aldosterone secretion is angiotensin, although increased plasma potassium concentration also contributes. Renin output, in turn, is regulated by sympathetic tone, blood pressure and tubular sodium concentration.

HORMONE PRODUCTION IN THE FASCICULATA AND RETICULARIS CELLS

Cortisol and the adrenal androgens are derived from the fasciculata and reticularis cells. The only known important control mechanism is by means of ACTH (Fig. 6.3). This anterior pituitary hormone regulates adrenocortical growth; it also mediates the rate at which steroid biosynthesis occurs. Other fragments of the ACTH precursor, pro-opiomelanocortin (POMC), may also have a trophic effect on the adrenal, and antidiuretic hormone (ADH or vasopressin) may act synergistically with ACTH to stimulate steroid biosynthesis. The effect of ACTH is rapid, occurring within a few minutes. The release of ACTH, and thus of cortisol and androgen secretion, occurs episodically through the twenty-four hour cycle in a circadian pattern. It is also released in response to stress (such as trauma, surgery, anxiety and emotional disturbance). ACTH release occurs in response to low circulating levels of cortisol (e.g. in Addison's disease) and is inhibited by high circulating levels of cortisol, or of synthetic glucocorticoids (e.g. in corticosteroid therapy). This negative feedback probably occurs at both hypothalamic and pituitary sites.

Mechanism of Action of ACTH

ACTH acts on the adrenal gland by binding to a specific receptor in the membrane of the cell (Fig. 6.4). This results in the stimulation of the membrane bound adenylate cyclase enzyme with the rapid production of intracellular cyclic AMP (cAMP), a mechanism which may also involve calcium entry into the cell. Other cyclic nucleotides, such as cGMP, may also be important. Cyclic AMP in turn activates a protein kinase (by dissociating an active subunit) which then stimulates a number of protein-phosphorylation processes using ATP. The role of the phosphoproteins formed is not yet clearly defined, but they appear to mediate cholesterol ester hydrolysis and side-chain cleavage of cholesterol to pregnenolone. The increased concentration of pregnenolone then leads to increased biosynthesis of cortisol and the androgens.

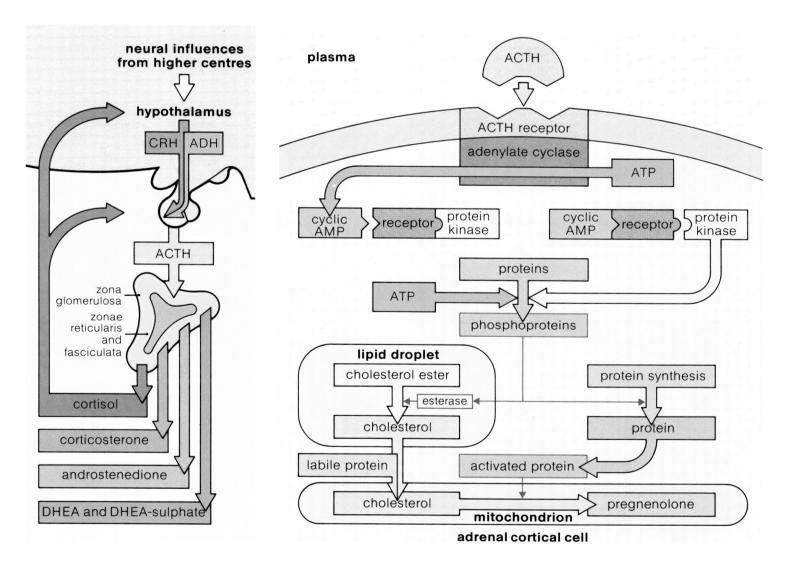

Fig. 6.3 Diagram showing the neuroendocrine control of steroid secretion from the adrenal cortex. Negative feedback in the hypothalamus and pituitary operates only in the case of cortisol. Thus high cortisol levels suppress ACTH output whereas low cortisol levels stimulate ACTH production by the release of corticotrophin releasing hormone (CRH).

Fig.6.4 Highly simplified diagram of the mechanism of action of ACTH on the adrenal cortical cell. The ACTH receptor is linked to the adenylate cyclase membrane enzyme system which is responsible for cAMP production. This 'second messenger' triggers the intracellular events responsible for steroid production and secretion.

Angiotensin II binds to specific high-affinity sites in the plasma membrane of the adrenal glomerulosa cell. Unlike ACTH, cAMP does not appear to be a 'second messenger' in aldosterone biosynthesis. Sensitivity to angiotensin is increased by sodium deficiency, with the formation of more angiotensin receptors and an increase in binding affinity. The diagrammatic representation of biosynthesis shown (Fig. 6.5) is probably the major pathway, although others almost certainly exist and may be important in particular conditions.

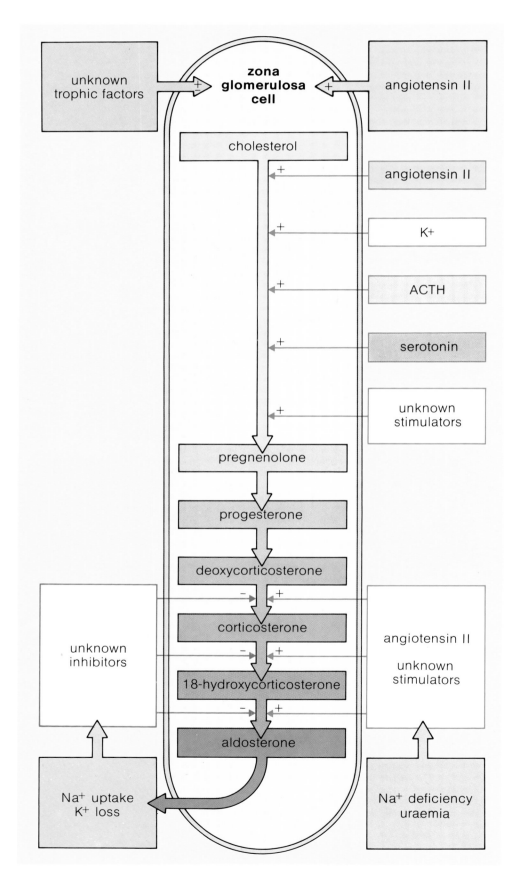

Fig. 6.5   Diagram indicating the physiological factors thought to be important in the control of mineralocorticoid synthesis. Angiotensin II appears to be the major stimulus to mineralocorticoid synthesis and secretion. Other factors play a minor role.

6.4

Cortisol and androgens are synthesised from cholesterol which is mainly derived from circulating cholesterol esters, although intracellular cholesterol biosynthesis also occurs (Fig. 6.6). Low density lipoprotein is an important source of cholesterol, especially during ACTH stimulation.

Specific enzymes and co-factors are required for glucocorticoid and androgen biosynthesis. These enzymes are located either in the smooth endoplasmic reticulum or the mitochondria within each cell. Movement of substrate between these organelles is therefore necessary and this mechanism of intracellular transport may require specific steroid-binding proteins. Thus intracellular feedback effects of intermediates in the earlier biosynthetic steps may be of importance in regulating cholesterol biosynthesis.

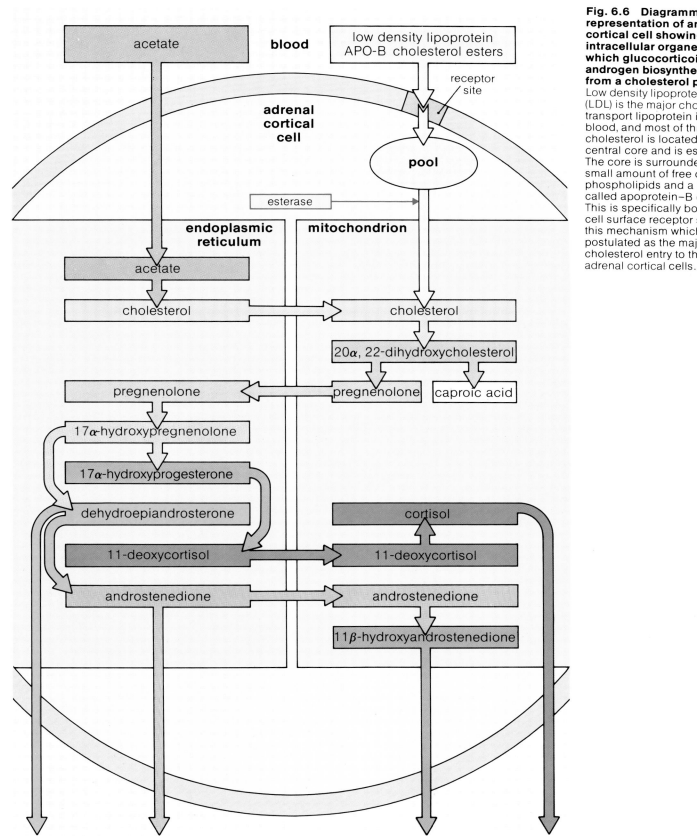

Fig. 6.6 Diagrammatic representation of an adrenal cortical cell showing the intracellular organelles in which glucocorticoid and androgen biosynthesis occur from a cholesterol precursor. Low density lipoprotein (LDL) is the major cholesterol transport lipoprotein in human blood, and most of this cholesterol is located in a central core and is esterified. The core is surrounded by a small amount of free cholesterol, phospholipids and a protein called apoprotein–B (APO–B). This is specifically bound to the cell surface receptor site. It is this mechanism which is postulated as the major route of cholesterol entry to the adrenal cortical cells.

Hydroxylation steps in the biosynthesis of adrenal steroids (Fig. 6.7) require NADPH, molecular oxygen and also an enzyme complex. This complex consists of a flavoprotein dehydrogenase, a non-haem iron-containing protein (adrenodoxin) and a cytochrome, called P_{450} because of the characteristic high absorption observed when this cytochrome is complexed with carbon monoxide. This oxidase system is essentially similar for 11β-, 20,22-, 17α- and 18-hydroxylation, and it appears that specificity is achieved through differences in the respective P_{450} cytochromes. Hydroxylation is mediated by the introduction

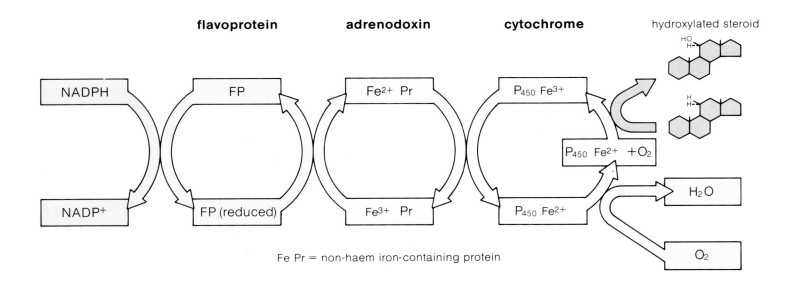

Fig.6.7 Diagram illustrating the roles of NADPH, a flavoprotein and cytochrome P_{450} in the hydroxylation of steroids. All hydroxylation steps share this common pathway.

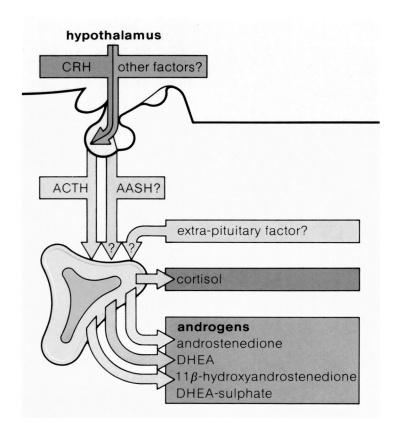

Fig. 6.8 Diagram showing the possible control mechanisms involved in the secretion of adrenal androgens. Although ACTH seems to be an important physiological regulator of adrenal androgen production, there is evidence supporting the existence of a separate adrenal androgen stimulating hormone (AASH), as yet unidentified, which stimulates DHEA-sulphate production.

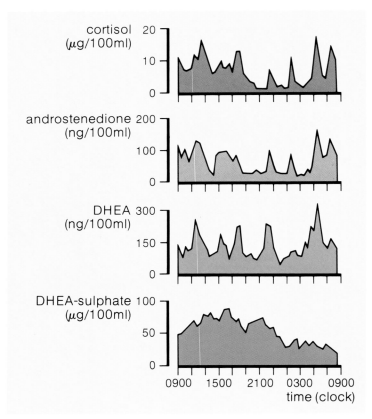

Fig. 6.9 Graphs showing the episodic nature of adrenal steroid secretion in plasma.

of one electron into the electron transport chain, with the introduction of one atom of oxygen into the steroid. The remaining oxygen atom combines with hydrogen to form water. This system is called a 'mixed function oxidase'.

Control of Androgen Secretion

The major adrenal androgens are androstenedione, dehydro-epiandrosterone (DHEA), 11β-hydroxyandrostenedione and DHEA-sulphate. The possible control mechanisms involved in the secretion of these androgens are shown in Figure 6.8. Although ACTH is capable of stimulating adrenal androgen secretion, there are several well-documented situations in which cortisol and androgen secretion appear to be dissociated. This has resulted in the concept of an additional factor, adrenal androgen stimulating hormone (AASH – as yet undefined), which can specifically stimulate adrenal androgen secretion. Prolactin has been invoked as such a factor since hyperprolactinaemia is associated with increased production of DHEA-sulphate in some patients, but this appears to be only a pathological phenomenon. Other largely discredited agents are growth hormone, oestrogen and gonadotrophins. It is possible that non-ACTH peptides derived from the precursor to ACTH may be involved, but the problem is still unresolved.

CIRCADIAN VARIATION

ACTH is secreted episodically through the twenty-four hour period. There are between seven and thirteen episodes, most of which occur during sleep, and which are largely reproducible from one twenty-four hour period to another. Since cortisol and all the adrenal androgens, with the exception of DHEA-sulphate,

are responsive to ACTH, there are also episodic changes in the peripheral plasma levels of these steroid hormones through the day (Fig. 6.9). It is not known what factors cause this pattern of ACTH release and the physiological advantage, if any, is not clear. The rhythm is shifted by an alteration in the sleep-wake pattern, such as occurs after travel across time zones, and five to seven days are required to complete the shift. Alterations of circadian rhythm also occur in disease states, particularly in adrenal hyperfunction (Cushing's syndrome) and in depressive illness.

Aldosterone is also secreted episodically, and the pattern closely resembles that for cortisol (Fig. 6.10). The mechanism and purpose of this episodicity are unknown. It is not caused by ACTH since aldosterone secretion continues to follow an episodic pattern of release in the absence of ACTH, and neither is it due to changes in plasma potassium or sodium; nor is it entirely established whether this periodicity is caused by changes in angiotensin. Whatever mechanism is involved, it is apparently closely co-ordinated with that which causes ACTH release. As with cortisol, the pattern appears to be disrupted by disease.

Stress also causes the release of ACTH and other pituitary hormones (e.g. human growth hormone and prolactin). Chronic stress (anxiety or trauma) produces prolonged elevation of ACTH and thus cortisol secretion. In the investigation of patients with suspected hypopituitarism, it is clinically advantageous to be able to provoke ACTH release by producing controlled hypoglycaemia. The integrity of the hypothalamo-pituitary-adrenal axis may thus be examined by measuring the plasma concentration of cortisol (Fig. 6.11) and, if necessary, other pituitary hormones released by stress (e.g. growth hormone).

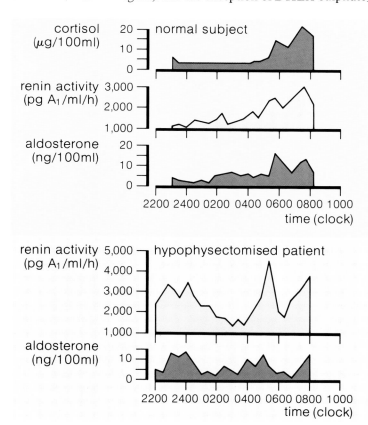

Fig. 6.10 **Graphs of aldosterone and cortisol secretion with time.** The mechanism behind these closely co-ordinated patterns in plasma levels is unclear. Renin secretion is also shown.

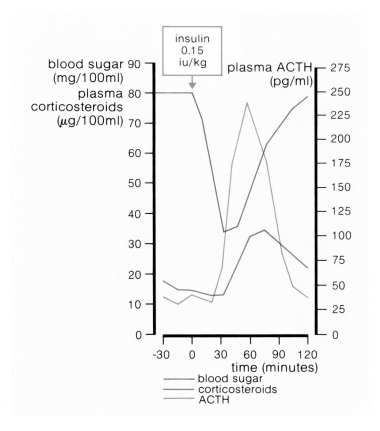

Fig.6.11 **Graph showing the changes in blood sugar, ACTH and cortisol secretion induced by the intravenous administration of 0.15 iu/kg soluble insulin.** Insulin-induced hypoglycaemia testing reveals the integrity of the entire hypothalamo-pituitary-adrenal axis.

BIOSYNTHESIS OF STEROID HORMONES

The overall scheme of biosynthesis is shown in Figure 6.12. Although the pathways are common to the various steroids shown, specificity is achieved by specific receptors for ACTH or angiotensin, and also by the location of specific enzyme systems. Thus the glomerulosa cells lack 17α-hydroxylase and do not participate in the synthesis of cortisol or androgens, for which this enzyme is essential. Conversely, fasciculata and reticularis cells lack the enzyme 18-hydroxylase and thus cannot synthesise aldosterone. However, all cells can produce deoxycorticosterone, since the proximal pathway is common to both these enzyme systems.

Steroid Production

At normal plasma concentrations approximately ninety per cent of the cortisol is bound to the specific binding protein –

corticosteroid binding globulin (CBG). An average cortisol production rate is 20 mg/day. It is metabolised rapidly, mainly by the liver, with a plasma half-life of approximately two hours; the metabolic clearance rate is 200 1/day. The major metabolites are formed by reduction of the double bond and ketone groups to produce tetrahydrocortisol, tetrahydrocortisone, cortol and cortolone (Fig. 6.13). These are excreted in the urine in conjugation with glucuronic acid, and account for about sixty to seventy per cent of the total cortisol produced. Estimation of these steroids in a twenty-four hour urine sample thus provides an estimate of the secretion rate of cortisol. A small amount of cortisol (up to 150 μg/day) is excreted unchanged and represents the unbound cortisol in plasma which is filtered through the kidney.

The average secretion rate of aldosterone is 100-200μg/day (Fig. 6.14). It is only weakly bound to plasma proteins and thus has a relatively short half-life (twenty minutes) and a high

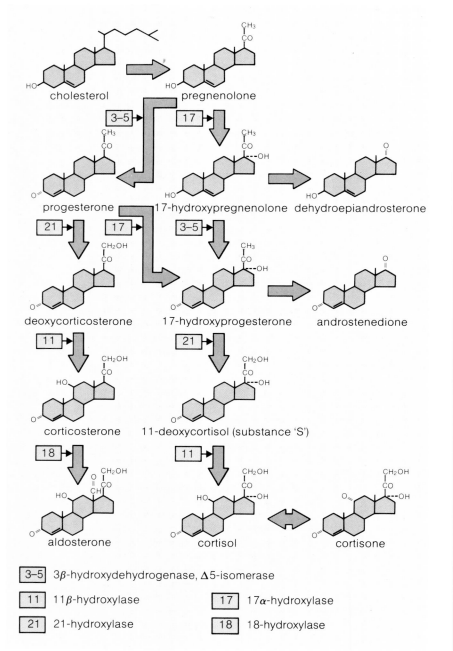

Fig.6.12 Diagram of the biosynthetic pathways and enzymes involved in the synthesis of glucocorticoids, mineralocorticoids and adrenal androgens from a cholesterol precursor.

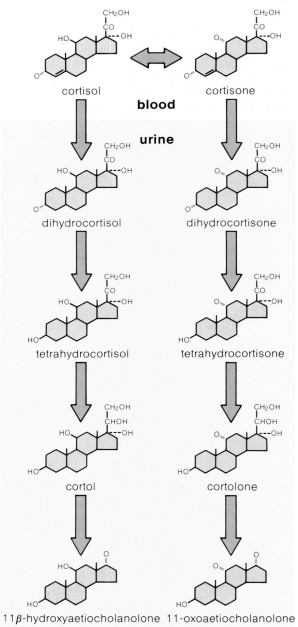

Fig.6.13 Diagram showing the origin of cortisol metabolites.

metabolic clearance rate (1500 1/day). Both liver and kidney are sites of metabolic clearance, and only a small percentage of aldosterone is excreted unchanged in the urine. Plasma aldosterone measurement, or an estimation of a metabolite 18-glucuronoside are commonly used in clinical situations. Diet, posture and time of day affect aldosterone secretion and must be adequately controlled to permit interpretation of results.

The major androgens produced by the adrenal cortex are DHEA-sulphate, androstenedione, DHEA, 11β-hydroxyandrostenedione and small amounts of testosterone (Fig. 6.15). Androstenedione and testosterone are also secreted by the ovary and the testis, and a small amount of DHEA arises from the ovary. Androgen metabolism is therefore complex because of these dual sources, and also because androgens undergo extensive interconversion and metabolism. The major metabolic pathway proceeds via the reduction of ring A, and the resulting metabolites are conjugated and excreted into the urine as sulphates and glucuronosides. Formerly, the conjugated urinary metabolites DHEA, aetiocholanolone, and androsterone, were measured collectively as 'urinary 17-oxosteroids'. Although the assay has been used extensively, it is now little employed because of the difficulty of interpretation. Currently, clinical investigations are predominantly based on the measurement of plasma androgen levels rather than urinary excretion products.

The peripheral interconversion of androgens has important physiological consequences. Androstenedione is a major precursor of testosterone and, in the female, it is a major source of this steroid. It is also converted to oestrone and in older women, when ovarian secretion of oestrogen is less important, the production of oestrone from androstenedione contributes significantly to the total production of oestrogen.

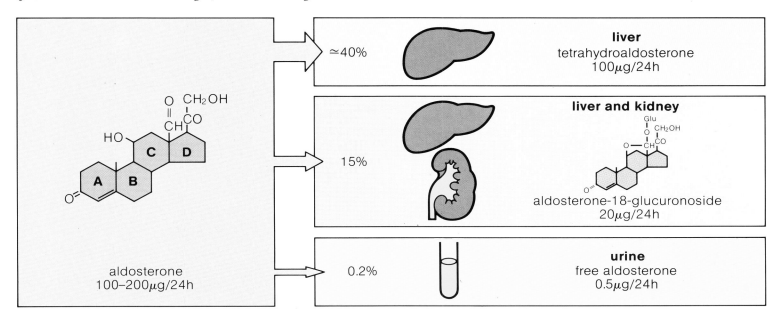

Fig.6.14 Diagram showing the metabolic fate of aldosterone. Only 0.2% of the daily aldosterone produced is directly excreted in the urine, whilst approximately 40% is converted to tetrahydro- aldosterone within the liver. The remainder of the aldosterone is converted into many other metabolites.

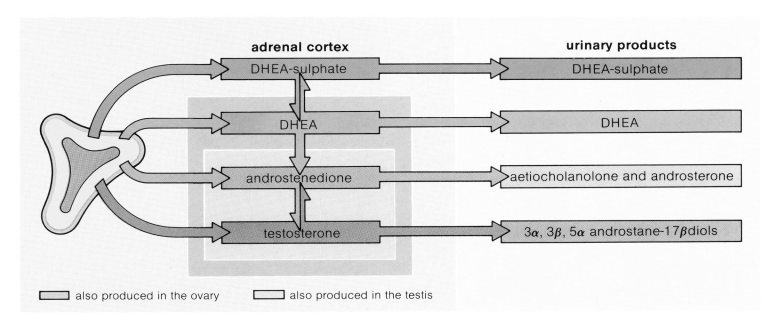

Fig.6.15 Diagram showing the metabolic fate of adrenal androgens. DHEA, DHEA-sulphate, aetiocholanolone, androsterone and the androstanediols are all excreted in the urine.

6.9

Inhibitors of Steroid Biosynthesis

Steroid biosynthesis can be blocked by a number of compounds which inhibit the activity of one or more of the enzyme systems involved in the pathway. These materials have been found to have clinical use in the investigation of pituitary-adrenal function, as an adjunct to the treatment of Cushing's syndrome, and as a method of reducing oestrogen synthesis in the treatment of women with breast cancer.

Metyrapone acts by interfering with the cytochrome P_{450} system, and mainly affects 11β-hydroxylation. This causes a relative increase in the production of the immediate precursor steroid, 11-deoxycortisol, with a concomitant decrease in cortisol synthesis. These actions have been exploited in the development of a test of pituitary-adrenal function which is used clinically. In a subject with intact pituitary-adrenal function, there is a fall in cortisol production with a subsequent fall in plasma cortisol following administration of metyrapone (Fig. 6.16). This causes a compensatory release of ACTH for as long as the drug is administered. ACTH, acting on the adrenal cortex, accelerates the early stages of steroid biosynthesis and therefore increases the production of all the steroids up to the step which is blocked by metyrapone.

The increased production of 11-deoxycortisol can be measured directly in the blood, or by measuring the metabolite, tetrahydro-11-deoxycortisol in urine, where it appears as a 17-hydroxy-corticosteroid. A patient with either hypothalamic, pituitary or adrenal insufficiency will show a diminished or absent response.

Aminoglutethimide also interferes with several of the biosynthetic steps in steroid biosynthesis, including the C20-, C22-, 11β-, 18-, 19-, 21-hydroxylases and also aromatase. Since it inhibits biosynthesis early in the pathway, it is useful as a blocking agent when alleviating the effects of excessive steroid production, as in the treatment of those patients with Cushing's syndrome resulting from adrenal carcinoma. The action on aromatase is useful in the treatment of breast cancer since it inhibits peripheral formation of oestrogens.

Trilostane inhibits steroid hormone synthesis by acting on 3β-hydroxysteroid dehydrogenase; it has been used to reduce cortisol and aldosterone production in the treatment of Cushing's syndrome and Conn's syndrome respectively, but its action is weak.

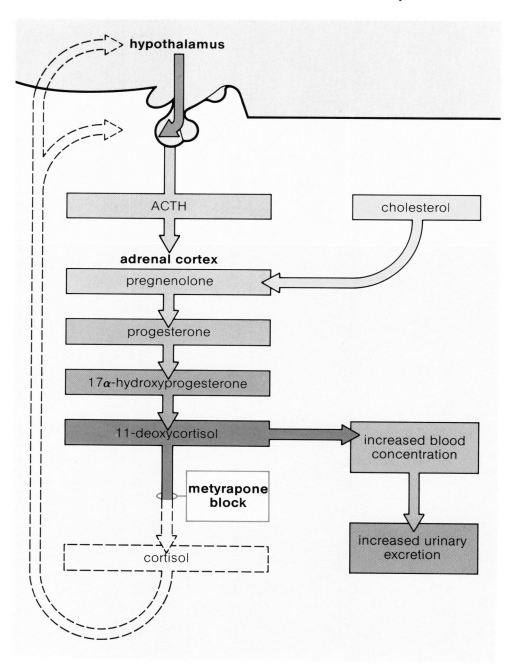

Fig. 6.16 Diagram illustrating the mechanism of action of metyrapone. Provided hypothalamic, pituitary and adrenal function are intact, the drug will cause an increase in the production of deoxycortisol and its urinary metabolites.

7 Cushing's Syndrome

Paul L Drury, MA, MRCP
Lesley H Rees, MSc, MD, FRCP

Cushing's syndrome is the clinical condition resulting from excessive, inappropriate exposure to glucocorticoids. It was first fully described clinically by Harvey Cushing in 1932 before the isolation of either the adrenal steroid hormones or the pituitary peptide hormones, although many earlier cases, often called 'diabetes of bearded women', had been recognised. Cushing's syndrome most commonly results from the therapeutic use of synthetic glucocorticoids or adrenocorticotrophic hormone (ACTH). Doses of steroids greater than replacement requirements (e.g. of 7.5mg prednisolone, 0.75mg dexamethasone or 30mg hydrocortisone daily in adults) may simulate the naturally occurring condition in most respects.

CLINICAL FEATURES

Virtually every system in the body may be affected by excessive exposure to glucocorticoids. A summary of the major clinical features in Cushing's syndrome is shown in Figure 7.1. The commonest presenting symptoms are weight gain and central obesity with muscular weakness (Fig. 7.2). General symptoms of weakness, especially in proximal muscle groups, and malaise as well as hirsuties and acne (Fig. 7.3), skin thinning, bruising and striae (Fig. 7.4) are all common, as are oligomenorrhoea or amenorrhoea in the female and decreased libido and possibly impotence in the male. Other musculoskeletal manifestations include osteoporosis and vertebral collapse, rib fractures (see Chapter 20), kyphosis and avascular bone necrosis, with proximal myopathy being almost universal. Depression is a frequent concomitant, while psychosis is less common. Symptoms of hypertension and diabetes mellitus also occur, and patients show an increased susceptibility to infection. In ACTH-

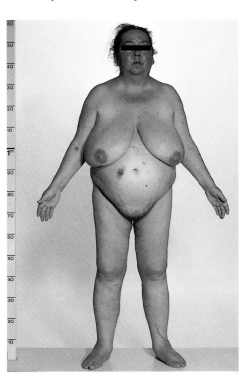

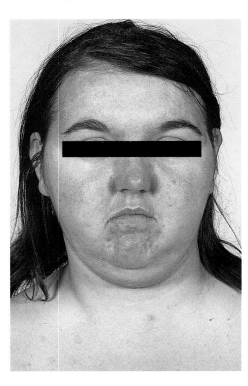

Major Clinical Features in Cushing's Syndrome

weight gain
central obesity
moon face and plethora
muscular weakness, especially
  proximal
malaise
depression or psychosis
oligomenorrhoea or
  amenorrhoea in females
hirsuties
striae
acne
skin-thinning
bruising
polyuria
nocturia
decreased libido and impotence
  in males
hypertension
diabetes or impaired glucose
  tolerance

Fig. 7.1 Table of the major clinical features in Cushing's syndrome. Patients with Cushing's syndrome gain weight but suffer muscular disability, malaise and depression. In addition, they are susceptible to various skin disorders such as acne and bruising; decreased fertility and libido may also be present.

Fig. 7.2 Photograph showing the typical clinical appearance of a patient with Cushing's syndrome. Central obesity with proximal muscle wasting can be seen.

Fig. 7.3 Typical 'moon face' appearance of a patient with Cushing's syndrome. A plethoric face with acne and hirsuties is characteristic, and there is evidence of temporal hair recession.

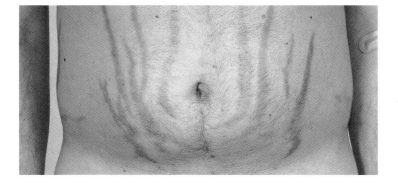

Fig. 7.4 Photograph of the abdomen of a male patient with Cushing's syndrome. The skin is stretched by underlying adipose tissue to such an extent that streaks of capillaries, or striae, can be seen.

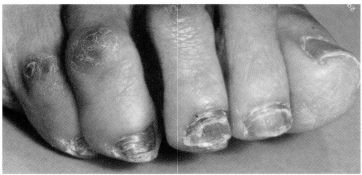

Fig. 7.5 Photograph of the nails in a patient with ectopic ACTH syndrome. The nails are grossly pigmented compared with a normal subject.

dependent disease, pigmentation may be present (Fig. 7.5) and, with pituitary-dependent disease, headaches and visual field defects are very occasionally found. All disease forms may be cyclical or intermittent, and pituitary-dependent disease may occasionally undergo spontaneous remission.

When the clinical features are unclear, examination of previous photographs of the subject may be very valuable. Rapid onset of the disease is more likely to result from an adrenal tumour or ectopic ACTH production than from pituitary-dependent disease, but the converse is not necessarily true. Overt pigmentation is more common with the ectopic ACTH syndrome, while marked virilisation is usually associated with adrenal tumours. The histological appearance of the adrenal gland in Cushing's syndrome reveals hyperplasia of the reticularis and fasciculata cells when compared with the normal gland (Fig. 7.6).

AETIOLOGY

Apart from the iatrogenic administration of either corticosteroids or ACTH, the main causes of Cushing's syndrome are listed in Figure 7.7; their effects on the hypothalamo-pituitary-adrenal axis are shown in Figure 7.8.

Pituitary-dependent disease (i.e. Cushing's *disease*) is four times more common in women than in men and occurs most often between the ages of twenty and forty years. Speculation about the pathogenesis of pituitary-dependent disease continues, particularly concerning the relative contribution of hypothalamic defects in the control of corticotrophin releasing hormone (CRH). There is also controversy about the proportion of cases resulting from the presence of intermediate lobe remnants.

Ectopic ACTH production may be associated with a large number of tumours, most commonly oat cell bronchial carcinomas

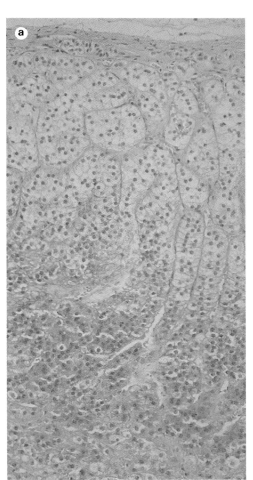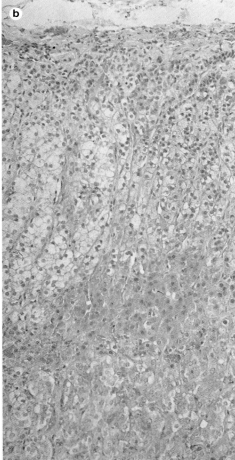

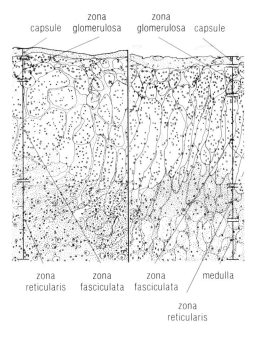

Fig. 7.6 **Histological section of the adrenal cortex.** View (a) is a section from a patient with Cushing's syndrome. Diffuse hyperplasia of the zona fasciculata with cords of cells can be seen, in contrast to section (b) where the less organised appearance of the normal cortex is shown. By courtesy of Prof. I. Doniach.

Fig. 7.7 **Table of the major causes of Cushing's syndrome.** Although the commonest cause, apart from steroid therapy, is pituitary-dependent disease (Cushing's disease), ectopic ACTH production is also important.

Major Causes of Cushing's Syndrome

cause	approximate incidence
pituitary-dependent disease (Cushing's disease)	60%
ectopic ACTH production	20%
adrenal adenoma	10%
adrenal carcinoma	5%
alcohol-induced pseudo-Cushing's syndrome	1–5%

(see Chapter 19), or bronchial and thymic carcinoids (Fig. 7.9), other gastrointestinal carcinoid tumours and islet cell tumours of the pancreas. Although ectopic ACTH production may produce a clinical picture identical to that of classical Cushing's syndrome, a severe wasting syndrome is often seen in which typical Cushingoid appearances are absent (Fig. 7.10).

Adrenal tumours may occur at any age, but predominate in children, particularly carcinomas. Their underlying aetiology is not known. Carcinomas are usually aggressive and large (>40mm diameter); they may be palpable abdominally. Adenomas are slower-growing and are usually of moderate size (15–60mm diameter) at presentation; they are also a rare manifestation of the Multiple Endocrine Neoplasia (MEN) syndrome type 1. Excess androgen production is common with adrenal tumours, but is usually only severe enough to cause virilisation with carcinomas.

The pathophysiology of alcohol-induced pseudo-Cushing's syndrome is poorly understood. It is, however, clear that it is not predominantly ACTH-dependent. Withdrawal of alcohol leads to remission of the biochemical abnormalities over a period of days, but the clinical signs take longer to abate.

The association of pigmentation and an enlarging pituitary tumour following bilateral adrenalectomy in a patient with Cushing's disease is known as Nelson's syndrome (Fig. 7.11). It is estimated that approximately thirty per cent of patients undergoing bilateral adrenalectomy without prophylactic radiotherapy will develop this condition.

BIOCHEMICAL FEATURES
When investigating a patient with suspected Cushing's syndrome two stages are necessary: (i) confirmation of the presence of Cushing's syndrome and (ii) if present, differential diagnosis of its cause.

Diagnosis of Cushing's Syndrome
The biochemical hallmark of the condition is inappropriate cortisol secretion. However, the simple biochemical features can also be caused by psychological or physical stress, alcoholism, depression and obesity, while Cushing's syndrome itself may also be intermittent or cyclical. Loss of the normal circadian pattern of cortisol secretion and lack of dexamethasone suppressibility (when administered as 0.5mg/6hrs for two days) are characteristic of the disease (Fig. 7.12), but can be mimicked by the conditions described above. Steroid measurements can be performed using either blood or urine samples, but care must be taken to ensure stress-free sampling. Failure of an increase in plasma cortisol after adequate insulin-induced hypoglycaemia (plasma glucose <2.2 mmol/l) is a strong indication of the presence of Cushing's syndrome since this response is usually intact in depressed and obese subjects. To exclude the possibility of alcohol-induced pseudo-Cushing's disease, ethanol consumption should also be rigorously banned since the resulting biochemical abnormalities revert to normal after several days of abstinence from alcohol.

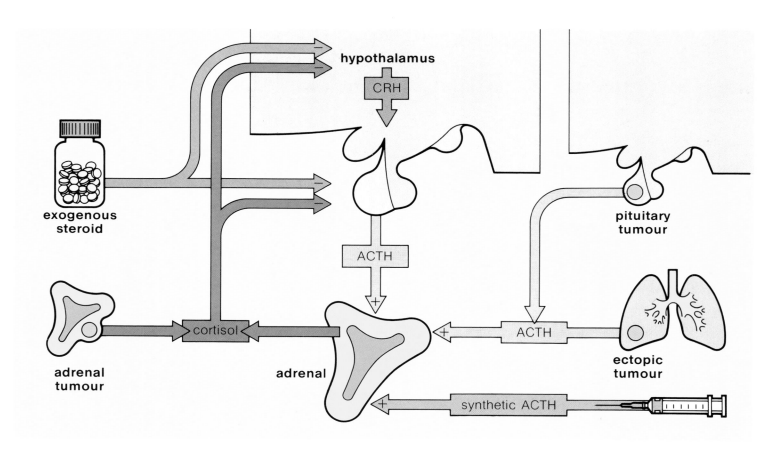

Fig. 7.8 Diagram illustrating the involvement of ACTH and cortisol in the hypothalamo-pituitary-adrenal axis. Cortisol produced in the adrenals, or by an adrenal tumour, has a negative feedback effect on ACTH production. Oral steroids have the same effect. Conversely, ACTH stimulates cortisol production and secretion, as do pituitary or ectopic tumours and intramuscular injections of ACTH.

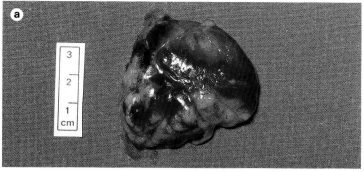

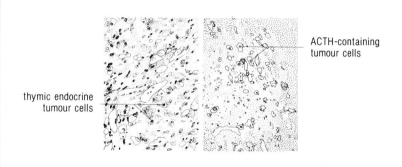

Fig. 7.9 Macroscopic and microscopic views of a thymic tumour. The whole tumour (a) is from a patient with Cushing's syndrome. The conventional histology of the tumour is shown in (b). The immunofluorescent staining in section (c), is used to reveal ACTH-containing tumour cells by staining them yellow with an anti-ACTH antibody. By courtesy of Mr. G.M. Rees and Prof. I. Doniach.

thymic endocrine tumour cells

ACTH-containing tumour cells

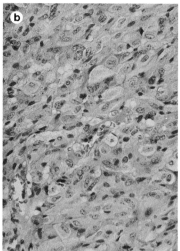

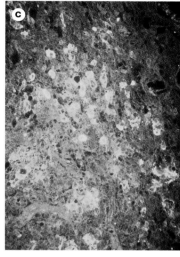

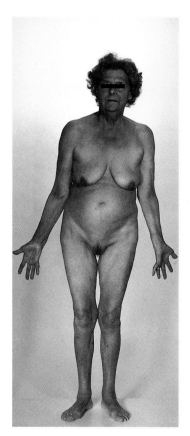

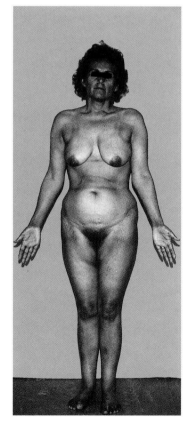

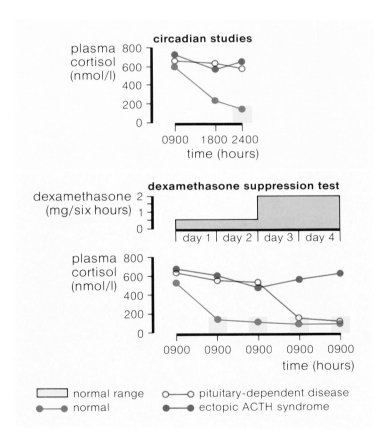

Fig. 7.10 Appearance of a patient with ectopic ACTH syndrome. Marked wasting and skin pigmentation are present.

Fig. 7.11 Appearance of a patient with Nelson's syndrome. The gross pigmentation that occurs in this syndrome is best seen on the flexural surfaces of the body.

Fig. 7.12 Graphs of plasma cortisol levels during circadian studies and a dexamethasone suppression test. In a healthy individual the plasma cortisol level falls naturally during the day, and administration of a low dose of dexamethasone (0.5mg six-hourly) will lead to complete suppression of cortisol. No such fall occurs in patients with ectopic ACTH syndrome, in contrast to pituitary-dependent disease in which partial suppression after administration of a high dose of dexamethasone (2mg six-hourly) is characteristic.

7.5

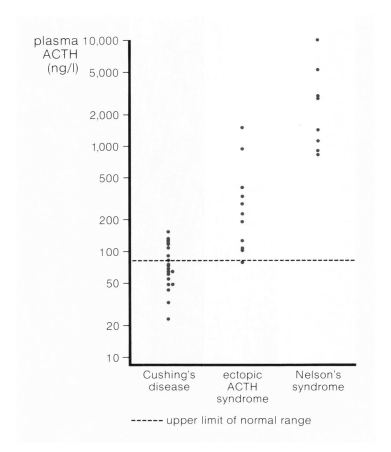

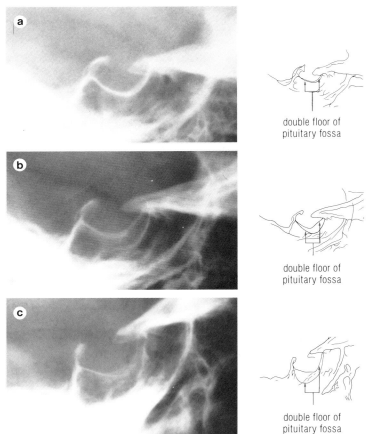

double floor of
pituitary fossa

double floor of
pituitary fossa

double floor of
pituitary fossa

Fig. 7.13 Graph of plasma ACTH concentrations at 0900h.
Each point on the graph represents one patient. Patients with
Nelson's syndrome have grossly elevated levels of ACTH, even when
levels are compared with those found in patients with ectopic ACTH
syndrome and Cushing's disease (pituitary-dependent disease).

**Fig. 7.14 Sequential skull radiographs of a patient with
Nelson's syndrome.** Nelson's syndrome developed in this patient
after bilateral adrenalectomy. The progression in the change in shape
of the fossa can be seen in views (a) pre-surgery, (b) two years post-
surgery and (c) eleven years post-surgery. The minor abnormality of
the fossa present before the operation became gross eleven years
after surgery.

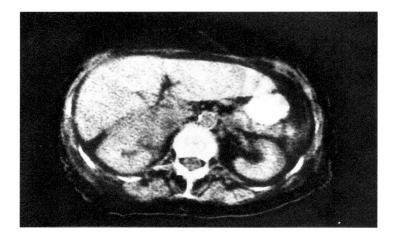

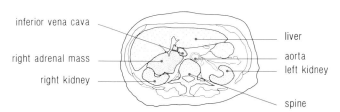

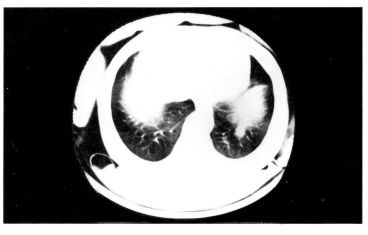

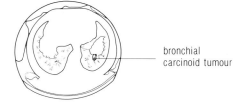

Fig. 7.15 CT scan of the abdomen in Cushing's syndrome. The
irregular lobulated mass in the position of the right adrenal was
confirmed at operation to be an adrenal carcinoma. By courtesy of
Dr. F.E. White.

Fig. 7.16 CT scan of the chest in Cushing's syndrome. The
small mass in the left lung was found to be a bronchial carcinoid
tumour. The resultant hypercortisolaemia was cured on removal of the
tumour. By courtesy of Dr. F.E. White.

Differential Diagnosis

No clinical features provide reliable differentiation between the causes of the syndrome, but unequivocal pigmentation, clinical diabetes and, especially, unprovoked hypokalaemia strongly suggest the presence of ectopic ACTH secretion.

The subsequent differential diagnosis is based upon both biochemical and radiological assessments. The syndrome may be conveniently classified into ACTH-dependent disease (pituitary or ectopic) and non-ACTH-dependent disease (adrenal tumours). These two types can usually be distinguished by the measurement of plasma ACTH, which is almost invariably undetectable with adrenal tumours. ACTH levels tend to be higher with ectopic than pituitary sources, but there is considerable overlap (Fig. 7.13).

The single most reliable test for pituitary-dependent disease is the high-dose dexamethasone suppression test (2mg/6hrs for two days), during which patients with Cushing's disease normally show suppression of urinary or plasma steroids. Cortisol levels in patients with ectopic sources or adrenal tumours are rarely suppressed by dexamethasone, although exceptions do occur. The metyrapone test, based on the urinary steroid or ACTH response to this 11β-hydroxylase enzyme blocker, has now been shown to be of no value. Abnormal, high molecular weight forms of ACTH ('big ACTH') are frequently seen with ectopic sources and in rare instances when pituitary-dependent Cushing's disease is caused by a large tumour.

RADIOLOGY

Advances in radiological techniques and computerised tomographic (CT) scanning have greatly aided the investigation of patients with this syndrome. However, the technique of choice depends upon the clinical circumstances and availability of high resolution scanners.

Plain Radiography

Even with proven pituitary-dependent disease, less than twenty per cent of pituitary fossae are abnormal on normal skull radiography. A small proportion of patients with abnormal fossae have locally invasive tumours, although this is more frequently seen with Nelson's syndrome (Fig. 7.14).

Careful plain chest radiography should be performed on all patients as 'small-cell' tumours are nearly always apparent using this technique. However, this is not the case for bronchial carcinoids or adenomas which may be less than 1cm in diameter.

Computerised Tomographic Scanning

CT scanning is now the most effective and rapid means of demonstrating an adrenal tumour causing Cushing's syndrome (Fig. 7.15). It allows definition of the site and size of the tumour.

Carcinomas are usually large (>40mm diameter), irregular or lobulated and may show local infiltration or metastatic deposits. Where an ectopic source of ACTH is suspected, enhanced high resolution CT scanning of the whole lung and mediastinum is mandatory (Fig. 7.16); very small bronchial and thymic tumours may thus be detected, even when the plain radiography is normal. Bronchoscopy is a complementary investigation when a possible abnormality has been identified.

Venous Catheterisation and Venography

These techniques may be of value in confirming a pituitary origin of ACTH and in locating some ectopic sources of the hormone (Fig. 7.17). Discrimination between ectopic ACTH and pituitary causes of Cushing's syndrome is enhanced by the technique of inferior petrosal sinus sampling, where high ACTH levels strongly suggest a pituitary origin of the ACTH. Though largely supplanted by CT scanning, catheterisation is still useful in the study of adrenal tumours where doubt exists as to the hormonal activity of a structural abnormality seen on a CT scan.

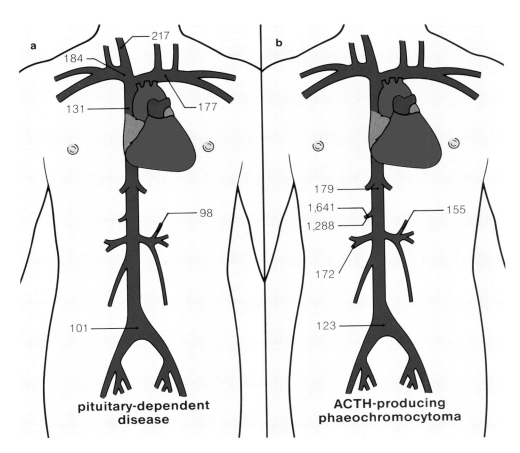

pituitary-dependent disease

ACTH-producing phaeochromocytoma

Fig. 7.17 Results of ACTH venous catheterisation studies. The results (in ng/l) obtained from a patient with Cushing's disease are shown in view (a). Peak ACTH levels are seen in the right high jugular vein. In view (b), peak ACTH levels were found in the right adrenal vein resulting from an ACTH-secreting phaeochromocytoma which was later removed. Two independent samples were taken from this vein and both showed abnormally high levels of ACTH.

TREATMENT

If left untreated, the life expectancy of patients with Cushing's syndrome is less than five years, death usually occurring from cardiovascular disease.

Where benign adrenal tumours or histologically benign ectopic sources of ACTH are present, successful removal of the tumour will cure the patient (Fig. 7.18). This is almost always possible for adrenal adenomas and for some ectopic sources, but adrenal carcinomas are rarely curable by surgery.

There is, however, no completely adequate therapy for pituitary-dependent disease. Pituitary surgery, radiotherapy and bilateral adrenalectomy are the three definitive options, but control of hypercortisolaemia with the 11β-hydroxylase blocker, metyrapone, is indicated before any definitive therapy.

Trans-sphenoidal surgery has become increasingly successful in the treatment of Cushing's syndrome by specialists and results in a high cure rate. However, long-term follow-up data on recurrence and subsequent pituitary function are not widely available. Immediate postoperative ACTH insufficiency is a valuable marker of successful removal of the pituitary lesion. This is usually transient but may take months or years to remit. Formerly, bilateral adrenalectomy was the most common definitive therapy: however, its significant mortality and morbidity have been greatly reduced by pre-operative preparation with metyrapone. Following adrenalectomy, patients require lifelong steroid replacement therapy and must carry steroid cards and Medic-Alert bracelets. Recurrent Cushing's syndrome from incomplete adrenalectomy or ectopic adrenal tissue is not uncommon. Such patients also require prophylactic pituitary irradiation to prevent the development of Nelson's syndrome.

Radiotherapy as a definitive therapy may be given conventionally or by local implantation with yttrium rods. Conventional external radiotherapy rarely produces an early cure, except in children who appear particularly sensitive to this form of treatment. This method of treatment is sometimes used in combination with metyrapone control of cortisol secretion. Local implantation of radioactive yttrium or gold into the pituitary, via the trans-sphenoidal route, has led to initial success in several centres, but long-term follow-up data remain limited.

Metyrapone (0.5–4g daily in two to four divided doses) is commonly used for short- and long-term control of excessive secretion of cortisol from any cause. Its mode of action is the reversible blockade of the 11β-hydroxylase enzyme involved in cortisol synthesis. It is reasonably tolerated by most patients and should be used to control the condition prior to adrenal or pituitary surgery or pending a final decision on definitive therapy. Metyrapone can also be used in conjunction with radiotherapy. When disseminated, adrenal carcinoma responds poorly to any therapy, but can sometimes be controlled by ortho-para-diethyl-diphenyl diethane (op'DDD) which reduces cortisol secretion by inducing necrosis of the adrenocortical cells. In pituitary-dependent disease a few patients respond to bromocriptine, cyproheptadine and sodium valproate; however, these drugs are rarely successful in the long-term reduction of ACTH secretion.

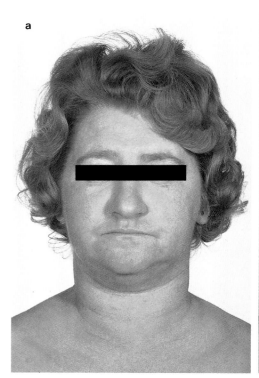 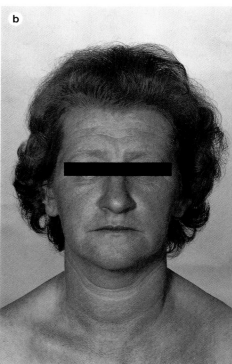

Fig. 7.18 Treatment of a patient with Cushing's syndrome. The facial appearance of the patient is seen (a) before and (b) after removal of an ectopic ACTH-secreting tumour.

8 Addison's Disease

Christopher R W Edwards, MA, MD, FRCP

Addison's disease results from primary adrenocortical failure. It was first described by Thomas Addison in his celebrated monograph, published in 1855, which contains an illustrated description of eleven cases of the disease. After qualifying at Edinburgh University, Addison worked with a well-known dermatologist, Bateman; this probably stimulated his interest in the skin pigmentation that is so characteristic of the condition.

AETIOLOGY

In Addison's original series, tuberculosis was the commonest cause of primary adrenal failure. With the decline in the prevalence of tuberculosis, the incidence of tuberculous Addison's disease has fallen and autoimmune adrenalitis is now the commonest cause, accounting for more than seventy per cent of cases. Other causes include metastatic tumour, amyloidosis, intra-adrenal haemorrhage (this is called the Waterhouse-Friderichsen syndrome when there is septicaemia due to meningococcus present), haemochromatosis, bilateral adrenalectomy, adrenal ischaemia or an extremely rare condition known as adreno-leukodystrophy. Congenital adrenal hyperplasia or hypoplasia are not normally included as causes of Addison's disease. Selective glucocorticoid deficiency can result from hereditary adreno-cortical unresponsiveness to adrenocorticotrophic hormone (ACTH).

Several diseases are associated with autoimmune Addison's disease and may thus suggest the diagnosis. These include Hashimoto's thyroiditis (see Chapter 13), pernicious anaemia, hypoparathyroidism, ovarian or testicular failure and diabetes mellitus.

CLINICAL FEATURES

The presentation is most readily classified into those features associated with acute adrenocortical insufficiency and those seen in patients with the chronic condition. In the acute stage the most obvious feature is shock. Most patients presenting with an acute adrenocortical crisis will be known to have the primary adrenal condition. In this situation, the crisis will have been precipitated by failure to absorb the drugs or because the glucocorticoid dose was not increased to cover intercurrent stress (e.g. in pneumonia or major surgery). In acute adrenal failure occurring *de novo* (e.g. as with a septicaemia) the patient will not be pigmented and the symptoms will usually be weakness, malaise, nausea (often with vomiting) and abdominal pain associated with constipation or diarrhoea. The most important physical sign is postural hypotension.

In chronic adrenal insufficiency, many of these features will be present, but the presentation is much more vague. Pigmentation is present in more than ninety per cent of cases. This results from increased melanin in the skin and mucous membranes, and is most readily seen in areas exposed to light or pressure. Thus the face (Fig. 8.1), back of hands (Fig. 8.2), elbows and knees, buccal mucosa, conjunctivae, nails, axillae and skin creases (Fig. 8.3) are commonly pigmented. Vitiligo, in which there is patchy and often symmetrical depigmentation of the skin surrounded by areas of increased pigmentation (Fig. 8.4), occurs in ten to twenty per cent of cases of Addison's disease. Its presence is almost invariably an indication that the cause of the adrenal failure is autoimmune adrenalitis. One of the cases described by Addison had extensive vitiligo; however, this was the only case in which permission for a post-mortem examination was refused.

The other clinical features of Addison's disease are less dramatic. Weakness and weight loss are almost invariable. Anorexia, nausea and vague abdominal symptoms including pain, diarrhoea or constipation are common. Symptoms suggestive of postural hypotension include dizziness and attacks of fainting on standing. However, it should be noted that postural hypotension may only occur late in the course of the disease, therefore its absence does not preclude the diagnosis. Occasionally hypoglycaemia may occur. The patient's ability to respond to stress is markedly impaired and thus the history may include a failure to recover normally after surgery or intercurrent illness.

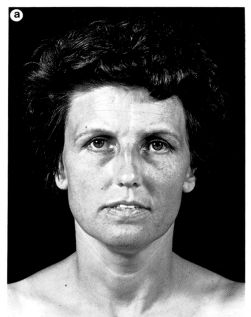 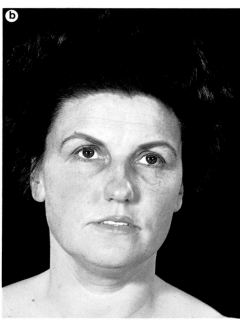

Fig. 8.1 Photographs of a patient with Addison's disease. View (a) is taken before treatment and view (b) whilst the patient is on glucocorticoid replacement therapy. The face is thin and pigmented before treatment; this resolves following treatment with glucocorticoids.

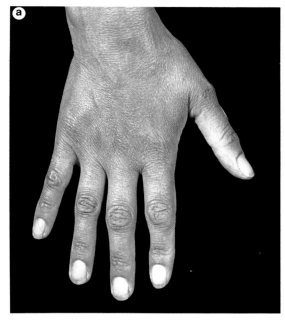
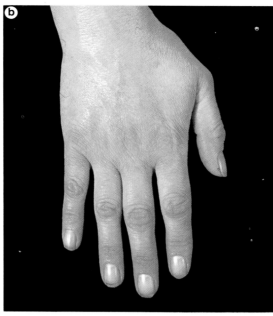

Fig. 8.2 Pigmentation of the dorsal surface of the hands in a patient with Addison's disease. View (a) is taken before treatment and view (b) whilst the patient is receiving glucocorticoid therapy; the normal hand colour is now restored.

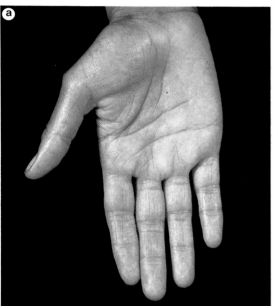
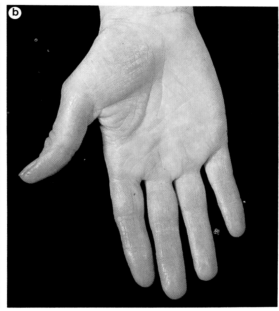

Fig. 8.3 Pigmentation of the palmar creases of the hands in a patient with Addison's disease. Pigmentation in Addison's disease commonly occurs in areas exposed to light and pressure. It is usually seen in the skin creases, as shown in view (a). During treatment (b) the normal colour returns.

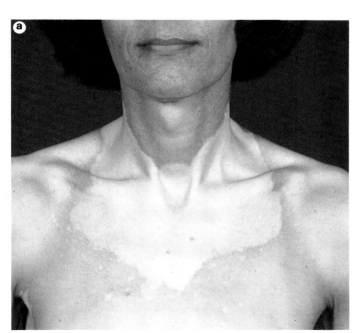
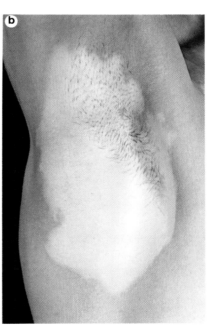

Fig. 8.4 Vitiligo in a patient with Addison's disease. In view (a) the depigmentation on the neck and chest is shown, whilst in view (b) the axillary region is shown. Increased pigmentation can be seen surrounding the areas of depigmentation.

DIAGNOSIS

In a patient with suspected adrenocortical insufficiency, the clinical sign of pigmentation will nearly always distinguish primary adrenocortical insufficiency from that which is secondary to either hypothalamic or pituitary disease (Fig. 8.5). Confirmation of the diagnosis of Addison's disease is normally made either by: (i) an early morning plasma cortisol and ACTH measurement, or (ii) plasma cortisol responsiveness to ACTH stimulation. Measurement of early morning basal cortisol alone is not satisfactory as it is often in the normal 0900h reference range; however, in Addison's disease this will be associated with an inappropriately high plasma ACTH level (i.e. above the normal 0900h reference range of 2.3–18pmol/l or 10–80ng/l). ACTH is derived from a large precursor molecule, pro-opiomelanocortin (Fig. 8.6). This precursor gives rise to three molecules which contain the melanocyte stimulating hormone (MSH) sequence; the NH_2 terminal sequence containing γ-MSH, ACTH with α-MSH and β-lipotrophin (β-LPH) with β-MSH. The relative importance of these molecules in the pigmentation of the disease is unclear. Assays have been developed for the NH_2 terminal sequence (N-POC) and for β-LPH. The levels of these molecules are high in Addison's disease, and since they are more stable in plasma than ACTH they may prove to be useful in clinical diagnosis, especially where sample handling facilities (e.g. cold centrifuge) are unavailable.

A variety of ACTH stimulation tests have been described in which either $ACTH_{1-39}$ or $ACTH_{1-24}$ is given. Only the first twenty-four amino acids of ACTH are required for full biological activity. Thus synthetic preparations such as tetracosactrin (Synacthen or $ACTH_{1-24}$) are usually used. In the 'short' tetracosactrin test a basal plasma cortisol sample is taken and then $250\mu g$ tetracosactrin are given either intramuscularly or intravenously. Further samples for cortisol assay are taken at thirty and sixty minutes after the injection. This test is best performed at 0900h and the patient does not need to be fasting. The normal increment in plasma cortisol is greater than 200nmol/l and the absolute level achieved should be greater than 580nmol/l (Fig. 8.7).

A lack of response to tetracosactrin does not distinguish between primary and secondary adrenocortical insufficiency. This can only be achieved by administering depot tetracosactrin – a zinc adsorbed preparation with a prolonged action, over approximately twenty-four hours. When this preparation is given (1.0mg intramuscularly) the plasma cortisol levels at thirty and sixty minutes after injection are virtually identical to the short acting preparation. With primary and secondary adrenocortical failure there may be no rise in cortisol at these times. With secondary failure, when blood samples are taken at eight hours and twenty-four hours, the cortisol level usually rises in contrast to the lack of response in primary failure. Further injections of depot tetracosactrin can be given at twenty-four or forty-eight hour intervals to restore the adrenal response to normal in secondary hypoadrenalism.

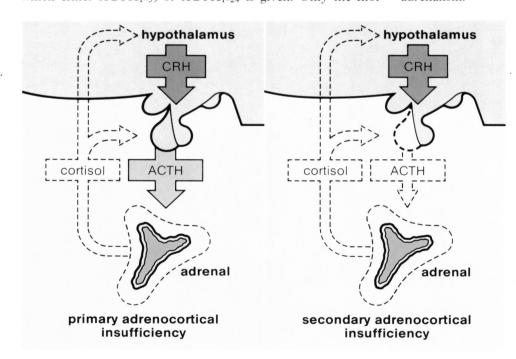

primary adrenocortical insufficiency

secondary adrenocortical insufficiency

Fig. 8.5 Diagram illustrating the hypothalamo-pituitary-adrenal axis in primary and secondary adrenocortical insufficiency. In primary adrenocortical insufficiency, circulating ACTH levels are elevated because of the negative feedback effects of low circulating cortisol. In secondary adrenocortical insufficiency, low circulating ACTH levels result from either hypothalamic or pituitary disease; as a consequence, cortisol levels are low.

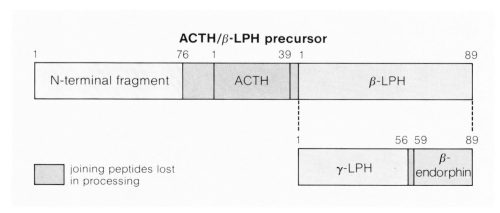

Fig.8.6 Structure of pro-opiomelanocortin (POMC). POMC is the ACTH/β-lipotrophin precursor molecule, therefore its cleavage results in ACTH and β-lipotrophin release. Precise residue lengths vary between species. While an MSH sequence recurs throughout the molecule, in normal man it is not liberated in the blood. (Takahashi et al., 1981; Whitfield et al., 1982).

Tests of adrenomedullary function are of no clinical relevance and are therefore not normally performed. Infusion of 2-deoxy-D-glucose has been shown to stimulate adrenaline output in idiopathic Addison's disease, but has minimal effect in tuberculous Addison's. This is in keeping with the histology (Fig. 8.8) which shows that, in the tuberculous disease, the whole gland is often destroyed. Plasma electrolyte concentrations are often normal but may show the classical picture of hyponatraemia, hyperkalaemia and elevated levels of urea. Serum aldosterone levels may be normal or low and levels of plasma renin are elevated.

The differential diagnosis usually lies between autoimmune adrenalitis and tuberculosis. In a patient with suspected auto-immune adrenalitis, evidence for other organ involvement should be sought; thus the presence of thyroid, gastric parietal cell and intrinsic factor antibodies should be tested, in addition to those directed against adrenal tissue. If adrenal antibodies are not found then evidence of tuberculosis should be sought. Often no active disease is found, but adrenal calcification usually indicates that tuberculosis was the cause of the adrenal failure. This is sometimes missed using conventional radiography and is most readily seen using computerised tomographic (CT) scanning of the adrenals (Fig. 8.9).

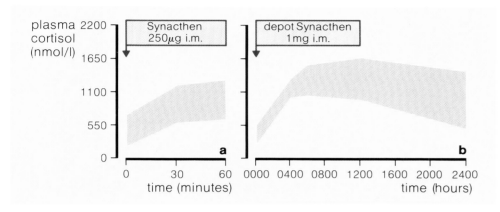

Fig. 8.7 Graph showing the normal responses to (a) tetracosactrin (Synacthen) and (b) depot tetracosactrin. Tetracosactrin is administered intramuscularly in doses of 250μg, whereas depot tetracosactrin is given in doses of 1.0mg.

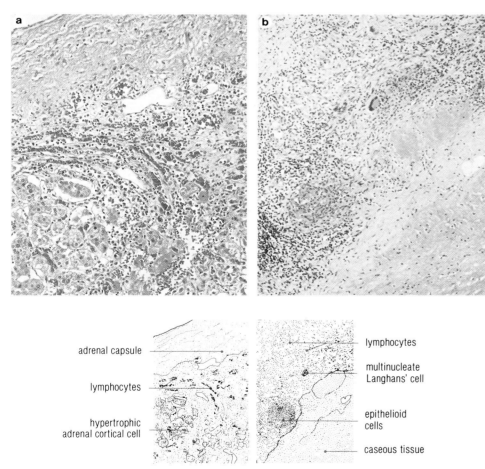

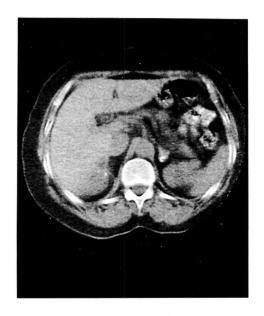

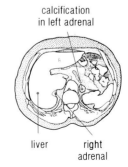

Fig. 8.8 Histological appearances in Addison's disease. The post-mortem histology of (a) autoimmune adrenalitis and (b) tuberculous adrenalitis in patients who died of Addison's disease is shown. In (a), the adrenal capsule is markedly thickened and the surviving cortex consists of scattered hypertrophied adrenal cortical cells heavily infiltrated with lymphocytes. Haematoxylin and eosin stain, magnification x 120. In (b), pink-staining amorphous, caseous necrosis can be seen in addition to tuberculous granulation tissue and a Langhans' giant cell. Haematoxylin and eosin stain, magnification x 80. By courtesy of Prof. I. Doniach.

Fig. 8.9 Computerised tomogram of the adrenal glands in a patient with tuberculous Addison's disease. Calcification of the left adrenal can be seen.

TREATMENT

All patients with Addison's disease require glucocorticoid replacement therapy and the majority also need mineralocorticoid treatment. Hydrocortisone (cortisol) is now regarded as the drug of choice since, unlike cortisone acetate, it does not need to be metabolised before it is metabolically active; it is also more readily absorbed. In an acute adrenal crisis, hydrocortisone hemisuccinate should be given (100 mg intravenously) together with saline to correct sodium losses and dextrose to treat hypoglycaemia. Intramuscular hydrocortisone should also be given (100 mg six-hourly) until the patient is able to take oral therapy, at which time hydrocortisone is given (40 mg on waking, 20 mg at 1800h). When the patient is well the latter dose is then halved. Since intercurrent infections often precipitate the crisis, evidence for this should be actively sought and the appropriate antibiotic treatment given.

For chronic adrenocortical failure, maintenance therapy of hydrocortisone is given, usually with 9α-fludrocortisone, to replace the mineralocorticoid deficiency. Most patients require 20 mg oral hydrocortisone on waking and 10 mg at 1800h. This should reverse the pigmentation (see Figs. 8.1–8.3) but should not produce Cushing's syndrome. Plasma cortisol levels should be measured during the day on replacement therapy to determine whether the dose is correct (Fig. 8.10). Mineralocorticoid replacement with 9α-fludrocortisone is given either daily, in single or divided doses, or on alternate days. The dose varies from 0.05 mg on alternate days to 0.2 mg daily. If the dose is excessive, oedema and hypertension may result. Adequacy of mineralocorticoid replacement can be monitored by measurement of plasma renin activity. Elevated levels of renin usually signify that inadequate mineralocorticoid replacement has been given. In practice, twice-daily 9α-fludrocortisone may give better suppression of renin than the once-daily therapy.

Patients should be told to double their dose of hydrocortisone in the event of intercurrent stress or febrile illness. If they cannot take their steroid by mouth (e.g. in the event of surgery or gastro-enteritis) then it should be given parenterally. All patients should carry a steroid card or preferably a bracelet or necklace giving details of their condition. For minor operations (e.g. dental extraction) 100 mg hydrocortisone hemisuccinate should be given with the premedication. For major surgery the steroid regime for acute adrenal crisis, outlined above, should be adopted.

Other autoimmune diseases may be present in patients with autoimmune adrenalitis and these should be treated if necessary. Patients with tuberculous Addison's disease usually require anti-tuberculous chemotherapy.

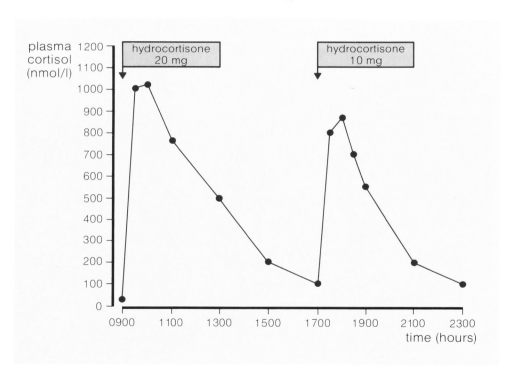

Fig. 8.10 Plasma cortisol profile of a patient with adrenocortical insufficiency on hydrocortisone replacement therapy. 20 mg of oral hydrocortisone was administered at 0900h with a further 10 mg at 1700h.

9 Endocrine Hypertension

Christopher R W Edwards, MA, MD, FRCP

Hypertension is one of the major medical problems of the world since it affects approximately fifteen per cent of the population in Western countries. It is defined as a persistent increase in systemic blood pressure above an arbitrary limit – often set at 140 mmHg systolic and 90 mmHg (phase V) diastolic – i.e. disappearance of sound. The lowering of blood pressure has now been shown to reduce the incidence of stroke, coronary artery disease (only in some studies) and also renal failure. However, as most patients with hypertension are symptomless for many years, there is a need for population screening. Since the diagnosis of hypertension may lead to life-long drug therapy, secondary causes of hypertension which may be remedied by surgery or respond to specific drug therapy should be excluded. A knowledge of the physiology and pathophysiology of the renin-angiotensin-aldosterone system and also catecholamines is therefore essential.

AETIOLOGY OF HYPERTENSION

The prevalence of various conditions resulting in hypertension is shown in Figure 9.1. In the majority of patients with hypertension no cause for the elevated blood pressure can be found and such patients are defined as having 'essential' or primary hypertension. A large number of secondary causes have been described (Fig. 9.2), although the prevalence of many of these conditions is debatable. The prevalence, however, depends upon a variety of factors. Primary hyperaldosteronism, for example, is approximately twice as common in non-Caucasian as in Caucasian hypertensive patients. The commonest secondary cause results from abnormalities of the renin-angiotensin-aldosterone system.

PHYSIOLOGY OF THE RENIN-ANGIOTENSIN-ALDOSTERONE SYSTEM

Renin is a proteolytic enzyme synthesised and stored by specialised cells in the wall of the afferent arteriole of the glomerulus of the kidney. These cells are anatomically and functionally associated with cells in the wall of the distal convoluted tubules which form the macula densa, and the whole structure is known as the juxtaglomerular apparatus. The release of renin activates a cascade system (Fig. 9.3) in which renin cleaves a leucine-valine bond in its specific substrate (angiotensinogen, an α_2 globulin produced by the liver). This results in the production of the decapeptide angiotensin I which is then converted by angiotensin converting enzyme (ACE) to the octapeptide angiotensin II (cf. Chapter 6). ACE is a dipeptidyl carboxypeptidase found in high concentrations in the pulmonary circulation, but also in the systemic vasculature and the kidney. Angiotensin II is a potent vasoconstrictor and can thus elevate blood pressure. It also directly stimulates aldosterone secretion which leads to sodium retention and potassium loss. The seven amino acid peptide, angiotensin III, is released by protease cleavage of angiotensin II. The role of this peptide in man is controversial. In many species angiotensin III has been shown to be at least as potent as angiotensin II in stimulating aldosterone secretion, but has less pressor activity.

Renin is produced in both an active and inactive form. Various *in vitro* techniques have been used to activate the inactive form including treatment with trypsin, pepsin or acid, or incubation at −4°C. The enzyme responsible for *in vivo* activation of renin is probably a serine protease, possibly kallikrein. The major trigger for renin release is a decrease in perfusion pressure. This may result from haemorrhage, hypotension or a reduction in the extracellular fluid volume after sodium depletion. The autonomic nervous system plays a role in renin release; catecholamines can also directly stimulate renin secretion. Conversely, hyperkalaemia,

angiotensin II and antidiuretic hormone (ADH or vasopressin) can all inhibit renin secretion.

Aldosterone is the principal mineralocorticoid secreted by the outermost zone of the adrenal cortex, the zona glomerulosa. The normal production rate is approximately 200 μg daily; this is critically dependent on sodium intake, being stimulated by sodium depletion and suppressed by salt loading. Plasma levels range from approximately 50–150 ng/l (140–420 pmol/l) when normal subjects are recumbent and from 150–300 ng/l (420–840 pmol/l) when standing upright. In addition, there is a circadian rhythm of aldosterone secretion. Thus posture, sodium intake and time of day all have to be taken into consideration when taking blood samples for aldosterone assay.

The three major factors which control the biosynthesis and release of aldosterone are angiotensin II, adrenocorticotrophic hormone (ACTH) and potassium. Of these, angiotensin II is probably the most important. Various factors can alter the adrenal responsiveness to this hormone; for example, sodium depletion increases the adrenal responsiveness to angiotensin II. Sodium deprivation is also involved in activating the renin-

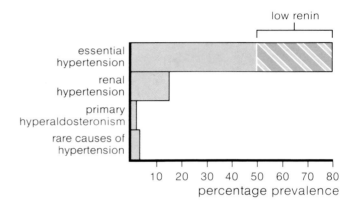

Fig. 9.1 Prevalence of the various causes of hypertension. Eighty per cent of patients have primary or essential hypertension with no apparent cause. Many secondary causes of hypertension have been described, but their prevalence is limited to a minority of hypertensive patients.

Secondary Causes of Hypertension

renal hypertension
renovascular
renal parenchymatous disease
primary reninism

primary hyperaldosteronism
unilateral adrenal adenoma
bilateral hyperplasia of the zona glomerulosa

rare causes of hypertension
phaeochromocytoma
Cushing's syndrome
coarctation of the aorta

Fig. 9.2 The secondary causes of hypertension. These can be classified as primary hyperaldosteronism, renal causes and rare causes of hypertension.

angiotensin system; this leads to elevated angiotensin II levels. Acute administration of ACTH stimulates aldosterone secretion, but chronic ACTH excess is associated with normal or even low levels of aldosterone. Thus, when the renin-angiotensin system is suppressed, for instance in patients with primary hyperaldosteronism, ACTH may play an important role. Aldosterone-secreting adrenal adenomas are extremely sensitive to ACTH stimulation and, as a result, plasma aldosterone levels have the same circadian rhythm as plasma cortisol in these patients. Hyperkalaemia can directly stimulate the zona glomerulosa; this can occur in patients with Conn's syndrome where aldosterone secretion may be markedly stimulated by potassium replacement therapy. Conversely, hypokalaemia may inhibit aldosterone release.

The primary effect of aldosterone is to increase the resorption of sodium by the distal convoluted tubule of the kidney in exchange for potassium and hydrogen ions. Therefore, if aldosterone levels are persistently elevated, hypokalaemia and alkalosis will ensue.

PATHOPHYSIOLOGY OF THE RENIN-ANGIOTENSIN-ALDOSTERONE SYSTEM

Hypertension may result from overactivity of one or more components of the renin-angiotensin-aldosterone system. Raised blood pressure may be associated with the excessive secretion of aldosterone due either to an adrenocortical abnormality, when it is termed primary hyperaldosteronism, or secondary to the excessive secretion of renin (e.g. in renovascular or renal parenchymatous disease). This would then be termed secondary hyperaldosteronism.

Primary Hyperaldosteronism (Conn's Syndrome)

The prevalence of this condition is not clear. Probably two per cent of all subjects with hypertension have primary hyperaldosteronism and, of these, approximately seventy per cent have a unilateral adrenal adenoma (Fig. 9.4) and approximately thirty per cent have bilateral hyperplasia of the zona glomerulosa (Fig. 9.5). Primary hyperaldosteronism is usually suspected when a hypertensive patient is found to be hypokalaemic. However, this diagnostic clue may be missed unless blood samples are taken

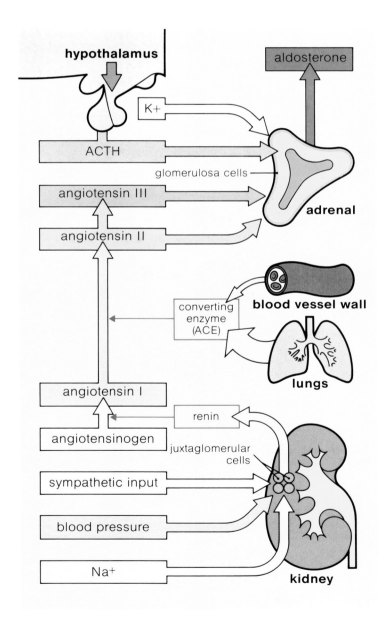

Fig. 9.3 The renin-angiotensin system. Following release, renin converts angiotensinogen to angiotensin I, which is then converted to angiotensin II by the enzyme ACE.

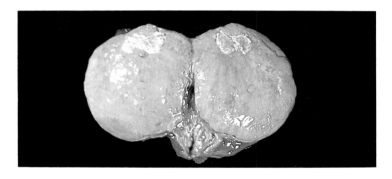

Fig. 9.4 Adrenal adenoma removed from a patient with primary hyperaldosteronism (Conn's syndrome). The canary yellow colour of the adenoma is typical.

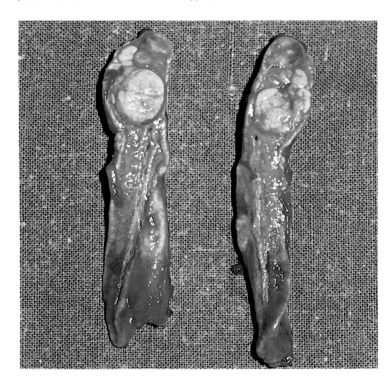

Fig. 9.5 Nodular hyperplasia associated with Conn's syndrome. Bilateral hyperplasia occurs in approximately thirty per cent of patients with hypertension which is caused by primary hyperaldosteronism.

9.3

properly: sampling without occlusion or muscular exercise is essential and the plasma must be rapidly separated from the red cells. In addition, the patient should be on an adequate sodium intake since, with a low sodium diet, there will be little sodium for distal tubular sodium-potassium exchange, and thus hypokalaemia will not persist. Once primary hyperaldosteronism is suspected, the diagnosis must be confirmed by demonstrating suppression of plasma renin activity and elevation of plasma aldosterone (Fig. 9.6).

Several methods are available to make the differential diagnosis between adenoma and hyperplasia. The simplest test is to take blood for aldosterone, plasma renin activity and cortisol at 0800h, with the patient recumbent, and then to repeat the blood sampling at 1200h after the patient has been standing upright for four hours. In patients with aldosterone-secreting adenomas, plasma renin activity is suppressed as the adenoma is sensitive to ACTH.

Thus when plasma ACTH levels fall between 0800h and 1200h, aldosterone levels will fall. Conversely, in patients with idiopathic bilateral hyperplasia, the hyperplastic adrenals are very sensitive to angiotensin II and the small amount of renin which is released on standing is sufficient to elevate aldosterone levels. The exception to this test is the rare condition of dexamethasone-suppressible hyperaldosteronism in which plasma aldosterone levels in the patient fall on standing. This diagnosis can be confirmed by demonstrating that the blood pressure is reduced to normal by ACTH suppression. If patients with adenomas are stressed by standing then ACTH, and hence cortisol levels, will rise during the course of the morning. In these patients, aldosterone levels will also rise.

The administration of radiolabelled cholesterol can be used to distinguish between adenomas and hyperplasia, since the labelled cholesterol is taken up only by the adenoma (Fig. 9.7). This is in

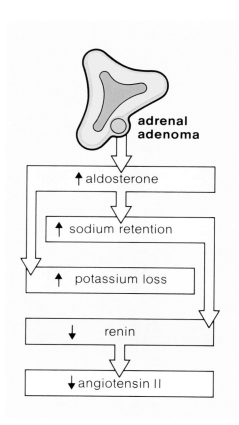

Fig. 9.6 Mechanism of pathophysiological changes occuring in primary hyperaldosteronism. The autonomous production and release of aldosterone from the tumour leads to excessive sodium retention and potassium wasting, largely by its effects on the distal tubule of the kidney. Renin release from the kidney is therefore inhibited and this leads to a fall in circulating angiotensin II.

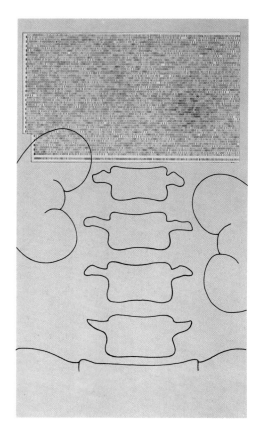

Fig. 9.7 Adrenal scan in patient with Conn's syndrome. Selective uptake of ^{131}I-cholesterol in a left adrenal adenoma is shown.

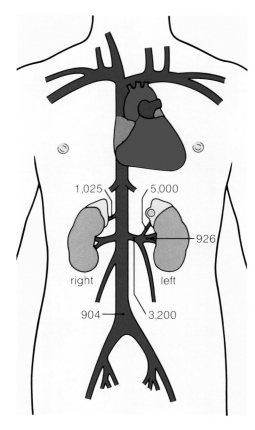

Fig. 9.8 Adrenal vein catheter study showing high levels of aldosterone in the left adrenal vein. The concentration of aldosterone (pg/ml) in the right adrenal vein is not significantly different from that found in the inferior vena cava. This patient had hypertension and hypokalaemia, and was subsequently cured after removal of his left adrenal adenoma.

contrast to the bilateral uptake found in patients with idiopathic hyperplasia. These scans may have to be performed after dexamethasone administration to suppress uptake by normal glucocorticoid-secreting cells. In some patients, misleading results can be obtained if spironolactone has been used as long-term therapy before the scan is performed. In such patients, adenomas can be missed as there may be bilateral uptake.

Adrenal vein sampling for aldosterone can be extremely useful in identifying whether there is a unilateral or bilateral source of aldosterone. Although cannulation of the left adrenal vein is relatively easy, it is a difficult procedure to enter the right adrenal vein. For this reason, blood samples for cortisol should always be taken in order to confirm that the catheter tip is actually in the adrenal vein. A typical example of an adrenal vein catheterisation in a patient with an adenoma is shown in Figure 9.8.

Renal Hypertension

Renal hypertension constitutes approximately fifteen per cent of all cases of hypertension. The causes can most readily be divided into three groups, renovascular, renal parenchymatous disease and primary reninism (Fig. 9.9).

The two most common causes of unilateral renal artery stenosis are atheromatous plaques and fibromuscular hyperplasia. Atheroma is most frequently found in the proximal third of the renal artery. It occurs in the middle-aged and elderly, in contrast to fibromuscular hyperplasia which involves the middle and distal thirds of the renal artery, and is the commonest cause of renal artery stenosis in young patients. In patients with malignant hypertension, the elevated blood pressure leads to fibrinoid necrosis of the small vessels of the kidney; this, in turn, stimulates excessive renin release and thus further exacerbates the hypertension by activation of the renin-angiotensin-aldosterone system. Thus these patients have secondary hyperaldosteronism (Fig. 9.10).

Renal Causes of Hypertension

renal parenchymatous disease

acute and chronic glomerulo-nephritis

chronic pyelonephritis – especially if calculi or obstruction with hydronephrosis

polycystic disease

interstitial nephritis e.g. with gout, hypercalcaemia or excessive analgesics (analgesic nephropathy)

radiation nephritis

amyloid

connective tissue disease e.g. with polyarteritis, systemic lupus erythematosus and diabetes mellitus

renovascular

coarctation of the aorta

renal artery stenosis e.g. with fibromuscular hyperplasia, atheromatous plaque, congenital

malignant or accelerated phase hypertension

primary reninism

reninomas (haemangiopericytoma)

some Wilms' tumours

ectopic renin secretion

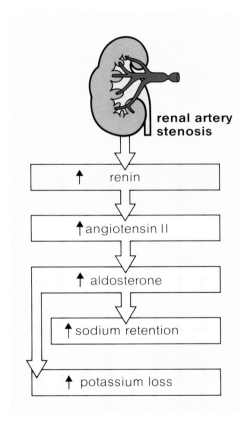

renal artery stenosis

↑ renin

↑ angiotensin II

↑ aldosterone

↑ sodium retention

↑ potassium loss

Fig. 9.9   Table of the renal causes of hypertension. These can be classified into renovascular, renal parenchymatous disease and primary reninism. Of these, renovascular hypertension is the most common.

Fig. 9.10   Diagram of the sequence of events in secondary hyperaldosteronism. In secondary hyperaldosteronism, circulating renin levels are elevated as a consequence of renal artery stenosis, renal hypoperfusion or volume depletion. High renin levels, in turn, lead to increased angiotensin II levels and hyperaldosteronism, with concomitant sodium retention and potassium wastage.

Renovascular hypertension may be implicated on finding a renal artery bruit, which is best heard over the long muscles of the back at the level of L1, or in the epigastrium. However, in many patients there are no clinical clues. Isotope renography reveals decreased uptake and delayed excretion of the isotope on the side of the lesion. Although this technique is less expensive, it is also less widely available than intravenous urography. On urography, a delayed nephrogram may be seen on the stenotic side in early films, with increased density and delayed excretion in later films (Fig. 9.11). Plasma renin activity may be normal in patients with

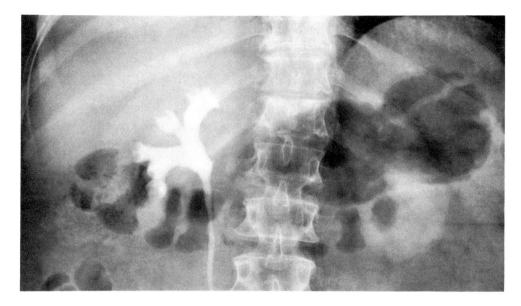

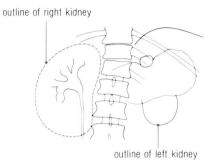

Fig. 9.11 Urogram in left renal artery stenosis twenty minutes after injection of contrast. Comparison of the left nephrogram with the right, where the contrast is in the calyceal system, demonstrates marked delay in excretion of contrast. This is caused by stenosis of the left renal artery.

outline of right kidney

outline of left kidney

Renal Vein Plasma Renin Activity (ng Aldosterone/l/h)

	supine	standing (6 min)
high inferior vena cava	7,400	12,800
left renal vein	6,160 (7,740)	12,700 (7,240)
right renal vein	>36,000 (7,040)	>36,000 (12,300)
low inferior vena cava	7,060	10,000

Fig. 9.12 Measurements of renal vein plasma renin activity in right renal artery stenosis. Figures in brackets are the renin concentrations in peripheral blood samples taken simultaneously. For a diagnosis of haemodynamically significant right renal artery stenosis, the renin level in the right renal vein should be markedly higher than the level in a synchronous peripheral blood sample, and there should be no gradient on the left side. Also, the ratio between left and right renal vein plasma renin activity should be greater then 1.5: 1.

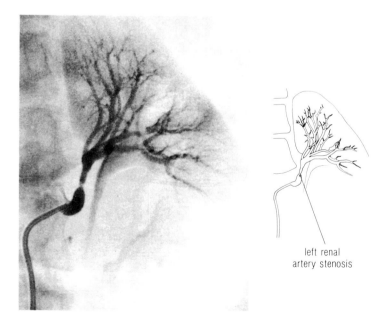

left renal artery stenosis

Fig. 9.13 Selective renal arteriogram showing left renal artery stenosis in an 18-year-old male with severe hypertension.

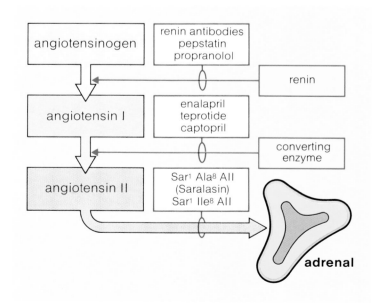

Fig. 9.14 Inhibitors of the renin-angiotensin system. Renin output may be reduced by beta blockade (e.g. propranolol), or its activity impaired by the presence of renin antibodies. The angiotensin converting enzyme (ACE), present in the lungs and blood vessels, can be inhibited by captopril, teprotide and enalapril. In addition, the drug saralasin is a competitive inhibitor of angiotensin II at its receptor site.

unilateral renal artery stenosis but, in some series, elevated peripheral venous levels of plasma renin activity have been found in up to sixty per cent of patients. Such patients may also have an exaggerated response of renin to dynamic function tests such as the diuretic administration test or sodium depletion test. The measurement of renal vein renin is important in the diagnosis of a haemodynamically significant renal artery stenosis (Fig. 9.12). The renin level in the renal vein draining from the kidney on the opposite side to the stenosis should mimic that in a peripheral blood sample taken simultaneously, thus indicating that the kidney is suppressed. There should be a gradient across the kidney on the affected side and the ratio between the renal vein plasma renin activity on the affected side and the renal vein plasma renin activity on the normal side should be greater than 1.5:1. In patients with this pattern of renin secretion, renal artery surgery or transluminal balloon dilatation will probably reduce the blood pressure. In patients with suspected renal artery stenosis, renal arteriograms will need to be performed to define the site and nature of the lesion. In addition to midstream aortography, selective renal arteriography will be required (Fig. 9.13).

The medical treatment of angiotensin-dependent hypertension has been revolutionised by the introduction of specific inhibitors of the renin-angiotensin-aldosterone system (Fig. 9.14). Of these, the most important has been captopril – the first effective and orally active inhibitor of the converting enzyme ACE. Transluminal angioplasty using a catheter with a balloon has been a major advance for the patient with renal artery stenosis. Good results have also been reported for both fibromuscular hyperplasia and atheromatous stenosis with low morbidity.

HYPERTENSION ASSOCIATED WITH ABNORMALITIES OF THE HYPOTHALAMO-PITUITARY-ADRENOCORTICAL AXIS
Genetic Defects of Cortisol Synthesis
Two types of congenital adrenal hyperplasia arising from enzyme deficiencies have been found to result in hypertension. In 1966,

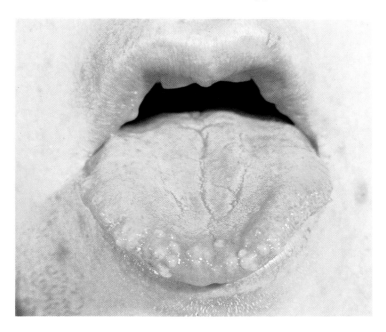

Fig. 9.15 Neuromas of lips and tongue in a patient with medullary carcinoma of the thyroid and adrenal phaeochromocytomas. This rare association is part of the Multiple Endocrine Neoplasia (MEN) 2b syndrome.

Biglieri and his colleagues described a new syndrome where defective 17α-hydroxylation was present in both the adrenals and the gonads. The resultant low levels of cortisol, acting via the negative feedback mechanism, stimulate ACTH release, with consequent bilateral hyperplasia and excessive secretion of corticosterone and deoxycorticosterone. This, in turn, causes sodium retention, potassium loss, hypertension and a hypokalaemic alkalosis. The absence of normal androgen secretion in the male causes male pseudohermaphroditism, while defective oestrogen secretion in the female results in primary amenorrhoea. Renin levels are also suppressed. Replacement therapy with glucocorticoids rapidly suppresses ACTH and hence corticosterone and deoxycorticosterone levels. This results in correction of the hypertension and electrolyte abnormalities.

In the presence of 11β-hydroxylase deficiency, defective cortisol secretion leads to secondary elevation of ACTH and bilateral adrenal hyperplasia. In addition, there are high circulating levels of 11-deoxycortisol and deoxycorticosterone present. Hypertension ensues, and also virilism as a result of the elevated androgen levels. The process can be reversed by glucocorticoid replacement therapy.

Cushing's Syndrome
Hypertension is commonly found in patients with Cushing's syndrome. The aetiology of high blood pressure is not well understood. Elevated levels of cortisol, which have mineralocorticoid as well as glucocorticoid effects, can increase vascular reactivity to pressor substances and also increase the production of angiotensinogen. (For the investigation and treatment of patients with Cushing's syndrome see Chapter 7).

Phaeochromocytoma
Hypertension is the commonest clinical feature in patients with phaeochromocytomas. Characteristically, the hypertension is labile and is often associated with a variety of symptoms. Patients may present complaining of attacks of palpitations, headache, excessive sweating, pallor or flushing which may be associated with anxiety. On examination most patients will be found to have hypertension. There is a significant fall in blood pressure on standing in about two thirds of patients. In approximately ten to twenty per cent of cases, phaeochromocytomas may be associated with other conditions such as Recklinghausen's disease, medullary carcinoma of the thyroid and hyperparathyroidism. The typical neuromas found on the tongue and lips in a patient with medullary carcinoma of the thyroid and multiple adrenal phaeochromocytomas are shown in Figure 9.15. These patients commonly present to psychiatrists with anxiety. Glucose intolerance may be provoked by the excess catecholamine secretion and such patients may therefore come under the care of the diabetologist. Some patients may have gastrointestinal complaints with abdominal pain, and constipation is common. The constipation may be caused by the very large amounts of met-enkephalin produced by these tumours.

Most clinicians rely on the clinical history to suggest the diagnosis and do not routinely measure catecholamines in all patients with hypertension. In a patient suspected of having a phaeochromocytoma, the first investigation is to measure the urinary excretion of vanillylmandelic acid (VMA). The urinary excretion of VMA is almost always elevated in patients with phaeochromocytomas. Very occasionally the level is normal. In such instances metanephrines should be measured in the urine; alternatively, plasma levels of adrenaline and noradrenaline should be measured.

A variety of pharmacological tests have been developed in an attempt to improve the diagnosis of patients with phaeochromocytoma. However, with advancements in biochemical diagnosis these have nearly all been discarded. The most commonly used test was that involving the administration of phentolamine, an adrenergic blocking drug. A positive response (Fig. 9.16) occurred within two to three minutes and resulted in a fall in blood pressure of at least 35/25 mmHg. Other pharmacological tests involved the administration of tyramine or glucagon; however, these tests yielded both false positive and false negative results.

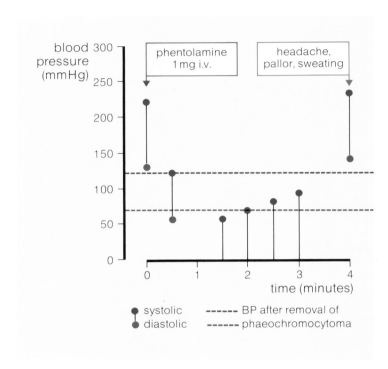

Fig. 9.16 Phentolamine test in a patient with a phaeochromocytoma. A positive response occurs within 2–3 minutes and results in a transient fall in blood pressure of at least 35/25 mmHg.

A variety of methods have been used to locate phaeochromocytomas. Eighty-five to ninety per cent of these tumours arise from the adrenal medulla and in ten per cent of cases the tumours are bilateral. Non-adrenal tumours may arise from sympathetic ganglia, usually alongside the aorta or its branches or, rarely, in the wall of the urinary bladder. Less than one per cent of phaeochromocytomas are found outside the abdominal cavity.

Plain radiography of the abdomen may reveal displacement of the kidney by a suprarenal mass, whereas intravenous urography associated with tomography may delineate the tumour itself. Historically, adrenal arteriography (Fig. 9.17) was commonly performed but not without risk. For this reason, computerised tomography of the adrenals is presently the method of choice (Fig. 9.18). In patients in whom a phaeochromocytoma cannot be localised by other means, it may be necessary to perform a venous catheter study and measure catecholamine levels in all the major veins to determine the source of catecholamine excess. Recently, however, a scanning agent, meta-iodo-benzyl-guanidine (MIBG), has been introduced. This compound is taken up by both benign and malignant phaeochromocytoma tissue and also by secondary deposits.

Surgery is the treatment of choice for all patients except those who are thought to be medically unfit, those in whom a tumour has not been localised or where there are multiple metastases. Prior to surgery, or any major investigative procedure, patients should be given a combination of alpha and beta blockade. The most commonly used alpha blocker is phenoxybenzamine which is usually used in conjunction with the beta blocker, propranolol: 0.5 mg/kg phenoxybenzamine over four hours by venous drip should be given daily for three days, with 40 mg propranolol three times daily starting after the first phenoxybenzamine infusion. Any delay in definitive surgery may be controlled by administration of 10 mg oral phenoxybenzamine four times daily or 40 mg thymoxamine four times daily with 40 mg propranolol three times daily. During surgery, sodium nitroprusside has proved to be extremely useful in controlling large swings in blood pressure which may occur even in patients who have been fully 'blocked' by alpha- and beta-blockers.

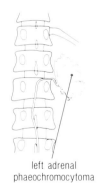

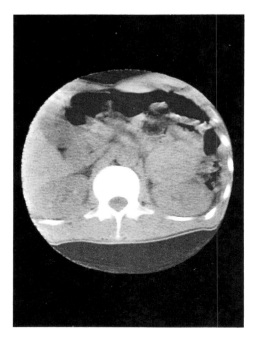

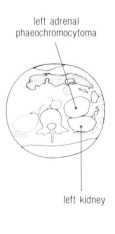

Fig. 9.17 Selective left adrenal arteriogram in a patient with a phaeochromocytoma. The abnormal vasculature and tumour blush are shown.

Fig. 9.18 Computerised tomogram of the upper abdomen showing a left adrenal phaeochromocytoma.

10 The Testis

Paul E Belchetz, MA, MD, MSc, FRCP

THE ADULT TESTIS

During sexual maturity the testis performs two distinct but related functions: spermatogenesis and androgen production. The seminiferous tubules are abundantly coiled and in man, in contrast to most mammalian species, different phases of spermatogenesis may be seen in the same cross section (Fig. 10.1). The seminiferous tubules constitute ninety-five per cent of the testis volume, and when spermatogenesis is impaired there is a corresponding degree of tubular atrophy. This is reflected clinically by diminution in testicular volume. Testicular dimensions are variously reported but since volume changes with the cube of linear change, measurement of length is a poor indicator of size. This can be seen in the indices of testis growth from infancy to adult life (Fig. 10.2). The accurate assessment of testis volume is greatly facilitated by using the orchidometer devised by Prader (Fig. 10.3), which simply involves comparing the patient's testis with a series of ellipsoids accurately manufactured to cover a range from 1 ml to 25 ml. Although the orchidometer was developed for use in paediatric and pubertal practice, this 'andrologist's rosary' should form an indispensable part of the clinicians's equipment for patients of all ages.

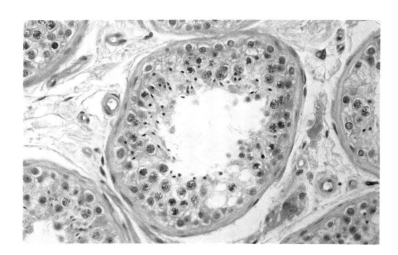

Fig. 10.1 Histological section of a normal testis.
Spermatogenesis takes place between the Sertoli cells in the seminiferous tubules. Different stages of spermatogenesis may be seen in the same cross-section, a feature particular to man and different from most other mammals. In the normal mature testis the Leydig cells appear in clumps between the seminiferous tubules. By courtesy of Prof. I. Doniach. H&E stain.

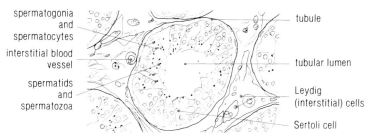

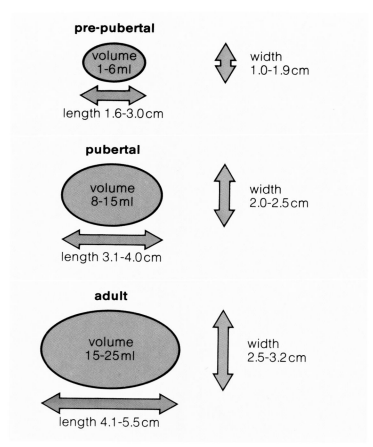

Fig. 10.2 Diagram showing testicular size and volume at three developmental stages from infancy to puberty.

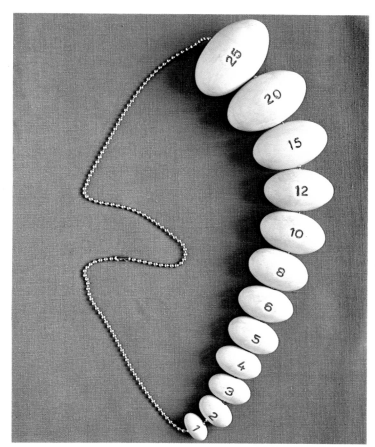

Fig. 10.3 Photograph of Prader's orchidometer. Testicular volume (ml) may be estimated by direct comparison with these ellipsoids. During measurement the epididymis should not be included in the assessment of testicular volume.

LEYDIG CELL FUNCTION

The role of Leydig cells is androgen production. In the normal adult testis, Leydig cells tend to appear in clumps between the seminiferous tubules (see Fig. 10.1), and Leydig cell mass tends to correlate well with androgen production. Thus with adult seminiferous tubular dysfunction and atrophy from any cause, there may be an illusion of Leydig cell hyperplasia (Fig. 10.4) if androgen secretion is normally preserved. Quantitative studies in Klinefelter's syndrome by Ahmad and colleagues (1971) have clearly revealed that there is no true hyperplasia.

Androgen secretion from Leydig cells is under the influence of gonadotrophins. The predominant androgen is testosterone. Its presence in fetal life is crucial to proper male sexual differentiation, and is indicated by the prominence of the fetal Leydig cells (Fig. 10.5). The important early peak of testosterone is in response to human chorionic gonadotrophin (HCG) whilst lower later levels of testosterone secretion are a result of luteinising hormone (LH) secretion from the fetal pituitary (Fig. 10.6). There is clear evidence of postnatal testosterone secretion continuing for several months and then declining, after which time Leydig cells cannot be recognised in the prepubertal child's testis (Fig. 10.7).

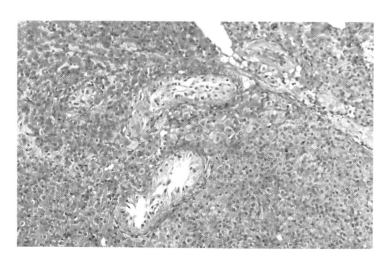

Fig. 10.4   Histological section of a testis in a patient with Klinefelter's syndrome. The dysgenetic seminiferous tubules are evident, and the clumps of Leydig cells give an illusory impression of hyperplasia. By courtesy of Prof. I. Doniach. H&E stain.

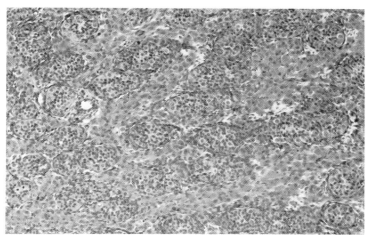

Fig. 10.5   Histological section of a fetal testis showing prominent Leydig cells. These cells are present at this very early stage of differentiation and are necessary for normal male sexual development. Primitive tubules can be seen in this section. H&E stain.

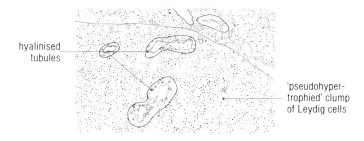

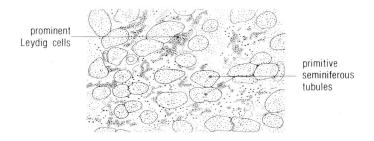

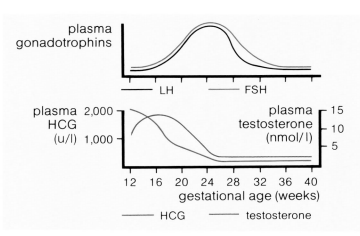

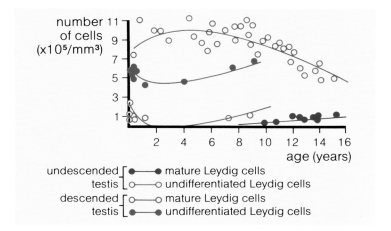

Fig. 10.6   Graph of plasma hormone concentrations in the fetus. LH and FSH concentrations follow a similar pattern during fetal life, with maxima at around 23 weeks of gestation. HCG causes the crucial early peak in plasma testosterone whilst secretion of lower levels of testosterone results from later fetal pituitary LH secretion.

Fig. 10.7   Leydig cell development during the first sixteen years. The distributions of undifferentiated interstitial cells and mature Leydig cells are shown for both the normal and undescended testis. Redrawn from Hayashi H and Harrison R G: The development of the interstitial tissue of the human testis. Fertil. Steril. 22:351, 1971. Reproduced with permission of the American Fertility Society.

SERTOLI CELL FUNCTION

It was thought for a long time that Sertoli cells only offered mechanical support and possibly nutrition to germinal cells. Subsequently several important functions have been discovered and are schematized in Figure 10.8. Early in fetal development the disappearance of Müllerian structures in males has been associated with local secretion of a peptide called Müllerian inhibitory factor (MIF) from the Sertoli cells. The important hormonal effects on spermatogenesis in the adult appear to be mediated by the Sertoli cells, which possess well-defined receptors for follicle stimulating hormone (FSH). Sertoli cells aromatise locally produced androgens to oestrogens, produce an androgen-binding protein, (similar to the sex-hormone-binding globulin, SHBG, in primates) and also produce cyclic AMP when stimulated by FSH. How these processes affect spermatogenesis remains unclear. FSH secretion is partially controlled by an incompletely characterised Sertoli cell product termed inhibin. A further, and clearly very important, function of Sertoli cells is the establishment of the blood-testis barrier. In general, the luminal milieu of seminiferous tubules differs sharply from extracellular fluid. During spermatogenesis the developing gametes cross into an immunologically secluded environment created by specialised tight junctions between Sertoli cells, thus separating the mature spermatocytes from meiotic spermatocytes and spermatids. The latter behave as if

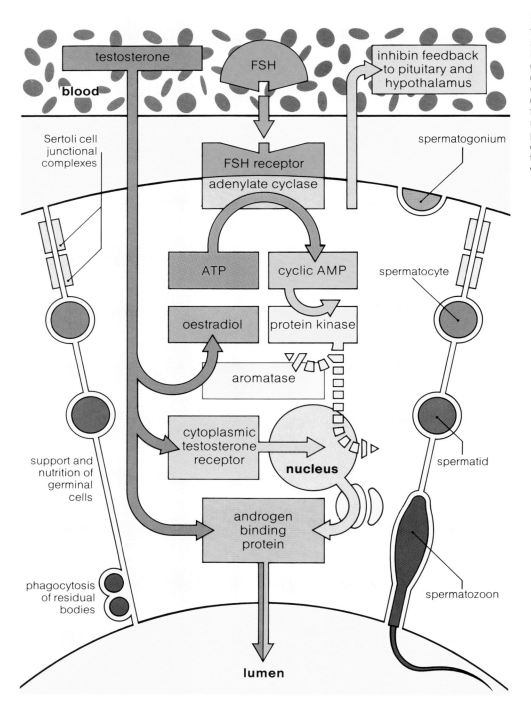

Fig. 10.8 Diagram illustrating the functions of Sertoli cells. These may be summarised as follows: (i) maintenance of blood-testis barrier by junctional complexes, (ii) nourishment of developing germ cells, (iii) phagocytosis of damaged germ cells, (iv) production of androgen binding protein (ABP) which is secreted by seminiferous tubules (ABP production is dependent upon FSH and testosterone action), (v) production of tubular fluid providing major drive for flushing sperm from the testis to the epididymis and (vi) production of inhibin which controls FSH secretion.

immunologically 'foreign', and breakdown of this blood-testis barrier probably underlies many cases of male infertility.

ANDROGEN SECRETION

The predominant androgen secreted by the Leydig cell is testosterone, the production of which averages 7 mg daily in adult men. Testosterone secretion follows stimulation of Leydig cells by LH (or, *in utero*, HCG) which binds to specific receptors. The free LH-receptor population may vary: excess LH 'down-regulates' their number and some FSH appears to be necessary for the acquisition of LH receptors by Leydig cells. LH activates the Leydig cell adenylate cyclase mechanism which ultimately enhances cholesterol conversion to pregnenolone, driving steroidogenesis (Fig. 10.9). Testosterone secretion is phasic, but in adult men this does not correlate clearly with LH pulses which on average occur every ninety minutes. There is a small circadian variation in testosterone with an amplitude of approximately thirty per cent, peaking in the early morning and lowest about 1800h. Androgen action at target organs involves the transport of the steroid by cytoplasmic receptors to the nucleus, where genomic activation leads to the synthesis of specific messenger RNA and proteins (Fig. 10.10). In many tissues the active androgen is the 5α-reduced metabolite of testosterone, dihydrotestosterone (DHT), which is largely generated *in situ* in the target tissues

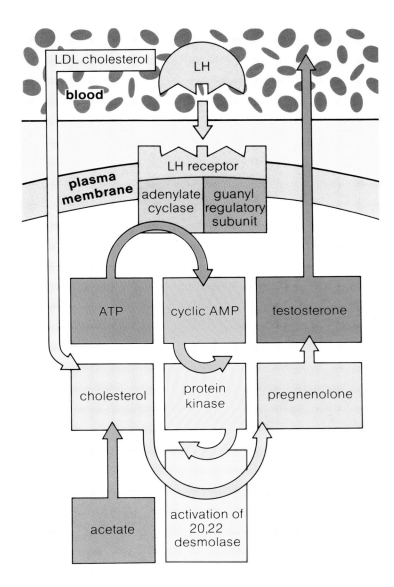

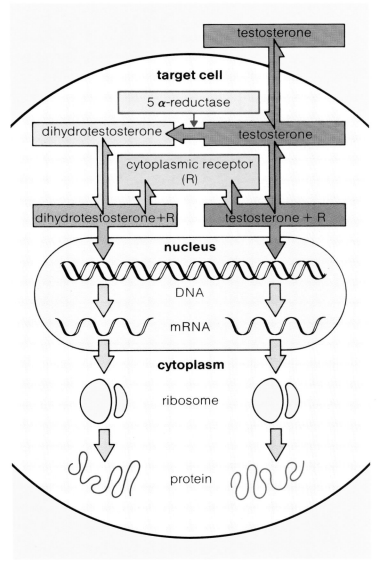

Fig. 10.9 Diagram illustrating the formation of testosterone in the Leydig cell from cholesterol substrate by LH. LH occupies a receptor site on the plasma membrane of the Leydig cell activating adenylate cyclase to catalyse the formation of cyclic AMP from ATP. Cyclic AMP binds to the regulatory subunit of protein kinase, leading to activation of a 20,22 desmolase enzyme which is responsible for the conversion of cholesterol to pregnenolone. Other enzymes then complete the synthesis of testosterone.

Fig. 10.10 Diagram showing androgen action on a target cell. Testosterone exerts its effect on target tissues by binding to a specific cytosolic protein receptor. The testosterone receptor complex is then transported to the nucleus where genomic activation leads to the synthesis of specific messenger RNA, and hence the translation of androgen-dependent proteins. In certain tissues the active androgen is the 5α-reduced metabolite of testosterone, dihydrotestosterone (DHT), which is generated largely *in situ*.

10.5

involved. The role of testosterone versus DHT at different stages of development is summarised in Figure 10.11.

CHROMOSOMAL DIFFERENTIATION OF THE GONAD

The normal human male karyotype is 46XY, and it has long been realised that the Y chromosome in some way determines testicular differentiation. It has also become clear that the major determinant of this process is a histocompatibility antigen, termed the H-Y antigen, disseminated from the primitive Sertoli cell. All cells possess so-called 'anchorage site' H-Y receptors but gonadal cells of both sexes also possess a second high-affinity receptor site. Experimentally, early exposure of gonads of either sex to sufficient H-Y antigen induces testicular differentiation. In nature, in mammals, only the male produces the H-Y antigen. The chromosomal locus for the H-Y antigen has been the subject of controversy but the consensus of the 1981 Workshop on Human Gene Mapping was that it resided on the Y chromosome. The developing testis can be distinguished from previously undifferentiated gonadal structures in the human fetus between forty-two days (12mm embryo) and forty-five days (15mm embryo) of gestation (Fig. 10.12).

MALE SEXUAL DIFFERENTIATION AND EMBRYOLOGY

By the early 1950's the pioneering work of Alfred Jost had conclusively demonstrated the active role of the fetal testis in determining male sexual differentiation from the earliest stages onwards. The experiments involving castration of rabbit fetuses at various stages and also additional manoeuvres, such as unilateral testis grafts or androgen implants, are summarised in Figure 10.13. The implications are that the fetal testis secretes two factors responsible for the inhibition of Müllerian structures and development of the Wolffian duct system respectively. The former may be the Müllerian inhibiting peptide of Sertoli cell origin, the latter testosterone, and both act locally. Subsequently the external genitalia differentiate under the true hormonal influence of testosterone which undergoes an indispensable local conversion to DHT in the genitalia and also in the prostatic precursor. Thus when the converting enzyme 5α-reductase is deficient the male genitalia are under-developed (Fig. 10.14).

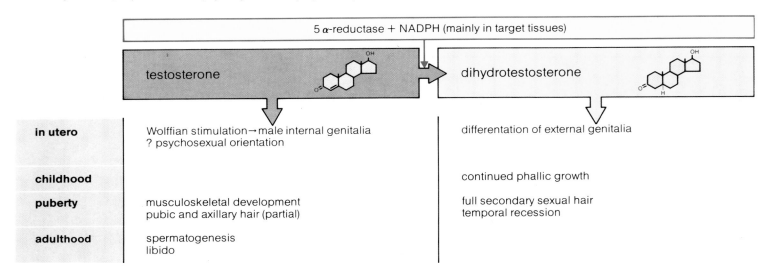

Fig. 10.11 Diagram showing the biological actions of testosterone and DHT in utero, early childhood, puberty and in the adult.

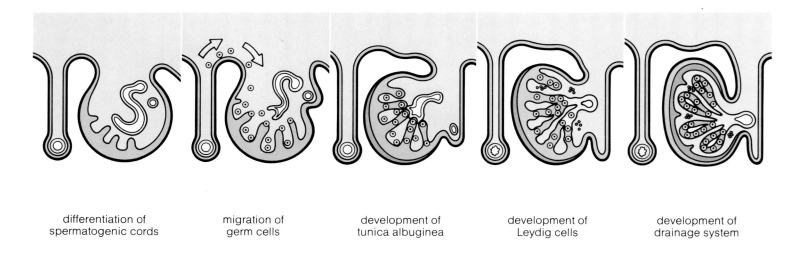

| differentiation of spermatogenic cords | migration of germ cells | development of tunica albuginea | development of Leydig cells | development of drainage system |

Fig.10.12 Diagram showing testicular differentiation within the first seven weeks of human embryonic life.

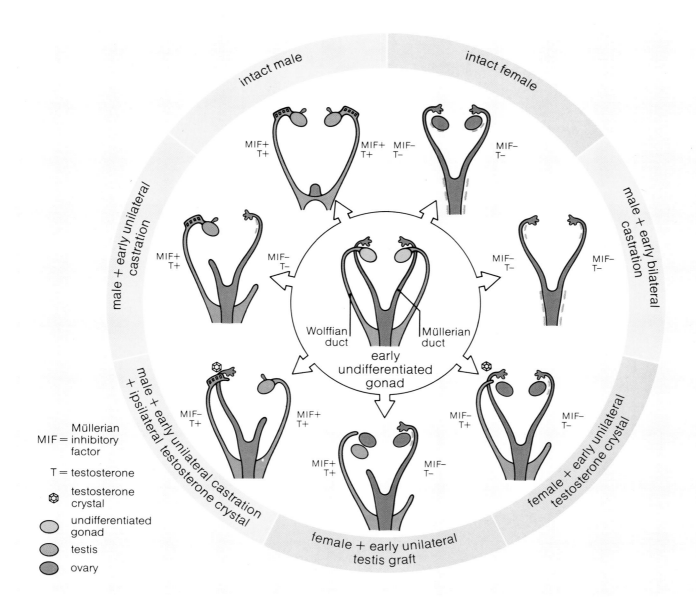

Fig. 10.13 Summary of the classical experiments of Alfred Jost. This work led to the discovery that the fetal testis secretes two factors: one, Müllerian inhibitory factor (MIF), which inhibits the development of Müllerian structures, whilst the other, testosterone (T), is necessary for the development of the Wolffian structures.

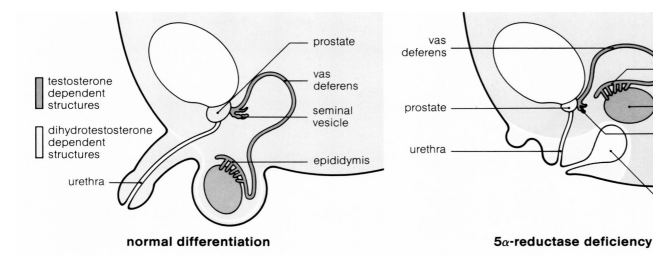

normal differentiation

5α-reductase deficiency

Fig. 10.14 The development of DHT dependent structures in utero. Development of the male external genitalia depends upon the hormonal effect of testosterone after conversion to DHT. Testosterone undergoes a 5α-reduction to DHT within the genitalia and within the prostatic precursor. DHT is therefore indispensable to the proper development of phallus, scrotum and prostate; these structures are under-developed in 5α-reductase deficiency. Redrawn from Imperato-McGinley et al. (1974) with permission of the AAAS.

10.7

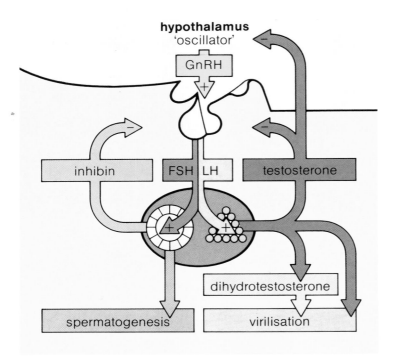

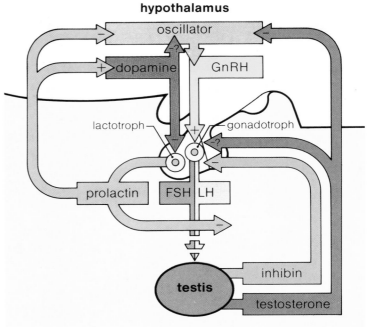

Fig. 10.15 Diagram of the hypothalamic regulation of gonadotrophin secretion. Episodic release of GnRH stimulates the gonadotrophs causing pulsatile release of LH and, to a lesser extent, FSH. LH acts on Leydig cells causing the production of testosterone which is responsible for virilisation (in some tissues through the production of DHT). LH release is suppressed by the negative feedback mechanism of testosterone action on the hypothalamus and pituitary. FSH acts on Sertoli cells and this results in spermatogenesis. Inhibin production by Sertoli cells has a negative feedback effect on FSH production in the anterior pituitary.

Fig. 10.16 Mechanisms controlling gonadotrophin secretion. In addition to control by the presence of inhibin and testosterone, GnRH production is also under dopaminergic and opioidergic control. In hyperprolactinaemia a partial blockade of the gonadotrophin action on testicular tissue may be caused by high circulating prolactin levels, but the normal pulsatile pattern of gonadotrophic secretion is also disrupted.

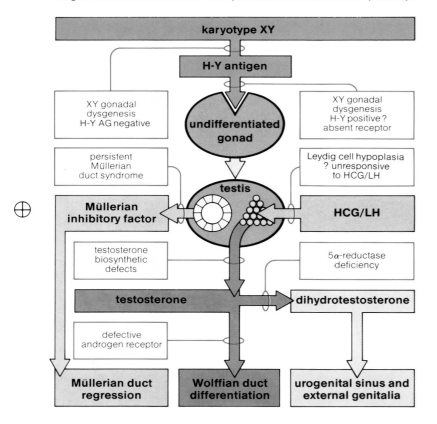

Fig. 10.17 Diagram showing the possible defects leading to male pseudohermaphroditism. This condition is most commonly caused by failure of androgen action, leading to the 'androgen resistance syndromes'.

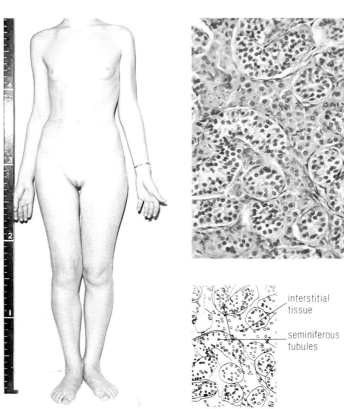

Fig. 10.18 Complete testicular feminisation. The female phenotype results from complete tissue insensitivity to circulating androgens.

Fig. 10.19 Histological section of the labial testis in complete testicular feminisation. H&E stain.

HYPOTHALAMO-PITUITARY-TESTICULAR RELATIONS

Hypothalamic regulation of both LH and FSH (Fig. 10.15) is currently believed to be controlled by a single decapeptide neurohormone, the gonadotrophin-releasing hormone(GnRH). The secretion of LH is pulsatile, but FSH appears less so, probably because the metabolic clearance of FSH appears much slower than LH. The pulsatility is probably caused by an oscillator mechanism within the medial basal hypothalamus, leading to episodic release of GnRH into the hypothalamo-hypophyseal portal vessels. This intermittency of pituitary exposure to GnRH is essential since, with unremitting delivery of the decapeptide, pituitary desensitisation ensues.

The target organs of the gonadotrophins secrete products which exert negative feedback control on the pituitary hormones. Thus testosterone secreted by Leydig cells tends to lower the secretion of LH, probably by reducing the frequency of GnRH release from the hypothalamus. The secretion of FSH tends to be selectively suppressed by the secretion of the Sertoli cell peptide hormone inhibin. The factors regulating the release of inhibin are obscure but seem to reflect the level or completeness of spermatogenesis.

Other factors also affect gonadotrophin secretion; for instance, FSH release is also influenced by testosterone levels. Oestradiol, which in the male is formed mostly by peripheral metabolism of androgens, inhibits gonadotrophins probably largely at a pituitary level. The pulsatile release of gonadotrophins is slowed by several other factors including exogenous and probably endogenous opiates and prolactin. Excess secretion of prolactin also inhibits testicular function by a partial blockade of gonadotrophin action on the testis (Fig. 10.16).

MALE PSEUDOHERMAPHRODITISM
Androgen Resistance Syndromes

Male pseudohermaphroditism most commonly results from failure of androgen action. The spectrum of disorders involved depends on the stage at which the defects become manifest and also the degree of their expression. Further categories include failure of Müllerian inhibition and the intriguing problems presented by true hermaphroditism. A classification is given in Figure 10.17. When either testosterone is absent from the earliest stages, or androgen receptors are totally missing, then, as predicted by Jost, the phenotype is female. The latter mechanism results in the condition generally known as complete testicular feminisation (Figs. 10.18 and 10.19), with female external features including full breast development; however, Müllerian structures and usually secondary sexual hair are absent, and the vagina ends blindly. The testes may be present in the abdomen, groins or labial folds and are liable to malignant change from the twenty fifth year onwards so castration and oestrogen replacement are indicated postpubertally. Although there is no germinal cell development there is ample Leydig cell activity. Variant forms are less strikingly feminised. Lesser degrees of androgen resistance are also encountered and a variety of eponymous subtypes have been described including (in order of increasingly masculine features) Lubs, Gilbert-Dreyfus, Reifenstein and Rosewater syndromes. Family studies have disclosed marked variation in phenotypes within kindreds possessing presumably single gene disorders. This suggests that the finer degrees of classification are artificial and merely reflect natural variation in range of expression of cytosolic gonadal steroid receptors. It has recently been suggested that idiopathic male infertility may result from extremely subtle degrees of androgen resistance, as suggested by the presence of high LH and testosterone levels.

Testosterone Deficiency due to Congenital Enzyme Deficiencies

This is a rare group of causes of male pseudohermaphroditism, and examples of each step in the synthesis of testosterone have been described (Fig. 10.20). Three of these steps are also obligatory for adrenal glucocorticoid and mineralocorticoid synthesis. Absence of any steps can therefore have major effects on the individual. Deficiency of the enzyme 20,22 desmolase leads to profound adrenal insufficiency and lipoid hyperplasia, with both sexes showing female external genitalia. In 17-hydroxylase deficiency low levels of cortisol and sex steroids occur. The resulting impairment of sexual differentiation varies according to the degree of enzymatic block, whilst the hypertension and

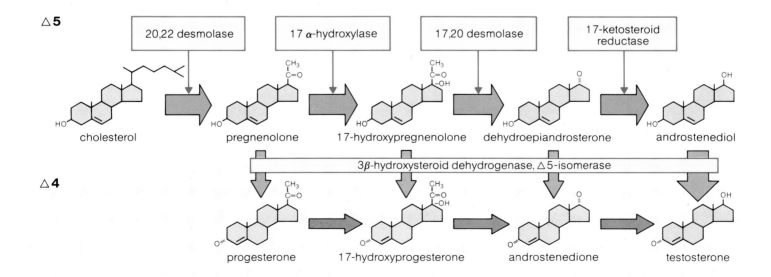

Fig. 10.20   Diagram showing major and minor routes of the testosterone biosynthetic pathway. Partial or complete deficiencies of any of these enzymes cause inadequate testosterone synthesis and may lead to inadequate virilisation resulting in male pseudohermaphroditism. The severity of the condition will depend on the enzyme concerned. A deficiency of any of the enzymes 20,22 desmolase, 17α-hydroxylase and 17,20 desmolase is also associated with adrenal insufficiency.

hypokalaemic alkalosis is caused by mineralocorticoid precursors. Deficiency of 3β-hydroxysteroid dehydrogenase, △5-isomerase leads to adrenal insufficiency but the defective masculinisation is of milder degree. The last two steps in testosterone synthesis do not affect glucocorticoid or mineralocorticoid pathways. Deficiency of 17,20 desmolase can cause a wide range of phenotypic appearances ranging from female (though lacking Müllerian duct derivatives) to male with perineal hypospadias; Wolffian duct derivatives vary from rudimentary structures to normal, but secondary sexual characteristics invariably fail to develop at puberty. The striking feature in 17-ketosteroid reductase deficiency is the degree of virilisation which occurs at puberty whereas prepubertally the genitalia are female or ambiguous in character. Despite the pubertal virilisation, however, gynaecomastia is commonly associated with this deficiency.

Defective Androgen Action due to 5α-Reductase Deficiency

The deficiency of △4-steroid-5α-reductase in tissues requiring high local concentrations of DHT rather than testosterone, for androgen action, has striking clinical consequences (Fig. 10.21). The tissues in question are the derivatives of the urogenital sinus and the urogenital tubercle, namely the prostate and external genitalia. Sporadic examples of this condition have been described from many parts of the world but an extraordinarily high incidence is found in an isolated community inhabiting the Dominican Republic (extensively studied by Imperato-McGinley and colleagues). Affected male individuals are born with ambiguous external genitalia, clitoral-like phallus, bifid scrotum, blind vaginal pouch and inguinal or labial testes but no Müllerian structures. They are raised as girls but at puberty undergo marked virilisation including phallic enlargement ('guevedoces' – penis at twelve), acquisition of male habitus and muscularity, testicular descent (occasionally with full spermatogenesis) and male psychosexual orientation. Beard growth is deficient and acne and frontal hair recession are absent. This constellation of findings graphically emphasises which processes of masculinisation are DHT- as opposed to testosterone-dependent.

GONADAL DISORDERS PRESENTING IN ADULT LIFE

There is probably no wholly satisfactory classification of gonadal disorders but an attempt to tabulate a number of clinical situations is shown in Figure 10.22. The major practical issue is that established primary gonadal disorders are largely untreatable

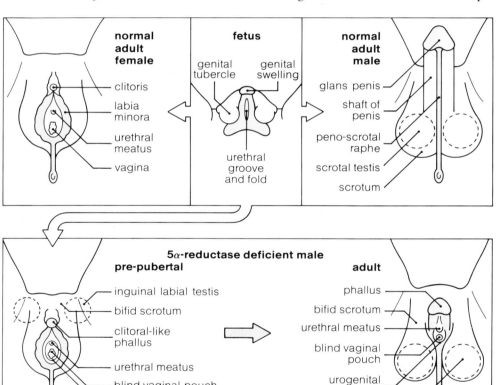

Fig. 10.21 Effect of DHT deficiency on sexual development. In the absence of 5α-reductase DHT-dependent structures (prostate and external genitalia) fail to develop. Affected individuals have ambiguous genitalia with a clitoral-like phallus and bifid scrotum. A blind vaginal pouch may be present and testes may be found in the labia or in the inguinal canals. At puberty limited development takes place, with some phallic enlargement and full testicular descent; but scrotal and urethral abnormalities remain.

Fig. 10.22 Classification of gonadal disorders in adult life.

Classification of Gonadal Disorders of Adult Life

primary gonadal dysfunction	hypogonadism/ feminisation	hypogonadotrophic hypogonadism
Klinefelter's syndrome	senescence	isolated gonadotrophin deficiency
cryptorchidism	liver disease	craniopharyngioma
myotonic dystrophy	thyrotoxicosis	pituitary tumours:
iatrogenic testicular damage	coeliac disease	functionless
idiopathic seminiferous tubule damage	renal disease	prolactinomas
	drugs e.g. spironolactone, oestrogens (see gynaecomastia)	acromegaly
	idiopathic androgen insensitivity	haemochromatosis

from the point of view of fertility whereas androgen deficiency is generally readily corrected. It should be noted that the view has recently been expressed that occult congenital adrenal hyperplasia is commonly responsible for infertility in the male, although this has not been the author's experience and the diagnosis can usually be made readily by measuring serum levels of 17α-hydroxyprogesterone.

Klinefelter's Syndrome

Klinefelter's syndrome is common, occurring approximately once in one thousand newborn males. The classical form (Figs. 10.23 and 10.24) is associated with a 47XXY karyotype (Fig. 10.26) and may present a range of appearances from the under-virilisation and excessive limb length with marked gynaecomastia of the typically eunuchoidal patient to one virtually indistinguishable from a normal male, except for small testes (Fig. 10.25). The usual size of the testis in those patients tending towards normal appearance is 2 ml except in some mosaic forms of Klinefelter's syndrome. Klinefelter's syndrome is associated with mental retardation, diabetes mellitus and pulmonary disease more often than in a control population.

A whole spectrum of variant forms of Klinefelter's syndrome

has been described. Many of these are mosaics and may have large numbers of excessive X chromosomes. In one uncommon variant there is, in addition to a supernumerary X, also a supernumerary Y chromosome. Some workers claim that there is a tendency for these patients to be tall (greater than six feet) and to have more marked problems with varicose veins. It is also claimed that they have more severe mental retardation, and a possible increased incidence of antisocial behaviour.

In Klinefelter's syndrome the testis is microscopically normal before puberty but later severe degeneration of the seminiferous tubules occurs with tubular hyalinisation and peritubular fibrosis; as mentioned earlier, the preserved Leydig cells clump together to give an illusion of hyperplasia whilst the Sertoli cells appear normal (cf. Fig. 10.4).

The clinical picture and testicular histology are paralleled by the endocrine findings, with uniformly high FSH levels but variable LH levels depending inversely on the state of Leydig cell reserve; nevertheless LH is often raised even in the twenty-five per cent of cases with normal testosterone levels. Increased oestrogen production and low androgen levels give rise to the gynaecomastia. Infertility is virtually universal and treatment is directed to androgen replacement and to the gynaecomastia where indicated.

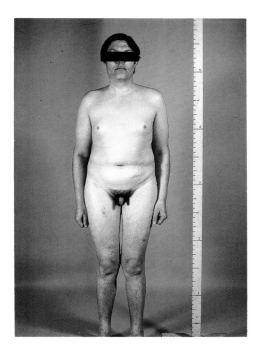

Fig. 10.23 Classical appearance of patient with Klinefelter's syndrome. The patient is hypogonadal, has a female habitus, is poorly virilised with gynaecomastia and eunuchoidism and has a small phallus. Body hair is sparse.

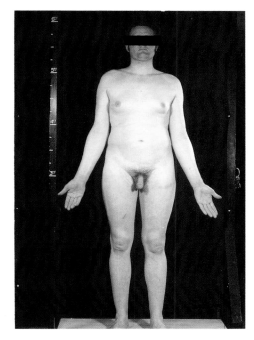

Fig. 10.24 Photograph of patient with Klinefelter's syndrome. He is eunuchoid but more virilised than in Figure 10.23 with a normal phallus but pea-sized testes. Gynaecomastia is present.

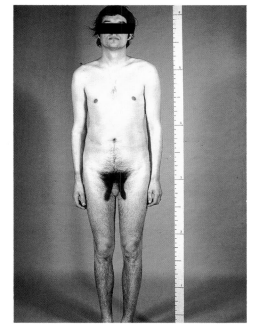

Fig. 10.25 Photograph of an unusual variant of Klinefelter's syndrome. This patient is well virilised; the only deviation from normality is the presence of small pea-sized testes. He presented with infertility and azoospermia.

Fig. 10.26 Typical karyotype of a patient with Klinefelter's syndrome.

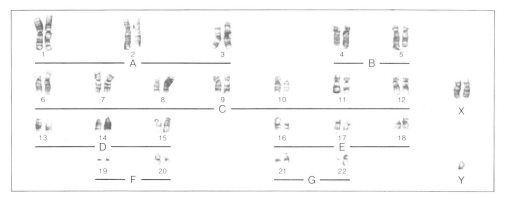

Varicocele

This condition is one of the most widely-cited treatable causes of male infertility (Fig. 10.27). Although varicoceles may frequently be found in fully fertile men, there is overwhelming evidence that varicoceles may impair fertility. The mechanism remains obscure but raised testicular temperature is probably important since, in the presence of a large varicocele, the abdominoscrotal temperature gradient may only be 0.1°C compared with a normal difference of 2.2°C. The blood supply to the testis is of major importance in securing this normal temperature gradient since the pampiniform plexus of veins surrounding the single testicular artery provides the basis for a counter-current heat exchange system. The abnormality in varicocele, however, is thought to involve primarily the cremasteric plexus of veins which lies outside the tunica rather than the pampiniform plexus. Other postulated factors operating to the disadvantage of the testis in the presence of varicocele include increased catecholamine concentration and also hypoxia due to venous reflux. Varicoceles almost exclusively occur on the left: this is because the left testicular vein drains into the left renal vein opposite the adrenal vein, in contrast to the right where the testicular vein enters the inferior vena cava directly. Patients must always be examined in the standing position when varicoceles are sought since they then fill by gravity.

In varicocele endocrine function may be normal although FSH may be high-normal or raised. Leydig cell function is usually normal in young men with varicocele but testosterone levels fall with increasing age.

Myotonic Dystrophy

This autosomal dominant condition leading to gonadal failure is characterised by progressive muscular weakness and myotonia, mental retardation, frontal baldness and cataracts (Fig. 10.28). The brunt of the testicular damage is borne by the seminiferous tubules with elevation of FSH being a constant feature. Leydig cell dysfunction is less marked although subnormal testosterone levels are not uncommon and exaggerated LH responses are seen in response to exogenous gonadotrophin-releasing hormone challenge.

Cryptorchidism

The permanently cryptorchid testis is associated with marked tubular damage and variable Leydig cell dysfunction (Fig. 10.29). The importance of the extra-abdominal position is demonstrated by the great salvage of fertility afforded by careful, early orchidopexy. Histological evidence of damage in the cryptorchid testis is apparent from the fifth year onwards. Intrinsic testicular abnormality is suggested by the impaired fertility associated with unilateral cryptorchidism, with the second testis being fully descended into the scrotum, and indeed often manifesting compensatory hypertrophy. Underlying causes are seldom discovered, although rare examples include varying pseudohermaphroditic states (dealt with earlier) and also disorders of the hypothalamo-pituitary system.

The cryptorchid testis is thirty-five times more likely to undergo malignant change than the scrotal testis, and surgical exploration may be necessary when the true situation is in doubt. The use of HCG to stimulate testosterone secretion may help distinguish bilateral cryptorchidism from the 'vanishing testis' syndrome, in which no response will be seen. The merit of HCG in securing testicular descent is hotly debated but this hypothesis certainly clarifies the situation in the case of readily retractile testes. Recently the non-invasive method of treatment with intranasal GnRH has been demonstrated as an effective method.

Seminiferous Tubular Damage

A heterogeneous group of situations may impair fertility through seminiferous tubular damage. Recognised examples include cytotoxic therapy, ionizing irradiation, severe mumps orchitis and trauma, although in the great majority of cases of male infertility the aetiology is quite unknown. In assessing the prospects for treatment, seminal analysis is of some, but rather limited, value. Much controversy surrounds the definition of 'minimal adequate ejaculate'. It is clear that normally fertile men may show markedly variable (ten-fold) sperm concentration for no apparent reason when studied frequently for prolonged periods. Similarly the evidence from pre-vasectomy specimens has led to a downward revision of the lower limit of normal sperm density to 20×10^6/ml. Other parameters of seminal quality are important, for instance, total sperm number per ejaculate, sperm motility and, probably of considerable value, sperm morphology since a marked increase in numbers of abnormal forms is prognostically poor despite adequate total sperm count (Fig. 10.30).

Severe damage to the germinal epithelium, generally associated with azoospermia or severe oligospermia ($<5 \times 10^6$/ml), leads to high FSH levels, presumably due to deficient inhibin secretion. Evidence of Leydig cell dysfunction is much less common, resulting either from a common injury which affects tubules more severely, or from interference with local feedback action from seminiferous tubules on Leydig cells. It has recently been claimed that forty per cent of men with azoospermia, or very severe oligospermia, display occult androgen resistance. This principally affects spermatogenesis with only minimally impaired virilisation and may be suspected if both LH and testosterone levels are elevated.

Seminal plasma fructose and hormone concentrations have not proved very informative. Seminal LH and FSH are reported to be lower than normal in azoospermia and oligospermia. The concentrations of androgens in seminal plasma are lower than in blood and azoospermics have markedly depressed seminal DHT. This may be an epiphenomenon since the presence of testosterone alone is adequate for spermatogenesis to occur whilst *in vitro* spermatozoa actively convert testosterone to DHT. Testicular biopsy cannot reveal the aetiology of testicular damage but can help quantify the damage and likely therapeutic dividend. A number of brief case reports together with their histology highlight the use and limitation of the technique (Figs. 10.31-10.35).

The treatment of azoospermia and oligospermia is largely empirical, poorly evaluated and unsuccessful. Discredited measures include tri-iodothyronine, vitamin E and arginine. Glucocorticoids may be of value when a distinct immunological disorder is demonstrated, such as high titre anti-sperm antibodies (agglutinatin) in blood and seminal plasma, and possibly at low doses in men with congenital adrenal hyperplasia; however, these can be detected by measuring 17α-hydroxyprogesterone levels, and are probably uncommon despite periodic assertions to the contrary. Although testosterone-rebound therapy has been advocated for over thirty years it has been evaluated inadequately. The use of mesterolone, an orally active, non-hepatotoxic androgen (an analogue of DHT) has been favourably reported but not universally so. Attempts to enhance spermatogenesis using gonadotrophin containing FSH have been unrewarding but some investigators have claimed success with anti-oestrogens such as clomiphene and tamoxifen. However the seventy-four day spermatogenic cycle, poor selection of patients, inadequate control data, known variability in sperm density in normal men and lack of proof of paternity render many trials in this area doubtful at the very least.

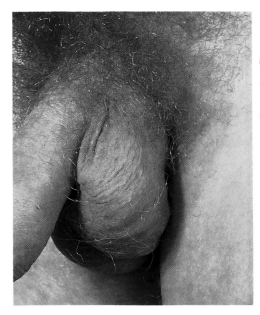
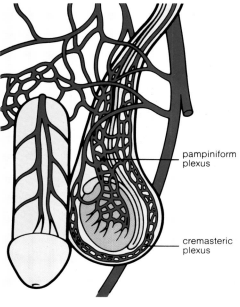

Fig. 10.27 Varicocele and diagram showing the venous drainage of the testis. Varicocele of the testis, shown on the left, may impair fertility since the abdomino-scrotal temperature gradient is reduced and spermatogenesis affected. The abnormality in varicocele is thought to involve primarily the cremasteric venous plexus rather than the pampiniform plexus. Varicoceles appear during or after puberty.

pampiniform plexus

cremasteric plexus

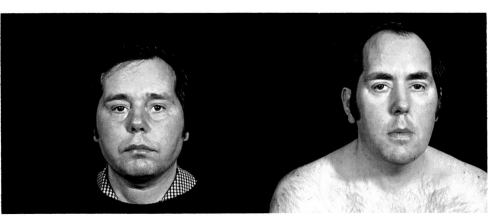

Fig. 10.28 Classical facial appearance of two brothers with familial dystrophia myotonica. Frontal baldness and bilateral ptosis may be seen in both men.
By courtesy of Prof. R.H.T. Edwards.

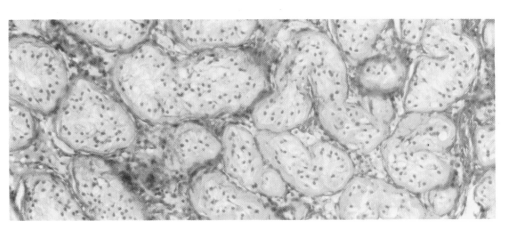

Fig. 10.29 Histological section of the cryptorchid testis. Marked tubular damage can be seen. This condition has a high incidence of malignant change.
Van Gieson stain.

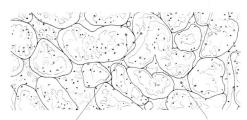

hyalinised tubules with marked basement membrane thickening   interstitial tissue

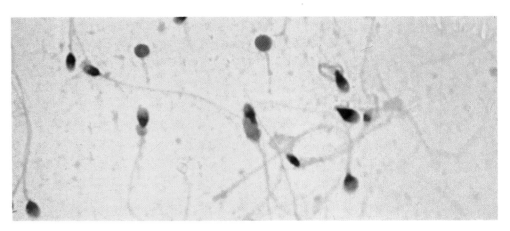

Fig. 10.30 Seminal specimen showing presence of abnormal forms of spermatozoa. This was taken from a patient with a high degree of infertility.
Papanicolaou stain.

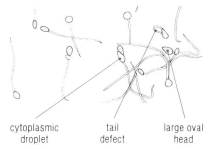

cytoplasmic droplet   tail defect   large oval head

10.13

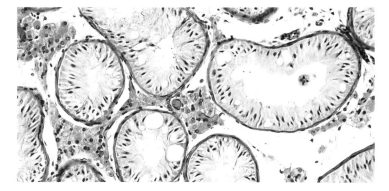

Fig. 10.31 Case 1: 'Sertoli-cells only' appearance. Bladder rupture and bilateral testicular haematomas caused by a road traffic accident. The patient presented with infertility some years later, where a left varicocele and an abnormally small left testis were found, together with elevated FSH and LH levels. On biopsy only Sertoli cells were found in the tubules; these extended from the basement membrane to the lumen. H&E stain. By courtesy of Dr. W.E. Kenyon.

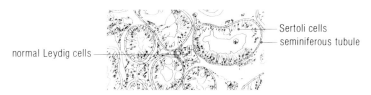

Fig. 10.32 Case 2: Focal atrophy. Patient presented with primary infertility, azoospermia and small testes: testicular biopsy revealed marked focal atrophy. There is heterogeneity of the histological appearance from area to area in the field shown. Much of this biopsy not shown in this photograph did, however, appear normal. H&E stain. By courtesy of Dr. W.E. Kenyon.

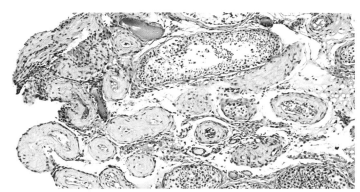

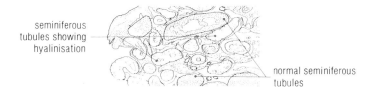

Fig. 10.33 Case 3: Maturation arrest. Patient with history of right testicular maldescent and left herniorrhaphy. The right testicular size was normal, but the left testis small and soft. A grade III left varicocele was present and the patient was azoospermic. The arrest of sperm maturation can be seen in the biopsy. H&E stain. By courtesy of Dr. W.E. Kenyon.

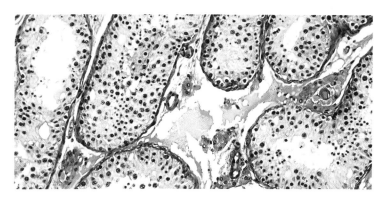

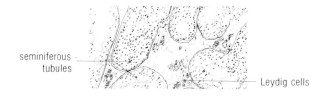

Fig. 10.34 Case 4: Maturation arrest. Patient with four years infertility with right testis in inguinal canal. Seminal analysis showed very occasional spermatozoa ($<10^5$/ml) although obstruction was excluded. Testicular biopsy revealed maturation arrest. Although more spermatozoa were present when compared with Case 3, none can be seen in this field. H&E stain. By courtesy of Dr. W.E. Kenyon.

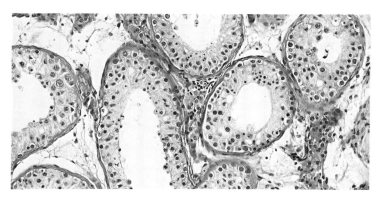

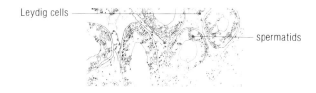

Fig. 10.35 Case 5: Hypospermatogenesis. Patient was obese with small testes. He was found to be azoospermic with high FSH but high LH and also testosterone suggesting possible androgen resistance. Hypospermatogenesis was revealed on biopsy. H&E stain. By courtesy of Dr. W.E. Kenyon.

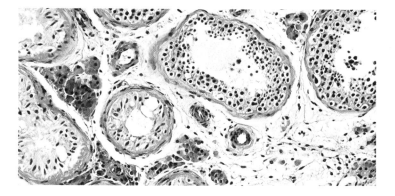

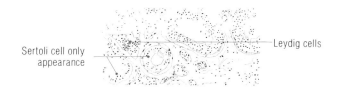

HYPOGONADOTROPHIC HYPOGONADISM

Hypogonadotrophic hypogonadism may arise from disorders of the pituitary or hypothalamus and the distinction may be difficult to make. Furthermore, other pituitary target organ axes may be impaired to an unsuspected degree and may only be revealed by formal testing of pituitary function. Conversely the occurrence of overt adrenal and thyroid dysfunction may lead to neglect of gonadal status.

The broad category 'isolated gonadotrophin deficiency' embraces at least four subclasses. Deficiency of both LH and FSH may occur in the absence of other clinical features, or may be associated with anosmia or hyposmia (Kallman's syndrome – Fig. 10.36) and other extragonadal features such as 'hare-lip' and cleft palate, neural deafness, colour blindness, cryptorchidism and renal tract dysgenesis. Absent septum pellucidum and corpus callosum are recognised in some patients. A variant with isolated LH deficiency, which has been graphically (if somewhat inaccurately) described by McCullagh as the 'fertile eunuch' syndrome (Fig. 10.37), combines the features of LH deficiency with variable spermatogenesis and a propensity to gynaecomastia. A further major variant occurs in association with growth hormone deficiency, which is apparent much earlier.

These conditions appear to share deficiency of hypothalamic GnRH. Fertility has been achieved by subcutaneous injections of synthetic GnRH self-administered eight-hourly, but this is a suboptimal regimen. Since unremitting exposure to GnRH desensitises the gonadotroph, chronic administration of superactive GnRH analogues with protracted binding to GnRH receptors is more likely to prove useful as a contraceptive method than as an aid to the promotion of fertility. The development of relatively cheap, portable syringe drivers (Fig. 10.38) which can be programmed to simulate the natural pulsatile release of GnRH holds promise. The hormonal response to hourly pulses of GnRH in Kallman's syndrome is brisk and sustained (Fig. 10.39).

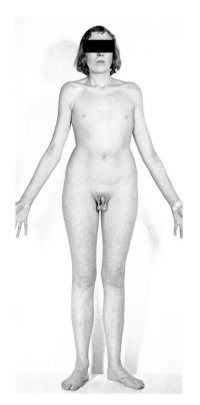

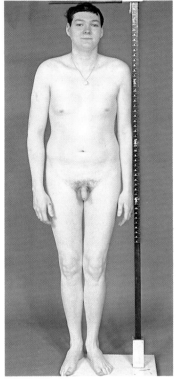

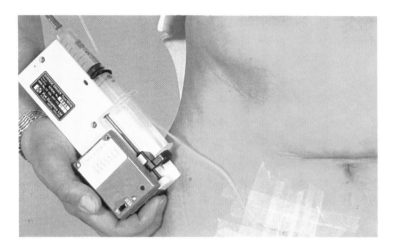

Fig. 10.36 Patient with hypogonadotrophic hypogonadism with anosmia (Kallmann's syndrome). This condition results from a deficiency of GnRH.

Fig. 10.37 Patient with 'fertile eunuch' syndrome. The features of LH deficiency with variable spermatogenesis are present in this syndrome.

Fig. 10.38 Photograph of programmable syringe driver used to deliver GnRH subcutaneously in a patient with Kallmann's syndrome. This device can be programmed to simulate natural pulsatile GnRH release which will lead to gonadotrophic secretion.

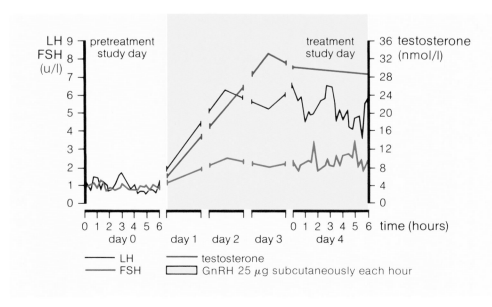

Fig. 10.39 Example of gonadotrophin and testosterone response to subcutaneous pulsatile GnRH therapy in a patient with Kallmann's syndrome. The hormonal response to this treatment is brisk and sustained.

Neuroradiological examination and screening for other pituitary hormone function is necessary to exclude pituitary tumours or other space-occupying lesions. Patients with craniopharyngiomas may present with gonadal dysfunction during or after puberty, in addition to the visual problems and raised intracranial pressure which dominate cases presenting in childhood or later in life (Fig. 10.40). Pituitary tumours are significant in that hyperprolactinaemia may complicate the situation by causing impotence. The conventional therapy for men with prolactinomas requiring potency is bromocriptine, as well as androgen replacement if there is gonadotrophin deficiency. However, the general treatment for reduced fertility is the use of exogenous gonadotrophins to stimulate the testis. Initially HCG alone is used to stimulate Leydig cell function, starting with 2,000 iu twice weekly. After two months the serum testosterone should be checked. This may suffice to achieve adequate spermatogenesis provided there is relative sparing of FSH secretion, which commonly occurs (Fig. 10.41). If not, the use of FSH-containing human urinary menopausal gonadotrophins should be added (Pergonal, four ampoules three times a week) after which the HCG dose can usually be lowered to 500 iu twice weekly.

Along with profound hypopituitarism there appear to be a number of conditions in which gonadotrophin lack is primary and thus do not respond to GnRH. A recently described example is the Laurence-Moon-Biedl syndrome.

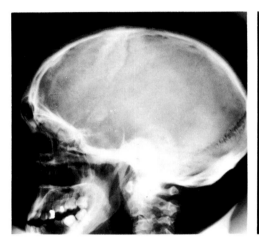 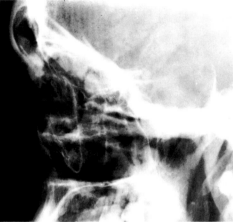

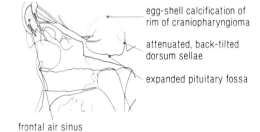

Fig. 10.40 Skull radiograph of a craniopharyngioma showing egg-shell calcification in the suprasellar region. The sella turcica is grossly ballooned. An enlargement of the ballooned sella turcica is shown on the right.

egg-shell calcification of rim of craniopharyngioma

attenuated, back-tilted dorsum sellae

expanded pituitary fossa

frontal air sinus

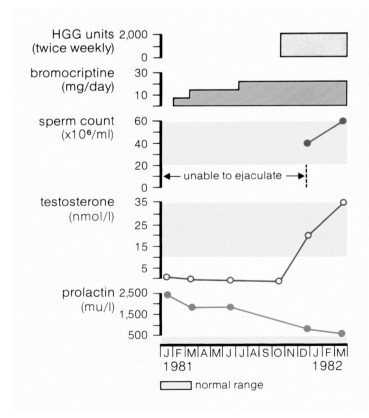
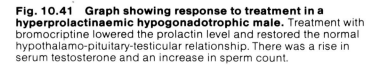

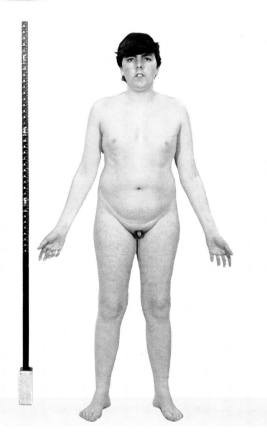

Fig. 10.41 Graph showing response to treatment in a hyperprolactinaemic hypogonadotrophic male. Treatment with bromocriptine lowered the prolactin level and restored the normal hypothalamo-pituitary-testicular relationship. There was a rise in serum testosterone and an increase in sperm count.

Fig. 10.42 Photograph of a patient with the 'vanishing testis' syndrome. These patients have evidence of hypogonadism, and no testicular tissue is found in the scrotum on surgical exploration. After HCG stimulation, testosterone levels do not rise. The term 'vanishing testis' derives from the presumption that testicular tissue was active in early fetal life in order to induce male phenotypic development. It is of unknown aetiology.

HYPOGONADISM

The differentiation of the male phenotype induced by fetal androgen action has already been described. Subsequent Leydig cell failure causes hypogonadism with features dependent upon the timing and severity of the disorder. Its early appearance is manifested by failure to enter puberty, with infantile genitalia and delayed epiphyseal fusion—giving rise to long limbs with span exceeding height—eunuchoidism (Fig. 10.42). There is also absence of secondary sexual hair growth and the voice will fail to 'break'. It should be noted that when the hypogonadism is central in origin (pituitary or hypothalamic) it may be associated with features of growth hormone deficiency leading to proportionate dwarfism (Fig. 10.43), or hypothyroidism where the infantile proportions are preserved with relatively short limbs. Post-pubertal gonadal failure leads to loss of libido, regression of secondary sexual characteristics and the typical finely-wrinkled skin, especially noticeable peri-orally, with vertical creases on the upper lip virtually bespeaking hypogonadism (Fig. 10.44). The speed with which these changes take place varies enormously and are most clearly seen in men castrated for treatment of prostatic cancer.

A feature commonly found in hypogonadal individuals is gynaecomastia, where it more often reflects a shift in balance of free sex steroid levels to oestrogen dominance rather than absolute excess in oestrogen secretion. The imbalance is accentuated by two features of sex-hormone-binding-globulin (SHBG): firstly that its production is enhanced either when androgen levels fall or oestrogen levels rise or both, and secondly, that androgens bind more avidly to SHBG than oestrogens. The failing testis, driven by high gonadotrophins, tends to produce relatively more oestrogen than testosterone; gynaecomastia therefore occurs more frequently in primary than in secondary hypogonadal states. There is insufficient space to consider causes of gynaecomastia in detail but many are recognised (Fig. 10.45). Various mechanisms involved, other than the one outlined above, may be:

(i) increased local oestrogen production from the pubertal breast caused by enhanced breast aromatase,

(ii) true excessive production of oestrogen, and

(iii) the action of drugs in binding to oestrogen or blocking androgen receptors.

Treatment of hypogonadism involves adequate testosterone replacement. Most commonly this is achieved by the action of testosterone esters releasing the steroid over the course of weeks, for example by using a preparation containing a mixture of esters (Sustanon) 250-500 mg intramuscularly every two to three weeks, or testosterone oenanthate (Primoteston depot). The 17-alkylated androgens such as methyl testosterone are active when taken orally; however, their use is barred since they are hepatotoxic. The use of oral testosterone undecanoate has recently been introduced. The early favourable reports are now typically being tempered by more cautionary views. There is often remarkably little suppression of gonadotrophins in primary hypogonadism suggesting that the measured 'normal' testosterone levels may be partly due to cross-reacting, undecanoate ester. Furthermore the DHT levels are disproportionately elevated, raising the need for caution in older men at risk of prostatic disease. Intramuscular pellets of testosterone are still given by some clinicians with satisfactory results.

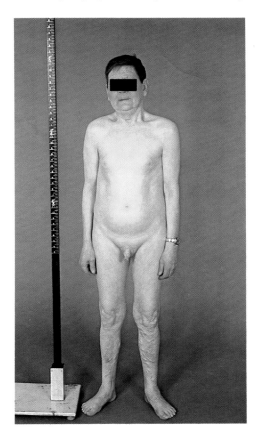

Fig. 10.43 Patient with proportionate dwarfism and hypogonadism. This may be caused by the concurrent presence of growth hormone deficiency, as found in this particular case.

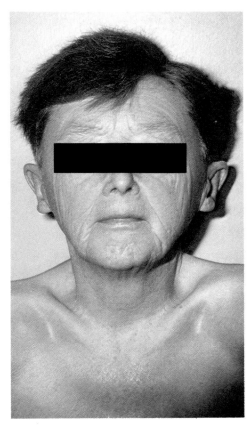

Fig. 10.44 Facial appearance in post-pubertal hypogonadism. The very characteristic peri-oral wrinkling of skin may be seen.

Causes of Gynaecomastia

physiological
puberty
old age

hypogonadism
Klinefelter's syndrome
incomplete androgen resistance
 (male pseudohermaphroditism, type 1)
isolated LH deficiency ('fertile eunuch')
chronic haemodialysis

chronic liver disease
cirrhosis
alcoholism
hepatitis
haemochromatosis

thyrotoxicosis

neoplasia
interstitial cell tumour of testis
bronchogenic carcinoma
adrenal carcinoma

drugs
spironolactone
digitoxin
oestrogens
HCG
testosterone
marijuana

Fig. 10.45 The causes of gynaecomastia.

MISCELLANEOUS CONDITIONS

Immunological Disorders

The realisation has grown that many men are infertile despite apparently normal sperm counts and, in some of these, autoimmune disturbances may be suspected. Non-specific indications include a negative post-coital test and agglutination between sperms, often of a uniform type in a given patient (e.g. head-to-head, or head-to-tail). A wealth of more specific tests have been developed to delineate the nature and intensity of the immune pathology (Fig. 10.46). The presence of antisperm antibodies in seminal plasma appears to be of much greater significance than their presence in blood. The easy experimental induction of autoimmune orchitis suggests that in nature this phenomenon may arise when the blood-testis barrier is breached following trauma, torsion of the testes, infection or vasectomy. High doses of prednisolone (20-40 mg/d) may improve fertility but the side-effects are considerable.

Immotile Sperm Syndrome

Several conditions lead to immotile sperm syndrome. They are found as part of Kartagener's syndrome along with situs inversus and sinusitis; in these conditions the normal dynein arms from cilia are missing (Fig. 10.47). In Young's syndrome sperm are immotile from radial spoke deficiency and this is presumably responsible also for the associated bronchiectasis and chronic sinus infections; with mucus in the vasa, sinuses and bronchi being pathologically viscid. Cystic fibrosis is associated with congenital absence of the vasa and also epididymal malformation.

Gastrointestinal Disorders

Coeliac disease has been associated with male infertility. Recently a reversible abnormality has been described in male coeliacs whereby DHT production is reduced in the untreated state but both LH and testosterone are high. The normal state is restored as jejunal morphology improves on withdrawal of dietary gluten.

Crohn's disease is commonly treated with long term sulpha-salazine which has been linked with infertility, although fertility returns when the drug is withdrawn.

Many liver disorders including alcoholism (with or without cirrhosis) and haemochromatosis can cause both testicular and pituitary dysfunction.

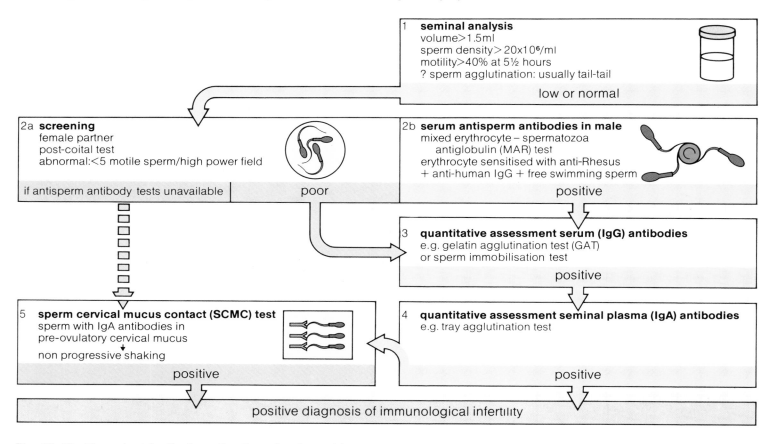

Fig. 10.46   Flow-chart for the investigation of patient with sperm antibodies causing 'immunological' infertility.

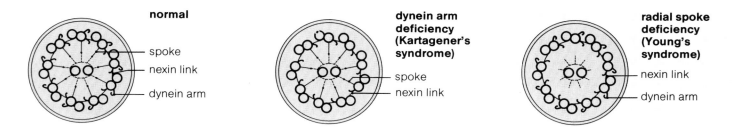

Fig. 10.47   Diagrammatic representation of cilia morphology.
Transverse sections showing the morphology of (a) normal spermatozoa, (b) spermatozoa from patients with Kartagener's syndrome and (c) spermatozoa from patients with Young's syndrome.

11 The Ovary

Richard J Lilford, MRCP, MRCOG
Timothy Chard, MD, FRCOG

EMBRYOLOGY

The gonad develops from the germinal ridge, near the meso-nephros, during the sixth week of embryonic life (Fig. 11.1). Germ cells migrate to the gonad from the yolk sac where they are easily recognised histologically by strong positive staining for alkaline phosphatase. The migration is thought to follow a chemotactic gradient. The early germinal ridge is in direct contact with the mesonephric ducts. In the developing testis this contact is maintained and the ducts persist as the rete testis. In the ovary such contact is lost at an early stage and the rete ovary disappears. The gender of the developing embryo can be recognised at eight weeks. Between three and seven months many oögonia enter the prophase of the first meiotic division and are then called primary oöcytes. They are surrounded by a single layer of spindle shaped granulosa cells forming primordial follicles (Fig. 11.2). The maximum number of germ cells, about seven million, inclusive of one million primary oöcytes, is reached at a fetal age of five months. By birth nearly all oögonia will have either developed into primary oöcytes or undergone atresia. The germinal vesicle or nucleus of the primary oöcyte has one or two large nucleoli. This appearance is maintained until shortly before ovulation.

GERM-CELL POPULATION OF THE OVARY

Many oögonia undergo atresia before oöcyte formation; many of the primordial follicles (Fig. 11.3) start to mature but development is arrested at an early stage and atresia follows. This process is very rapid during fetal life and at birth the number of germ cells is reduced to one or two million from seven million. Early follicular development leading to atresia continues at a lower rate during childhood and reproductive life, leaving 400,000 follicles at puberty and a few hundred by the menopause (Fig. 11.4).

ANATOMY OF THE OVARY

The ovaries are slightly flattened organs between three and four centimetres long, situated on the side wall of the pelvis between the external and internal iliac arteries. The ureter crosses the bifurcation of the common iliac artery and lies lateral to the ovary (Fig. 11.5). The ovary is an intraperitoneal structure attached to the side wall of the pelvis by a fold of peritoneum. The upper portion of this fold carries the ovarian artery and pampiniform plexus of ovarian veins and is called the infundibulo-pelvic ligament. The lower portion is continuous with the broad ligament. The fallopian tube curls up the anterior surface of the ovary and projects over its upper pole, whilst the inferior pole is connected to the cornu of the uterus by the ovarian ligament. The ovarian artery, a branch of the aorta, anastomoses with the terminal branch of the uterine artery before spiralling into the medulla of the ovary. In the human the ovarian contribution is greater than that of the uterine artery.

The fibrous *tunica albuginea* of the ovary lies beneath the covering peritoneal mesothelium. After the age of eight years, numerous spindle shaped cells accumulate in the ovary and make up the ovarian stroma. These are thought to arise from the dormant genital ridge mesenchyme and are the source of ovarian androgens. The stroma forms the thecal cells of secondary follicles. Numerous primordial and a few primary follicles are scattered throughout the stroma with the greatest concentration at the periphery of the cortex. A number of secondary follicles are seen in deeper layers; prior to ovulation one of these will grow towards the surface. The hilum contains numerous blood vessels and hilar cells which are of mesenchymal origin and equivalent to the Leydig cells of the testis.

FURTHER DEVELOPMENT OF PRIMORDIAL FOLLICLES

The spindle shaped granulosa follicles become cuboidal and proliferate to form the multi-layered primary follicles. Most such follicles undergo atresia but during a menstrual cycle some ten or twenty mature into secondary follicles. Small numbers of secondary follicles are also formed during late fetal life and childhood and tend to push the primordial follicles into the peripheral cortex.

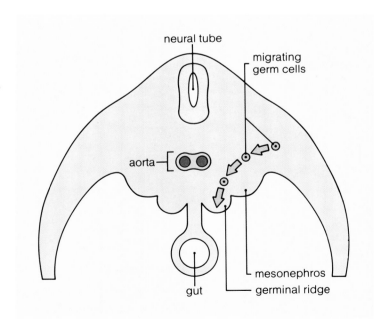

Fig. 11.1 Diagram showing the embryonic origin of the gonad. The gonad appears as a swelling in the medial surface of the mesonephros. This scheme shows the stage of development at the 5th to 6th week of embryonic life.

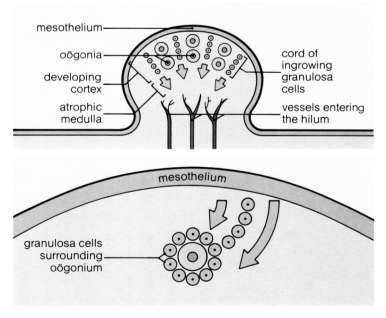

Fig. 11.2 Schematic representation of primordial follicle formation. The sex cords break up and the primordial germ cells divide to form oögonia which become scattered in the mesenchyme. These germ cells then become surrounded by a group of granulosa cells to form a primordial follicle. By this stage the oögonia will have entered the first meiotic division to become a primary oöcyte.

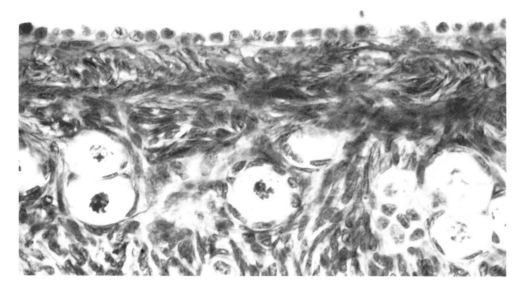

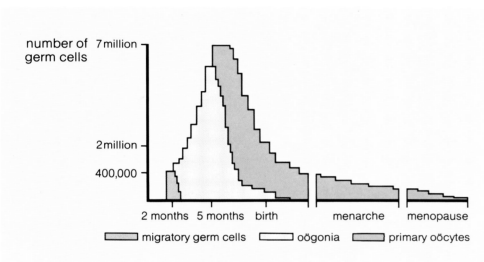

migratory germ cells ☐ oögonia ☐ primary oöcytes

Fig. 11.3 Histological section of the ovarian cortex showing developing primordial follicles. The primordial follicle consists of an oöcyte surrounded by a single layer of spindle-shaped cells. When these follicular granulosa cells become cuboidal and form more than one layer they are called primary follicles. By courtesy of Dr. P.R. Wheater.

germinal epithelium   cords of granulosa cells

primary oöcyte   surrounding granulosa cells

Fig. 11.4 Graph showing average number of germ cells throughout the female life. At puberty there are approximately 400,000 follicles present in the ovaries, contrasting with menopausal ovaries where only a few hundred remain.

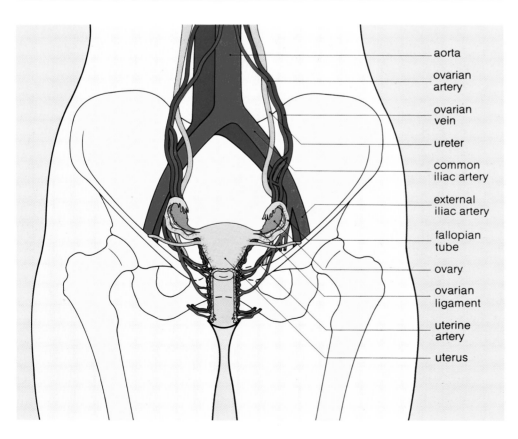

aorta

ovarian artery

ovarian vein

ureter

common iliac artery

external iliac artery

fallopian tube

ovary

ovarian ligament

uterine artery

uterus

Fig. 11.5 View of the female pelvis showing internal genital organs and their relations. The ovary is suspended in the pelvis chiefly by attachment to the infundibulo-pelvic ligament, a fold of peritoneum, in which run the ovarian artery and veins.

11.3

Secondary follicles are characterised by the formation of a large fluid-filled cavity, the antrum. This is accomplished through coalescence of many smaller cavities which appear among the granulosa cells (Fig. 11.6); these small cavities with their surrounding rosette of granulosa cells are called 'Call-Exner bodies'. The fluid, *liquor folliculi*, is formed by transudation and secretion from surrounding cells.

The granulosa cells project into the antrum in the area of the primary oöcyte forming a mound known as the *cumulus oöphorus* (Fig. 11.7). A homogeneous layer, the *zona pellucida*, is secreted around the oöcyte by the granulosa cells which nevertheless maintain contact by means of thin cytoplasmic processes which penetrate this layer. At this time substances preventing the premature resumption of meiosis, and which will promote the formation of the male pronucleus after fertilisation, cross to the oöcyte. The granulosa cells are linked to each other by means of numerous intra-epithelial bridges. The surrounding ovarian stroma cells form a compact layer, the *theca interna*, which is separated from the granulosa cells by a basement membrane. A loose layer of stroma cells, the *theca externa*, envelops the whole structure.

Only one or two follicles undergo further development in any cycle. This involves the rapid expansion of the antrum and thinning out of the follicle wall within forty-eight hours of ovulation to form the tertiary follicle. Fully grown follicles are about three centimetres in diameter.

Extensive changes occur on the cell surface of granulosa cells during the follicular cycle. Multiple microvilli containing microfilaments develop and these are believed to carry the rapidly increasing number of gonadotrophin receptors which amplify the follicular responses in the pre-ovulatory period. These microvilli are withdrawn in the luteal phase.

FURTHER DEVELOPMENT OF THE OÖCYTE

The primary oöcyte enlarges from 35 to 100 microns in diameter early in follicular development and undergoes no subsequent enlargement. The nucleus is displaced to the periphery of the expanding cytoplasm. Peripheral cortical granules are formed from the Golgi apparatus; these contain the substances which will block polyspermic fertilisation. Energy is provided by direct metabolism of pyruvate from the cumulus cells; the mitochondria

where this occurs are found in greatest concentration around a lamellar paranuclear structure called Babiani's vitelline body.

Reduction division which began with the formation of the oöcyte is resumed thirty-six hours before ovulation. The first polar body is extruded a few hours before ovulation. The secondary oöcyte thus formed immediately enters the second meiotic division and remains in metaphase until fertilisation. Division is then completed, the second polar body is extruded, and the female pronucleus formed. The very prolonged meiosis of the primary oöcyte is due to an inhibitory effect of the granulosa cells through their cytoplasmic extensions; and these are withdrawn before meiosis is resumed.

THE CORPUS LUTEUM

The corpus luteum (Fig. 11.8) is formed immediately after ovulation as a result of several changes. Firstly the follicle collapses after extrusion of the ovum and fluid, and the central cavity fills with blood and fibrin. Secondly the basement membrane separating the granulosa from the theca disappears and thecal capillaries enter the granulosa. Finally the cytoplasm of the granulosa and theca cells hypertrophies with accumulation of lipid droplets and proliferation of the smooth endoplasmic reticulum and mitochondria (granulosa lutein and theca lutein cells). Degeneration and formation of a corpus albicans (Fig. 11.9) begins after ten days unless a pregnancy occurs.

Luteinisation of human follicles without extrusion of the ovum is a rare event. Progesterone production begins before ovulation, increases rapidly after extrusion of the ovum and oestrogen production recovers within a day. Both hormones peak six to eight days after ovulation.

Small amounts of LH are required to maintain the corpus luteum and administration of small amounts of HCG in the mid-luteal phase delays menstruation. Oestrogen also promotes progesterone synthesis, an example of the 'servo' mechanisms which seem to characterise ovarian hormone production.

Luteolysis begins with shunting of blood away from the corpus luteum, following which lysosomes initiate a process of lipolysis.

A specific luteolytic factor has not been isolated in primates, but prostaglandin $F_2\alpha$ from the endometrium may fulfil this function in other species.

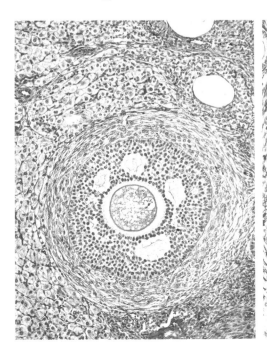
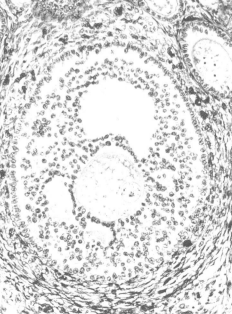

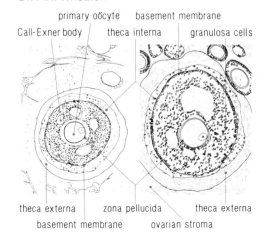

Fig. 11.6 Histological section showing secondary follicles in the ovarian cortex. The cells surrounding the primary follicle divide to form a multilayered stratum granulosum. Fluid filled antra, Call-Exner bodies, develop within this layer, and later coalesce to form the antrum. By courtesy of Dr. P.R. Wheater.

primary oöcyte   basement membrane
Call-Exner body   theca interna   granulosa cells

theca externa   zona pellucida   theca externa
basement membrane   ovarian stroma

HORMONE PRODUCTION BY THE OVARY

The two principal ovarian steroids, oestradiol and progesterone, are produced by the developing follicles (Fig. 11.10). Luteinisation coincides with the surge in progesterone production and secretion from the granulosa cells (which had begun shortly before ovulation). Furthermore, the enzyme 3β-hydroxysteroid dehydrogenase, which converts the parent compound pregnenolone to progesterone, is found in highest concentrations in granulosa cells.

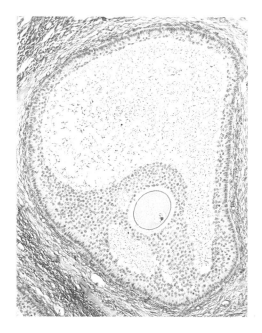

Fig. 11.7   The mature tertiary or Graafian follicle. The Call-Exner bodies have now coalesced and contain *liquor folliculi*. The ovum has been surrounded by a mound of cells known as the *discus proligerus* or the *cumulus oöphorus*.

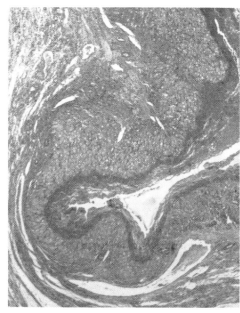

Fig. 11.8   The corpus luteum shown in histological section. Once ovulation has occurred the walls of the ruptured ovarian follicle collapse and become folded. Cells of the stratum granulosum increase in size and also become eosinophilic and luteinised. These cells form the major part of the corpus luteum. By courtesy of Prof. I. Doniach.

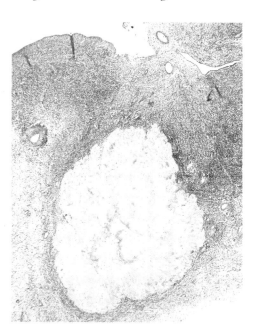

Fig. 11.9   Section through the corpus albicans. If fertilization has not occurred, the corpus luteum degenerates over the succeeding months and the cells undergo colloid, then fatty and finally hyaline degeneration to produce the corpus albicans.

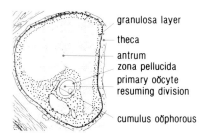

granulosa layer
theca
antrum
zona pellucida
primary oöcyte resuming division
cumulus oöphorous

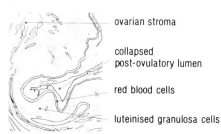

ovarian stroma
collapsed post-ovulatory lumen
red blood cells
luteinised granulosa cells

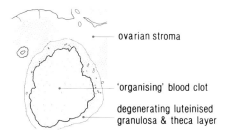

ovarian stroma
'organising' blood clot
degenerating luteinised granulosa & theca layer

Fig. 11.10   Summary of events in the menstrual cycle showing hormonal changes and stages of development of the germ cells. In the primordial and primary stages of development the follicle is independent of hormonal influences; thereafter gonadotrophins play an important part in follicular development.

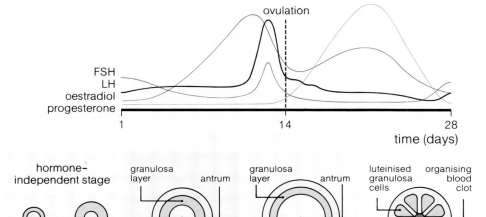

The source of oestrogen is more difficult to determine. Significant progesterone production by the granulosa cells only occurs after ovulation and vascularisation. Prior to this, enzyme levels in the granulosa are low suggesting that these cells are relatively quiescent. The original two-cell theory proposed that oestrogen is manufactured by the theca throughout the cycle, whilst progesterone is synthesised by granulosa cells after ovulation. In many species, however, the theca cells have little of the aromatising ability necessary for oestrogen formation. Granulosa cells are capable of performing this transformation and this, together with the very high oestrogen levels in follicular fluid, has led to the two-pathway theory (Fig. 11.11). Androgenic precursors produced in theca cells by the delta-5-pathway are transferred across the basement membrane to the granulosa layer for aromatisation.

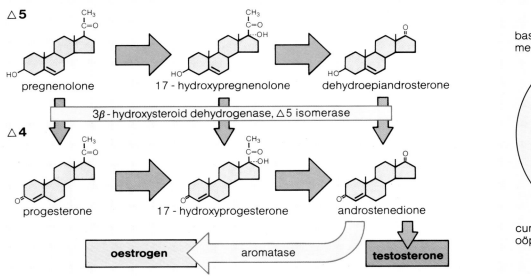

Fig. 11.11 Scheme showing pathways of steroid biosynthesis within the ovary. Under LH stimulation the theca cells produce delta-5 products. Within the granulosa cells the delta-4 pathway is more active under the influence of FSH.

Fig. 11.12 Diagram of receptor sites within a theca cell. Note that the LH receptors are situated in both the theca interna and granulosa cells whereas the FSH receptors are only found within the granulosa cells.

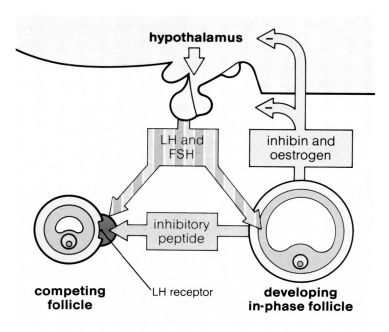

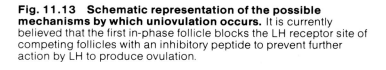

Fig. 11.13 Schematic representation of the possible mechanisms by which uniovulation occurs. It is currently believed that the first in-phase follicle blocks the LH receptor site of competing follicles with an inhibitory peptide to prevent further action by LH to produce ovulation.

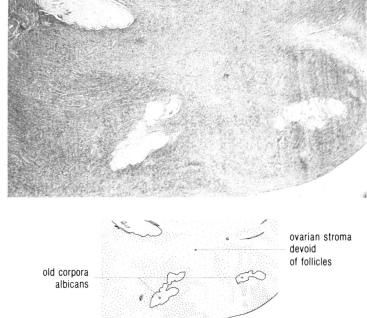

Fig. 11.14 Histological section of the postmenopausal ovary. Not only is there a massive reduction in the number of primordial follicles contained within the ovary, but the follicles are now unresponsive to gonadotrophins. By courtesy of Dr. J.W. Keeling.

These cells, however, do not produce progesterone from the parent pregnenolone until the delta-4-pathway is activated around the time of ovulation.

Androgens are produced by stromal cells using the delta-5-pathway and the ovary is responsible for twenty-five per cent of testosterone and forty per cent of androstenedione output. Stromal cells, however, respond to variations in gonadotrophin levels so that these proportions are increased at mid-cycle.

CONTROL OF FOLLICULAR GROWTH

Initiation of follicular activity and early atresia is independent of gonadotrophins. This occurs during fetal life and childhood and quiescent periods of adult life such as pregnancy, lactation, and amenorrhoea. Follicles probably begin their early development in the same sequence as they arrived as germ cells in the embryonic ovary; the 'first in, first out' theory.

When follicles reach the sixty-cell stage (early primary follicles) further growth becomes gonadotrophin dependent. At the beginning of each menstrual cycle a few primary follicles respond to the relatively high levels of gonadotrophins at this time and develop further. The factor determining which of these follicles becomes dominant is unknown but a blood-borne message is likely since usually only one ovary contains the dominant follicle in any cycle. Cell membrane receptors (MW 20,000-30,000) respond to these gonadotrophins. The hormone-receptor complex activates adenylate cyclase in the cell membrane, generating cyclic AMP from ATP. The cyclic AMP then initiates a sequence of intracellular events leading to activation of cholesterol synthetase and subsequent steroid formation.

FSH receptors are found only in granulosa cells and show a small increase during follicular growth; LH receptors are found on granulosa and theca cells and increase more dramatically (Fig. 11.12). Oestrogen leads to an increase in FSH receptors and FSH to an increase in LH receptors. LH on the other hand depletes gonadotrophin receptors leading to a temporary refractory period after the LH peak. Oestrogens have important effects within the

ovary itself (similar to testosterone in the testis) and are able to sustain follicular growth for several days after hypophysectomy. Amongst other actions they increase the concentration of FSH and oestrogen receptors and stimulate formation of gap junctions between granulosa cells.

Oestrogen builds up rapidly in mature follicles and this is reflected in follicular fluid where the oestradiol content of one follicle in the ovary may exceed that in the rest of the body. Only those follicles which are completely 'in phase' with the menstrual cycle can fully exploit and amplify changes in gonadotrophin levels. They make further use of their advantageous position to hasten atresia of 'competing' follicles by secretion of an inhibitory peptide of molecular weight 4,000 which impairs the binding of LH to receptors (Fig. 11.13). They also inhibit FSH by means of negative feedback from (a) oestrogen and (b) inhibin (a protein of molecular weight 710,000 which is found in high concentration in follicular fluid).

Extensive follicle development takes place not only during the menstrual cycle, but also during fetal life, some reaching the tertiary stage. Gonadotrophins from the fetal pituitary are probably the stimulus for this. A summary of hormonal events during the menstrual cycle is shown in Figure 11.10.

MECHANISM OF OVULATION

The dominant tertiary follicle forms a protrusion, the stigma, on the surface of the ovary. The cell layers rupture and the ovum, surrounded by the 'corona radiata' of granulosa cells, is released. The process takes place within a period of two minutes: it is *not* an instantaneous rupture resulting from a rise in follicular pressure. The oöcyte and corona are sloughed off into follicular fluid shortly before ovulation.

Prostaglandin synthesis by granulosa cells increases rapidly prior to ovulation and may play a part in the release of collagenase and lysosomal enzymes which are important in the erosion of the superficial layers of the ovary.

Ovulation is a direct result of the LH surge and occurs some fifteen hours after the LH peak. The LH surge is thought to be responsible for oöcyte maturation, the early progesterone secretion which precedes ovulation by approximately twenty-four hours and also prostaglandin production which leads to rupture of the follicle. The surge also decreases the affinity of gonadotrophin receptors resulting in desensitisation to LH within a few hours of its initiation; this in turn leads to a transient decrease in oestrogens which may be important in promoting subsequent luteinisation.

THE MENOPAUSAL OVARY

The menopause usually occurs between the ages of forty-five and fifty-five years and refers, by definition, to the last menstrual period. The cessation of uterine bleeding is a consequence of withdrawal of oestrogens as a result of depletion of competent ovarian follicles (Fig. 11.14). Apart from certain strains of rodent, the menopause is confined to the human species and does not occur, for example, in other primates.

Failure of gonadal steroid production leads to a great increase in trophic hormone secretion; FSH levels by a factor of ten and LH by a factor of five (Fig. 11.15). Although several hundred primordial follicles remain in the ovary, these are insensitive to the action of gonadotrophins and development is arrested at an early stage.

Oestradiol production is low after the menopause. However, the ovarian stroma continues to secrete androstenedione and circulating oestrone levels are maintained by peripheral conversion.

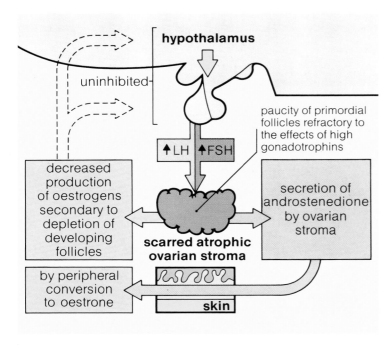

Fig. 11.15 Schematic representation of the feedback mechanisms in the menopausal ovary.

DISTURBANCES OF OVARIAN HORMONE PRODUCTION
Polycystic Ovarian Syndrome (PCO)

This term is used to describe a spectrum of abnormalities characterised by excessive androgen production but excludes congenital adrenal hyperplasia (CAH), Cushing's syndrome and hormone-producing tumours. The ovary is often enlarged (Fig. 11.16); however, the most characteristic feature is the presence of numerous small cystic follicles 0.5-1.0 centimetres in diameter (Fig. 11.17) situated beneath a thickened capsule. Histologically there is hyperplasia of the theca cells and the interstitial stroma, and attenuation of the granulosa cell layer. Some of the milder biochemical and clinical abnormalities may occur in the absence of these characteristic morphological features, though these are often included in the definition of PCO.

The clinical features of this syndrome are very varied (Fig. 11.18). Oligomenorrhoea with heavy menstrual bleeding is characteristic, and cycles are typically anovulatory. Primary or secondary infertility is therefore a common mode of presentation. Some patients suffer from a mild degree of virilism with acne (Fig. 11.19), greasy skin and hirsutism (Fig. 11.20); others however, may display more severe features of androgen excess and have marked hirsutism, capital hair loss with temporal hair recession (Fig. 11.21). Mammary hypoplasia (Fig. 11.22) and clitoromegaly may be present (Fig. 11.23). Many patients are obese, however this is not universal. Typically there is signficant endometrial hyperplasia. In accordance with the original description, the term 'Stein-Leventhal' syndrome is best reserved for those patients manifesting the complete spectrum of these features. Any one clinical feature together with one of the biochemical abnormalities listed below (Fig. 11.24) is considered sufficient to make the diagnosis of polycystic ovarian syndrome.

The biochemical features may occur singly or in combination and include increases in testosterone secretion and urinary 17-oxosteroid excretion and also in the ratio of LH to FSH. In patients with testosterone levels in the upper end of the normal range the excessive androgenisation may be explained by a reduction in levels of the specific testosterone binding globulin in blood, known as sex-hormone-binding-globulin. Thus the unbound free testosterone, the metabolically active portion, is increased despite the normal levels of total testosterone (protein bound plus unbound). In contrast to other endocrine causes of amenorrhoea, the oestrogen levels are not substantially decreased and a short course of a progestogen drug will provoke a withdrawal bleed. The menstrual disturbance is therefore the result of an imbalance rather than a deficiency of hormones.

Despite these well-documented changes in hormone levels the underlying cause or causes are uncertain. The ovary, hypothalamus and adrenal glands have all been suggested as the primary site of the defect.

Some workers have found deficiencies in ovarian aromatase activity with reduced 3β-hydroxysteroid dehydrogenase activity. Thus raised LH levels may be a response to reduced oestrogen secretion; these high LH levels will then stimulate excessive androgen

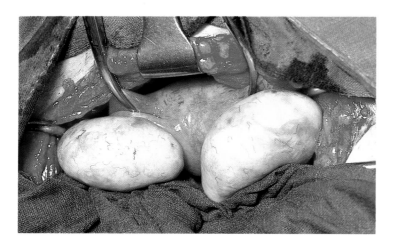

Fig. 11.16 Macroscopic appearance within the pelvis of enlarged, pearly white ovaries of a patient with polycystic ovarian syndrome (PCO). The ovarian capsule is thickened.

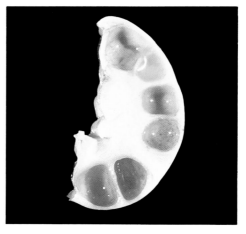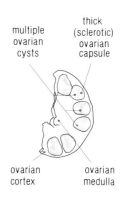

Fig. 11.17 Section through an ovary excised from a patient with PCO. The yellow colouration of the cyst is evidence of the luteinisation which has occurred. By courtesy of Dr. J.W. Keeling.

Principal Symptoms of Polycystic Ovarian Syndrome	
feature	frequency (% of all cases of PCO)
amenorrhoea	60
dysfunctional bleeding	25
hirsutism	70
infertility	70
obesity	30
palpable ovaries	20

Fig. 11.18 Table showing the clinical features of the polycystic ovarian syndrome.

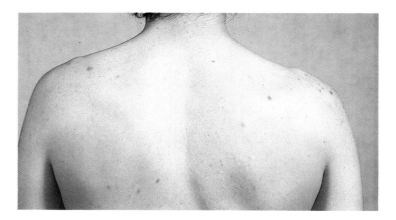

Fig. 11.19 Photograph showing acne on the back of a patient with PCO.

production by the stromal cells. However the rapid surge in oestrogen production, which follows ovulation induction with clomiphene or gonadotrophins, contradicts this theory. Other workers maintain that the disturbance in gonadotrophin secretion is the primary defect. Indeed the histological appearance of the ovary in PCO has many features in common with pregnancy since high levels of human chorionic gonadotrophin (HCG) bind to the ovarian LH receptor and this may account for the changes in ovarian morphology.

Support for an adrenal aetiology comes from the dramatic clinical and biochemical improvement which is produced by suppression of ACTH during treatment with glucocorticoids.

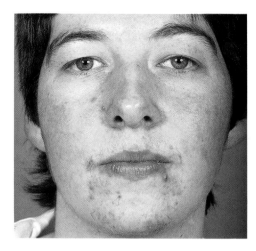

Fig. 11.20 Photograph showing facial acne, greasy skin and hirsutism in a patient with PCO. The extent of hair growth in this patient is minimal.

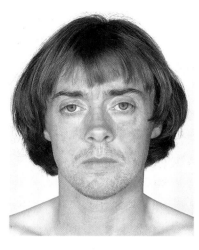

Fig. 11.21 Photographs of a patient with an androblastoma with associated PCO before and after treatment. Before treatment (left), the patient had marked facial hirsutism. On the right the patient is shown

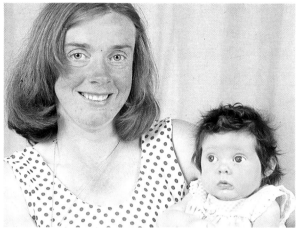

successfully treated. The androblastoma was resected and regular menstruation was initiated with reversed circadian rhythm prednisolone therapy, and ovulation ensued with clomiphene and HCG therapy.

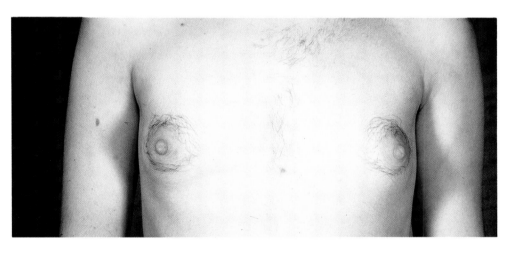

Fig. 11.22 Periareolar hirsuties and mammary hypoplasia in a patient suffering from an androgen-secreting ovarian tumour.

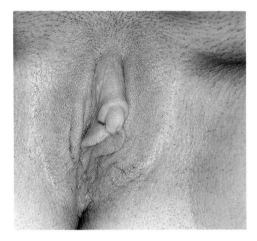

Fig. 11.23 Photograph of an enlarged clitoris in a patient with an androgen-secreting tumour.

Biochemical Abnormalities in Polycystic Ovarian Syndrome

raised adrenal and ovarian androgens	normal or raised prolactin
raised testosterone	raised LH/FSH ratio
lowered sex hormone binding globulin (SHBG)	raised urinary oxosteroid excretion

Fig. 11.24 Table of the biochemical events leading to the polycystic ovarian syndrome.

Furthermore the classical changes in the ovary are also found in association with primary adrenal disturbances such as congenital adrenal hyperplasia and androgen-secreting tumours.

Whatever the initiating abnormality the condition is self-perpetuating and a proposed model for this positive feedback loop is shown (Fig. 11.25). The ovarian disturbance abolishes the normal hormone fluctuations of the reproductive cycle, leading to the so-called 'steady-state syndrome'. The resulting anovulation may be manifest as dysfunctional bleeding or amenorrhoea.

Treatment is dependent upon the primary complaint (Fig. 11.26). If infertility is the most important consideration anti-oestrogens (clomiphene or tamoxifen) will induce ovulation in the majority of patients. However, only half of these will become pregnant. The initial response to this treatment is frequently an increase in ovarian androgen production. This may be prevented by suppressing androgen production and restoring ovulation with glucocorticoids before starting the clomiphene. This is normally accomplished by administration of 5mg prednisolone on retiring, and 2.5 mg on waking. This 'reversed circadian regime' suppresses ACTH and endogenous glucocorticoid production and hence adrenal androgen production; also, since it is a physiological re-placement dose, it does not cause side-effects. Both these therapies are relatively ineffective in reducing excessive hair growth and, where this is the predominant symptom, the addition of cyclical oestrogen therapy to prednisolone may be effective, although it may take six to nine months for improvement to occur. In cases where glucocorticoid and cyclical oestrogen therapy fail to resolve the hirsutism, the anti-androgen cyproterone acetate may be added. This treatment prevents conception, which is beneficial since cyproterone potentially inhibits the normal development of a male fetus.

Where dysfunctional bleeding is the predominant complaint cyclical oestrogen and progesterone treatment alone may be effective but some would recommend an initial course of gluco-corticoids to reverse the underlying defect.

Cyclical therapy in patients with polycystic ovarian syndrome has the further advantage of reducing the risk of developing endometrial hyperplasia and subsequent endometrial carcinoma by regularly stripping the endometrium.

Functional Ovarian Tumours

These are much less common than non-functional epithelial tumours. The most important examples are the oestrogen-secreting tumours (granulosa and theca cell tumours, Fig. 11.27) and androgen secreting tumours (androblastomas and Hilus cell tumours and Leydig cell tumours, Fig. 11.28). Gonadoblastomas

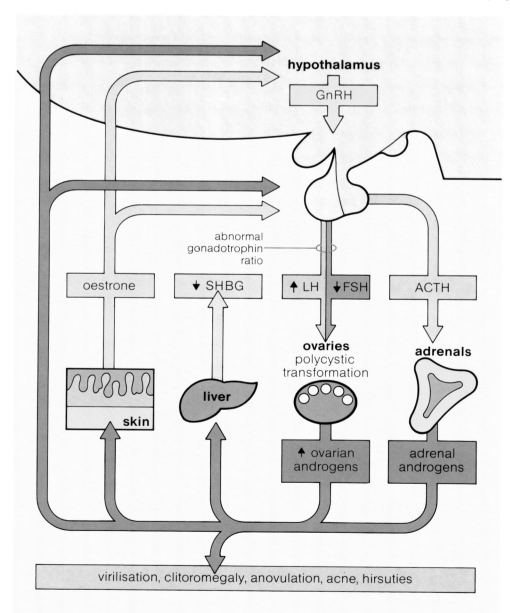

Fig. 11.25 Diagram depicting the positive feedback model of events during PCO. An important abnormality in PCO may involve the abnormal production of adrenal androgens under ACTH stimulation. Androgens of both adrenal and ovarian origin will suppress SHBG production in the liver; this results in a rise in 'free' androgens which is responsible for virilisation. Androgens are also converted in the skin to oestrone throughout the cycle. The persistent oestrogen levels feed back in the hypothalamus and the pituitary causing high LH levels (positive feedback) and low FSH levels (negative feedback). The high LH:FSH ratio is responsible for polycystic transformation and increased androgen output from the ovarian stroma. This perpetuates the viscious cycle. The pituitary is therefore exposed to oestrogen effect at all times and is therefore unable to restore the appropriate FSH:LH ratio at the beginning of the cycle.

(a tumour involving germ cell and stromal elements) and neoplastic adrenal cell rests may also be implicated, but these are even less common. The functional activity is not always true to the histological classification; for example, granulosa cell tumours may produce androgens. Non-steroidal hormones are produced by various germ-cell tumours. Thus *struma ovarii*, a usually benign form of teratoma, secretes thyroid stimulating hormone (TSH) whilst the highly malignant choriocarcinoma and endodermal sinus (yolk sac) tumours frequently produce HCG and alphafetoprotein.

Fig. 11.26 Table of the methods of treating patients with PCO.

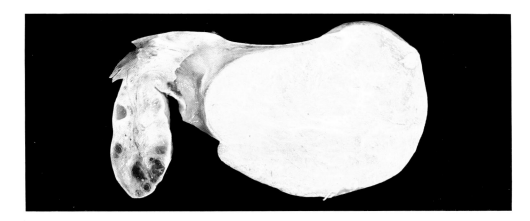

Fig. 11.27 Section of an ovary showing a theca cell tumour. This tumour is oestrogen-secreting and is probably the most common type of functional ovarian tumour.

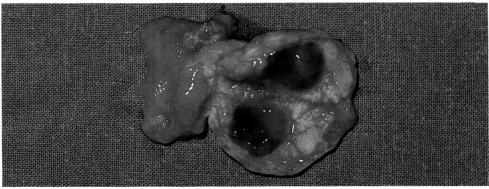

Fig. 11.28 Excised Leydig cell tumour (upper) with histological appearance (lower). Leydig cell tumours, as well as Hilus cell tumours, secrete androgens, although the functional activity of tumours does not always correlate with their histological classification. By courtesy of Dr. J.W. Keeling and Prof. I. Doniach.

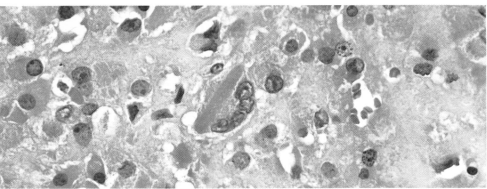

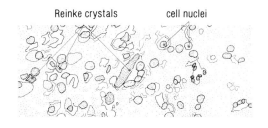

11.11

Whilst theca cell tumours are invariably benign, ten per cent of granulosa cell tumours are malignant. The number of mitoses gives some indication of their malignant potential but this diagnosis cannot be made reliably by histological means; only the subsequent biological behaviour can distinguish the malignant tumours with certainty. About one third of androblastomas, previously called arrhenoblastomas, are malignant. The clinical effects of oestrogen-secreting tumours depend upon the patient's age. They are most common in postmenopausal women and give rise to bleeding, whereas in young girls they cause pseudo-precocious puberty and cause menorrhagia in women of reproductive age. The endometrium becomes hyperplastic due to the prolonged effects of high oestrogen levels, and carcinoma may ensue.

Androgen secreting tumours tend to arise in younger age groups. They produce more profound virilisation than PCO: in addition to hirsutism there may also be considerable enlargement of the clitoris, temporal hair recession, increased musculature and deepened voice. Testosterone levels are higher, usually half the normal male value, and are not significantly suppressed by dexamethasone administration (0.5 mg six hourly for forty-eight hours). The tumour can sometimes be localised by measurement of steroids in blood samples obtained from a catheter at different sites in the inferior vena cava and from the ovarian veins. Physical methods such as ultrasound and laparoscopy are less useful in this respect since ovaries containing small androgen-secreting tumours may look normal or polycystic and often have to be split open before the tumour can be found.

12 Normal and Abnormal Sexual Development and Puberty

Edward O Reiter, MD

PUBERTAL DEVELOPMENT AND MATURATION

Puberty is the transitional period between the juvenile state and adulthood during which the adolescent growth spurt occurs, secondary sexual characteristics appear, fertility is achieved and profound psychological changes take place (Fig. 12.1). The events characterising pubertal maturation of the reproductive endocrine

Fig. 12.1   The definition of puberty

Definition of Puberty

The process by which and the period of life during which sexual maturation occurs and reproductive capacity is attained.

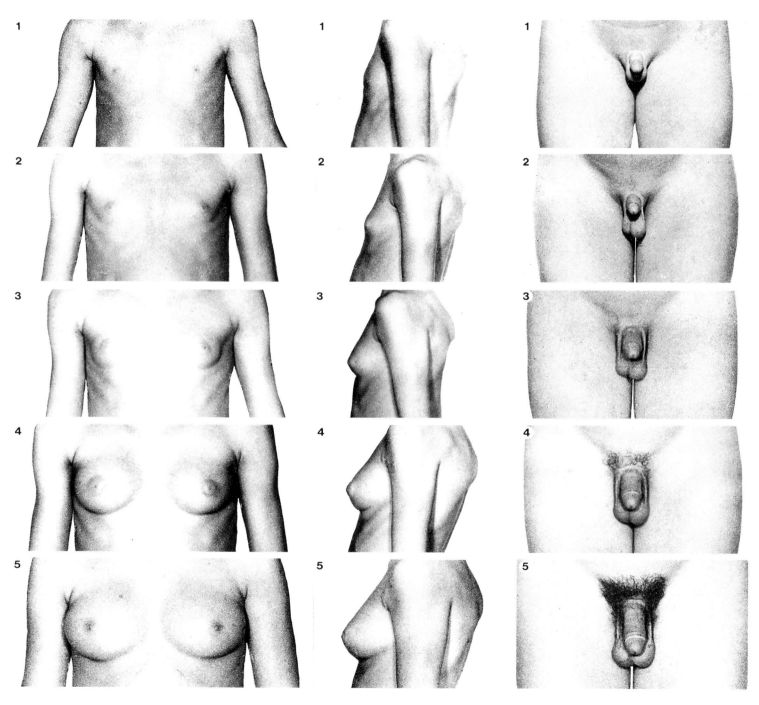

Fig. 12.2   Stages of pubertal breast development. The five stages are characterised as follows: stage 1 – no discernable breast tissue; stage 2 – areolar widening and pigmentation with some subareolar tissue; stage 3 – further growth of breast and areolar tissue; stage 4 – further breast enlargement and stage 5 – adult breast size has been achieved and the areola has now receded into the contour of the breast. From Tanner (1962), by courtesy of the publishers, Blackwell Scientific Publications.

Fig. 12.3   Stages of pubertal maturation of male genitalia. Enlargement, thinning and reddening of the scrotal skin is present in stage 2, but darkening and enlargement of the scrotum, together with substantial increase in phallic width and length are not apparent until stage 4. From Tanner (1962), Blackwell Scientific Publications.

system should be viewed as part of a continuum, extending from sexual differentiation and the development of the hypothalamo-pituitary-gonadal system in the fetus to the attainment of full

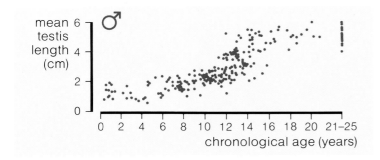

Fig. 12.4 Changes in testicular size from early childhood to adolescence. Testicular size is the mean of the longest diameter of both testes and is less than 2.2cm prior to puberty. Testicular size may also be evaluated as testicular volume (see Chapter 10). Redrawn from Winter and Faiman (1972), by courtesy of the publishers, Williams and Wilkins Company.

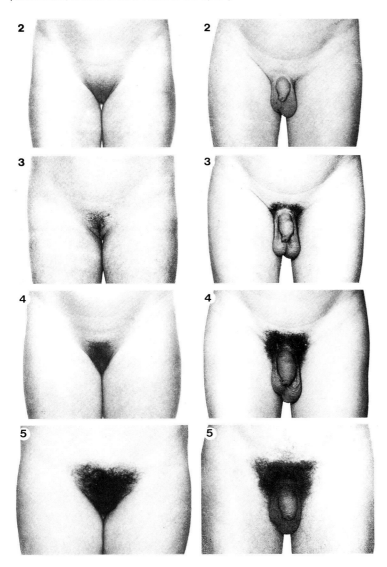

Fig. 12.5 Pubertal stages of pubic hair growth and development. From Tanner (1962), by courtesy of the publishers, Blackwell Scientific Publications.

sexual maturation and fertility, and then ultimately to senescence. Failure to achieve sexual maturation at an age and time similar to that of one's peers, whether early or late, is often accompanied by significant concern and possibly anxiety, which sometimes interferes with the child's ability to progress effectively within his peer group.

Breast Development

In females, secretion by the ovaries of oestrogens appears to be the major controlling factor of breast growth. The stages of breast development described after a longitudinal British study (Tanner, 1962) are those most widely used to characterise breast development from the prepubertal period to adulthood (Fig. 12.2). Stage 1 is the prepubertal girl with no discernable breast tissue. In stage 2 there is areolar widening and pigmentation has taken place with the development of a small amount of subareolar breast tissue. Further growth of breast and areola occurs in stage 3; during stage 4, there is further breast enlargement, with mounding of the areola above the plane of the breast (this latter stage may not occur in all individuals). Finally, stage 5 is the adult breast in which the areola recedes into the general contour of the breasts. Size or inherent shape of the breasts do not appear to be directly under hormonal control, but are determined by genetic, nutritional and other diverse factors.

Development of the Male Genitalia

The initial manifestation of male pubertal development is enlargement of the testes to a length greater than 2.2cm. The normal development of male genitalia up until puberty is shown in Figures 12.3 and 12.4. In stage 1, there has been no increase in testicular size, with a testicular length of less than 2.2cm and an immature phallus. In stage 2, testicular length is between 2.2–3.0cm with enlargement, thinning and reddening of the scrotal skin and a slight increase in phallic size. Testicular length is between 3.1–4.0cm in stage 3, with further enlargement of the scrotum and more substantial growth of the phallus. This is followed in stage 4, by darkening and enlargement of the scrotum, a substantial increase in phallic width and length, and an increase in the size of the glans; testicular length being between 4.1–4.9cm. Finally, stage 5 is characterised by adult male genitalia in which testicular length is generally greater than 5.0cm with the scrotum pigmented and thickened and adult phallus size attained.

Pubic Hair Development

In females, pubic hair growth appears to be under the hormonal control of the adrenal androgens; in males, both gonadal and adrenal androgens appear to play a role. The importance of pubic hair as an indicator of sexual maturation is less than that of either breast development or of gonadal and phallic growth. Again, the stages of pubic hair growth introduced by Tanner are used. In the prepubertal individual (stage 1), there is absence of hair over the pubic area other than the vellus hair of the abdominal wall. In stage 2 (Fig. 12.5) there is sparse, long, slightly curly and pigmented hair at the base of the phallus or scrotum, or the labia majora or mons veneris. There is an increased quantity of coarsely pigmented curled hair in stage 3 and in stage 4, the coarse hair now fully covering the pubic symphysis. Finally, in stage 5, the hair is of adult quality and quantity covering the entire pubic area with spread to the medial surface of the thigh. In females, the hair is distributed as an inverse triangle, whereas in men, there is further spread of pubic hair up the linea alba forming the male escutcheon.

Sequence of Pubertal Events in Females

A relationship exists between the height spurt, the age of onset of breast development and the age of the first period, or menarche (Fig. 12.6). In American children, the ages of pubertal development for any given stage are somewhat earlier than the British data by four to twelve months. The first pubertal event is the onset of the growth spurt, which may precede the onset of breast development by as much as one year. Peak height velocity in girls coincides with stage 3 of breast growth and usually with stages 2 to 3 of pubic hair development. Menarche occurs after the time of peak height velocity has passed; indeed, only 5–8cm of growth will occur after the first period. Breast growth is usually complete four years after initiation and menarche will occur approximately two years after the onset of breast growth. Menarche coincides with breast stage 2 in approximately five per cent of girls, stage 3 in twenty-five per cent, stage 4 in sixty per cent and stage 5 in ten per cent. In ninety-nine per cent of females, menarche occurs within five years after the onset of breast growth. Also, in approximately one out of six girls, pubic hair growth may begin before breast growth begins, but rarely are stages 3 or 4 of pubic hair growth achieved without some breast development.

Sequence of Pubertal Events in Males

The initial manifestation of male pubertal development is enlargement of testicular volume (Fig. 12.7). The onset of the adolescent growth spurt occurs approximately one year after the increase in gonadal volume; the peak height growth velocity being attained after a substantial amount of growth of the genitalia has already occurred. In striking contrast to the female, in whom the adolescent growth spurt is a rather early event of puberty, the male peak linear growth velocity does not occur until mid to late

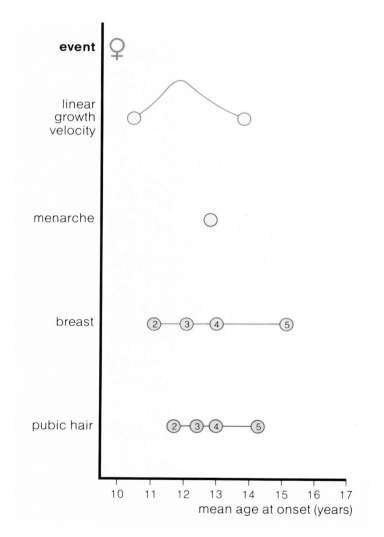

Fig. 12.6 Schematic representation of events during pubertal maturation in females. Redrawn from Marshall and Tanner (1969), by courtesy of the publishers, the British Medical Association.

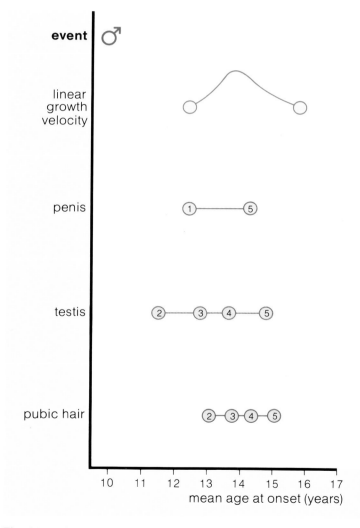

Fig. 12.7 Schematic representation of pubertal changes in males. Redrawn from Marshall and Tanner (1970), by courtesy of the publishers, the British Medical Association.

puberty. In addition, the increase in muscle mass, bone size and the general appearance of the adult torso are late characteristics of male puberty.

Secular Trend of Puberty

The specific mechanisms involved in the timing of puberty are complex and poorly understood. The average age at onset of puberty shows a secular trend over the past one hundred and fifty years toward earlier occurrence, regardless of race or geography (Fig. 12.8). This progressive decline in the age of puberty is thought to result from improvements in socioeconomic conditions, nutrition and general health. In developed nations, such a trend appears to have slowed or ceased over the last twenty years.

The relationship between the age of menarche and weight at menarche has been examined by Frisch and her co-workers (1973). Data from three different studies reveal that, in large numbers of healthy girls between ten and sixteen years of age, the slope of the regression line of the weight on age does not differ significantly from zero. This suggests that there is an 'invariant mean weight' (approximately 48kg) associated with the age of menarche. Further, they have found 'critical weights' associated with the initiation of the pubertal growth spurt and with the time of maximum growth rate. Using these cross-sectional data, together with an indirect measure of total body fat (total body water/body weight %), Frisch and her co-workers have suggested that the percentage of total body fat more closely relates to the age of menarche than simply body weight; there appears to be a decreased range around the regression line of total body water/body weight (TW/BW) versus age at menarche. They have constructed a nomogram, based on TW/BW as an index of fatness, to determine the minimal height for weight necessary for menarche (Fig. 12.9).

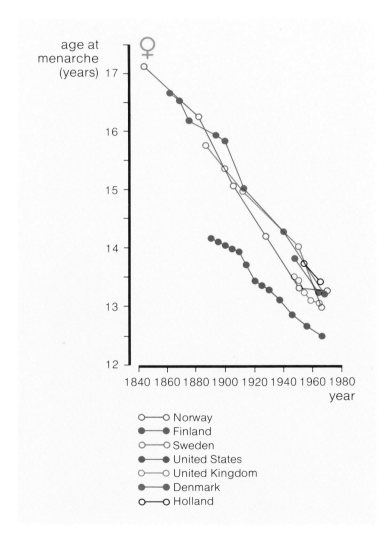

Fig. 12.8 Age at menarche from 1840 to 1970. Over the past century and a half, a general trend of girls to have menarche at earlier ages can be seen. The menarchal age has decreased by three to four months per decade during this time interval. Redrawn from Tanner (1975), by courtesy of the publishers, W.B. Saunders Company.

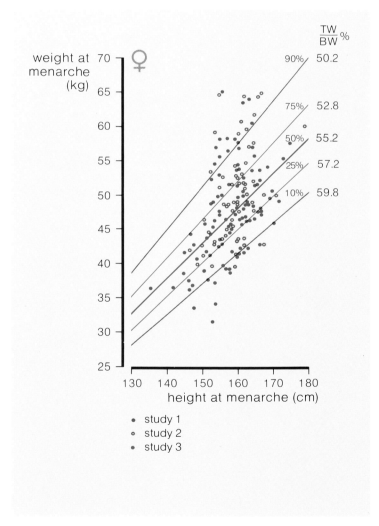

Fig. 12.9 Graph of girl's weight versus height in relation to menarche. The diagonal lines represent centiles of the ratio of body water to total body weight. Thus for example, only 10% of girls who are 160cm in height with a weight of 42.5kg or less will have had menarche, whereas 50% of girls of this height will have reached menarche with a weight of 47.5kg. Redrawn from Frisch and McArthur (1974), by courtesy of the AAAS.

12.5

Critical Fat Hypothesis

1   There is a similar mean weight at the time of onset of puberty, peak growth velocity and menarche

2   The body fat:weight ratio expressed as a percentage more closely defines these pubertal events.

Fig. 12.10   The critical fat hypothesis. Weights at differing ages at each of three major pubertal events and the percentage of fat of total body weight even more closely relates to these pubertal events.

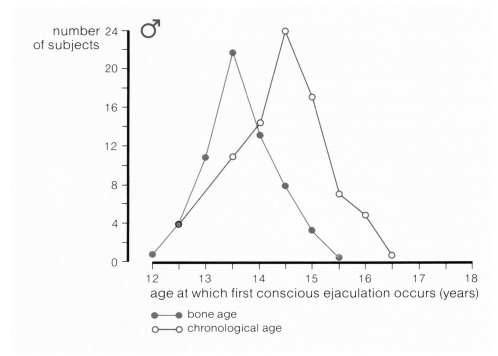

Fig. 12.11   Graph showing the age at which the first conscious ejaculation occurs. Chronological and skeletal ages are shown. Redrawn from Laron et al. (1980), by courtesy of the publishers, Schwabe and Company.

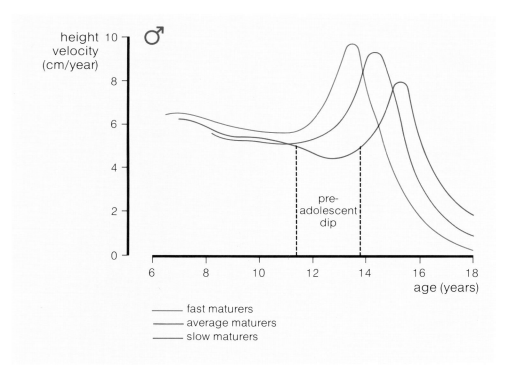

Fig. 12.12   Height velocity curves of normal boys with variable onset of pubertal maturation. These data were shown by Smith (1977) as an example of the striking discrepancies between slow and fast maturing boys. Redrawn by courtesy of the publishers, W.B. Saunders Company.

These considerations, though difficult to evaluate, appear to be significant, and this has led to the critical fat hypothesis (Fig. 12.10). However, the effect of nutritional factors and body composition upon the time of onset of puberty is certainly supported by the earlier age of menarche in moderately obese girls and by delayed maturation of the reproductive endocrine system in states of malnutrition and chronic illness or following early athletic or ballet training. It is also supported by the relationship of amenorrhoea to such states of diminished body fat as anorexia nervosa, voluntary weight loss and vigorous physical exercise. Although menarche is a relatively late pubertal event, and is thus removed from those neural factors that influence both the gonadotrophin-gonadal sex steroid change and physical changes at the beginning of puberty, the possibility exists that some alteration of body metabolism, including the ratio of fat to lean body mass, may affect the higher centre restraints on pubertal onset.

In the male, there is no event so striking as the female menarche. However, Laron and his associates (1980) in Israel have studied the age of first conscious ejaculation (Fig. 12.11). There is a relatively narrow period during which this event occurs; the bone age at which the majority of subjects experience ejaculation for the first time (13.5 years) is similar to that of British girls having their menarche. No extensive endocrine studies have been undertaken to examine boys around the time of first ejaculation, but it appears to be a mid-pubertal event when circulating testosterone levels have reached approximately forty to fifty per cent of adult concentrations.

There may be substantial variability in the growth curves of normal boys during the adolescent growth spurt (Fig. 12.12). Indeed, the growth rate of boys who are slow to mature (i.e. with a growth velocity of approximately 4cm per year during the age range from eleven to fourteen years) greatly contrasts with the velocity of 9–10cm per year in those who mature quickly. The growth process is fully achieved at a much earlier age in the 'fast maturers', while the boys who have a more delayed adolescent growth spurt may still be growing for several years longer.

HORMONAL DEVELOPMENT AND THE REPRODUCTIVE ENDOCRINE SYSTEM
Components of the Reproductive Endocrine System
The regulatory systems that control human male and female reproduction are listed in Figure 12.13. A complex network of factors from the higher central nervous system modulates the function of the hypothalamus. The fundamental components of the reproductive endocrine system include the hypothalamus, the pituitary and the gonads.

The arcuate nucleus of the medial basal hypothalamus and its neurosecretory neurons translate neural signals into a periodic oscillatory chemical signal, gonadotrophin-releasing hormone (GnRH). GnRH is synthesised by the neurosecretory peptidergic neurons. It is subsequently released from axon terminals at the median eminence into the primary plexus of the hypothalamo-hypophyseal portal circulation, where it is carried to the anterior pituitary gland. Recent evidence suggests that catecholaminergic and opioidergic neuronal networks, together with sex steroids, modulate the release of GnRH. The pituitary gonadotrophs then, in response to the rhythmic GnRH signal, release luteinizing hormone (LH) and follicle stimulating hormone (FSH) in a pulsatile manner at periodic intervals; these hormones then influence the gonads.

This control system, with its three principal components – the arcuate GnRH neurosecretory neurons, the pituitary gonadotrophs and the gonadotrophin responsive elements of the gonads – is common to all mammalian species. It is at each of these loci that modulating factors exert their effects. Furthermore, in the pituitary and gonads, the target cells contain specific cell surface receptors for the peptide hormones that mediate the cellular response to the signal.

Components of the Reproductive Endocrine System

higher central nervous system
cerebral cortex, limbic system; complex neurotransmitter system modulating hypothalamic function

hypothalamus
site of synthesis and storage of the gonadotrophin-releasing hormone (GnRH); in several nuclei

anterior pituitary
site of synthesis and storage of luteinizing hormone (LH) and follicle stimulating hormone (FSH); in the gonadotrophs

gonads
ovaries: site of sex steroid production in follicles and thecal tissue; production of ova
testes: site of sex steroid production in Leydig cells; production of spermatozoa

organs of reproduction
female: vagina, cervix, uterus, fallopian tubes
male: penis, testes, seminal vesicles, vasa deferentia

Fig. 12.13 **Components of the reproductive endocrine system.** These include the higher central nervous system, hypothalamus, anterior pituitary, gonads and reproductive organs.

In the female (Fig. 12.14), FSH increases proliferation of granulosa cells and induces them to acquire an aromatising enzyme; this permits conversion of androgen to oestrogen (primarily, oestradiol). It appears that the oestrogens themselves act at the ovary to increase granulosa cell stimulation. The ovarian androgen is produced by the theca interna cells which surround each of the ovarian follicles. Oestradiol then influences higher central nervous system sites, and also the hypothalamus and pituitary, to modulate gonadotrophin secretion.

In the male, gonadotrophins act upon the testes to stimulate Leydig cells to produce sex steroids, primarily testosterone, and to stimulate the germinal epithelium to produce spermatozoa (Fig. 12.15). There is an intimate interaction between gonadal testosterone and the development of the seminiferous tubules. Indeed, in early pubertal development the increased gonadal volume results from both an increase in volume of the seminiferous tubules and also from an increase in size and number of Leydig cells. The sex steroids, especially testosterone,

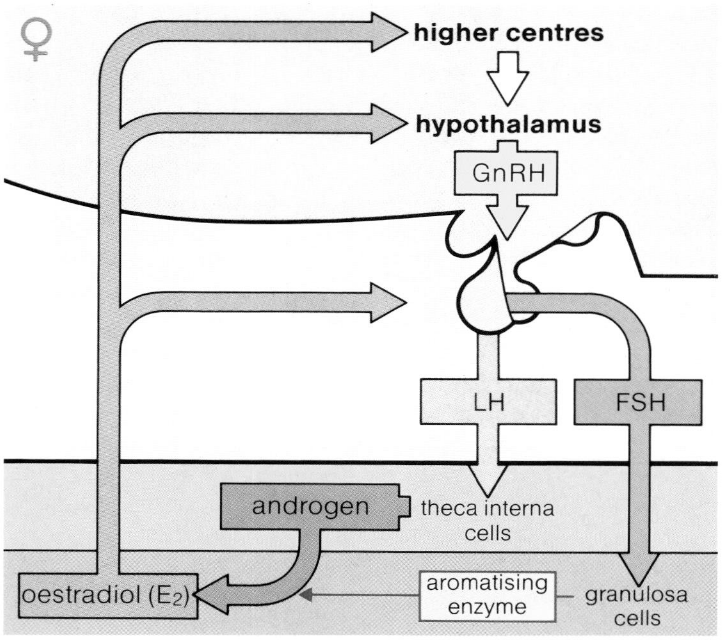

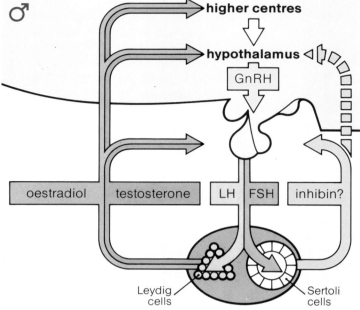

Fig. 12.14 Diagrammatic representation of the hypothalamo-pituitary-ovarian axis. The interaction of gonadotrophins and the components of the ovarian follicles are shown. Sex steroid feedback effects upon the brain, hypothalamus and pituitary can also be seen.

Fig. 12.15 Diagram of the hypothalamo-pituitary-testicular axis. The testes differentiate into steroid-producing tissue (Leydig cells) and germinal epithelium (seminiferous tubules). The effects of gonadotrophins upon the two gonadal components, as well as feedback of steroids and inhibin upon the brain, hypothalamus and pituitary are indicated.

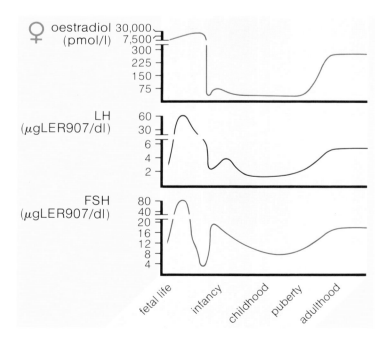

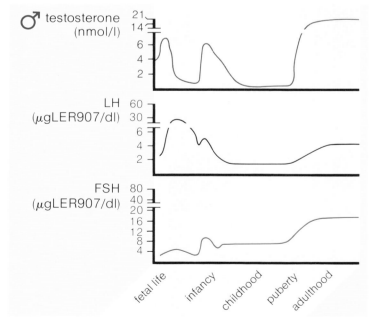

Fig. 12.16 Changes in serum FSH, LH and oestradiol during life in normal females. Redrawn from Winter et al. (1976), by courtesy of the publishers, Williams and Wilkins Company.

Fig. 12.17 Changes in serum FSH, LH and testosterone during life in normal males. The rather striking increment of testosterone during the first six months of life, into the mid-pubertal range, should be noted. Redrawn from Winter et al. (1976), by courtesy of the publishers, Williams and Wilkins Company.

modulate the brain, hypothalamus and pituitary to control gonadotrophin secretion. In addition, a recently described peptide, inhibin, produced by the Sertoli cells of the seminiferous tubule, appears to significantly influence FSH secretion.

Hormonal Changes at Puberty

There are rather substantial changes in levels of pituitary gonadotrophins and of the major sex steroids (oestradiol in females and testosterone in males) during the life cycle. The

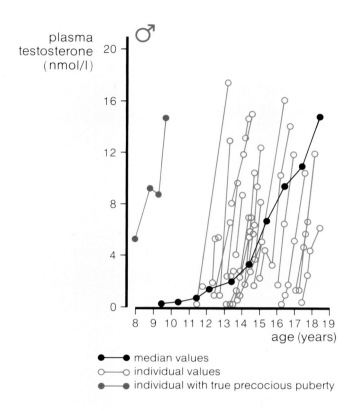

Fig. 12.18 Changes in plasma testosterone during pubertal years. The levels of testosterone rise abruptly in individual subjects in contrast to the shallow slope of the median curve. Redrawn from Knorr et al. (1974), by courtesy of the publishers, Periodica.

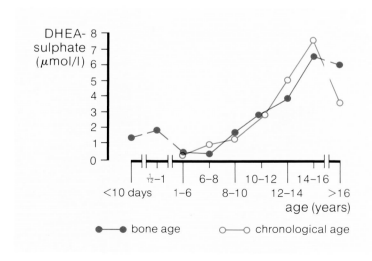

Fig. 12.19 Serum DHEA-sulphate concentrations throughout childhood related to both chronological and skeletal age. Redrawn from Reiter et al. (1977), by courtesy of the publishers, The C.V. Mosby Company.

human fetal pituitary gland can synthesise and store FSH and LH by the tenth week of gestation and secretes these hormones by the eleventh or twelfth week. The pattern of changes of FSH and LH concentrations in pituitary glands, and also the serum of fetuses, is consistent with the sequence of increased synthesis and secretion in which peak serum concentrations reach adult castrate levels, followed by a decline after mid-gestation that persists to term. In the data of Winter and colleagues (Figs. 12.16 and 12.17), fetal FSH levels are higher in female infants than in male infants, while LH levels during fetal life tend to be similar in both sexes.

After the fall in sex steroids, especially oestrogens, following birth, the concentrations of FSH and LH increase and exhibit wide fluctuations during the first months of life; intermittent, high gonadotrophin concentrations are associated with increased levels of testosterone in male infants and oestradiol in females. The infantile increment of testosterone in males to levels comparable with the mid-pubertal range is more striking than that of oestradiol in the female. By approximately six months in the male and one to two years of age in the female, the concentrations of gonadotrophins have already decreased to the low levels present during childhood, until the onset of puberty.

In the peripubertal period, gonadotrophin concentrations rise. In girls, FSH levels rise during the early stages of puberty and then plateau, whereas LH levels tend to rise in the later stages. In boys, LH concentrations rise progressively during puberty, whereas FSH levels increase sharply in early pubertal development and then more gradually throughout the remainder of pubertal maturation. As a consequence of the gonadotrophin changes at the time of puberty, testosterone and oestradiol levels also rise rather sharply to adult levels. Biologically-active LH has been quantified throughout fetal life and at all stages of extra-uterine life in human studies. In general, bioactive LH levels are usually undetectable during prepubertal years, then rise dramatically during pubertal maturation. Qualitative changes in the LH molecule may possibly occur during pubertal maturation.

During the pubertal years, median values of testosterone only gradually increase from the prepubertal levels to adult levels, especially during the first half of pubertal development. However, when individual subjects are examined (Fig. 12.18) the incremental change in testosterone is rather striking. There may be rises of testosterone of 3 to 14 nmol/l over a period of six to eighteen months in a given boy. The adolescent growth spurt follows closely behind the very rapid upsurge of plasma testosterone levels.

In addition to changes in gonadotrophin, testosterone and oestradiol levels, there are also changes in secretion of the adrenal androgen, dehydroepiandrosterone sulphate – DHEA-sulphate (Fig. 12.19). A significant increment in DHEA-sulphate secretion by eight years of age in both boys and girls has been defined from both cross-sectional and longitudinal studies. In normal full-term infants, the mean DHEA-sulphate concentrations are significantly higher than in the one- to six-year-old age group. Levels during the first year of life also tend to be higher than in later prepubertal years; however, when DHEA-sulphate concentrations are viewed in relation to skeletal maturation, a significant increment occurs in the six- to eight-year-old combined group of boys and girls. In our studies no significant sex differences were present within varied age groups, although a greater increment occurred in girls during the eight to ten year chronological age period, whereas, in boys, a rise of comparable magnitude required a four year period from eight to twelve years of age.

Patterns of Gonadotrophin Secretion

There are two patterns of gonadotrophin secretion: tonic and cyclic. Tonic, or basal, secretion appears to be largely regulated by negative or inhibitory feedback mechanisms. Thus changes in the concentration of circulating sex steroids, and possibly inhibin, result in reciprocal changes in secretion of pituitary gonadotrophins. The levels of the gonadotrophins shown in Figures 12.16 and 12.17 are largely dependent upon such regulation. Tonic secretion is the general pattern of secretion in males and one of the control mechanisms in females. FSH and LH are probably always secreted in a pulsatile or episodic manner at periodic intervals. In adult men, and women during the follicular and early luteal phases, discrete episodic or pulsatile bursts of LH occur approximately once every ninety minutes.

In prepubertal children, some investigators, but not all, have found secretory episodic bursts of LH; the pulses being of a lower amplitude than in pubertal children or adults. The pattern of pulsatility of LH release during childhood years is demonstrated in Figure 12.20. Boyar first described the predominantly sleep-associated release of LH in early and mid-puberty; only late in puberty were prominent LH pulses noted during the day which stimulated the adult pattern. In addition to episodic (ultradian) fluctuations of gonadotrophin release, a circadian rhythm with

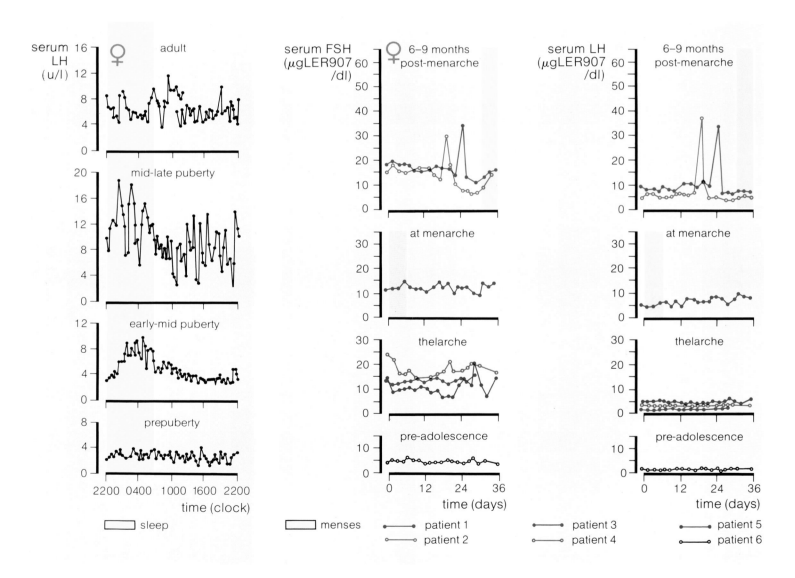

Fig. 12.20 Patterns of LH secretion during pubertal development. Episodic pulses and circadian rhythms of secretion can be seen. Redrawn from Weitzman et al. (1975), by courtesy of the publishers, Academic Press Inc.

Fig. 12.21 Serum FSH and LH concentrations in six perimenarchal girls. The evolution of cyclicity in each girl can be seen. Redrawn from Winter and Faiman (1973), by courtesy of the publishers, Williams and Wilkins Company.

nocturnal peaking develops during late childhood and adolescent years. During puberty, there is further maturation of sleep-enhanced LH secretion; this is presumably related to alterations in hypothalamic GnRH pulses that initiate increased gonadotrophin production.

The second pattern of gonadotrophin secretion is cyclic. Cyclic secretion involves positive or stimulatory feedback mechanisms. Thus an increment in circulating oestrogens to a critical level and of sufficient duration, initiates a synchronous pulsatile burst of LH and FSH (the mid-cycle surge). This surge is characteristic of the pattern in normal adult females prior to menopause. There is evidence of high spikes of gonadotrophins in several peri-menarchal patients in Figures 12.21 and 12.22. In these patients, high levels of oestradiol were associated with the gonadotrophin spikes, and in one patient there was a typical post-ovulatory rise of progesterone, suggesting the development of a corpus luteum. In normal women, the mid-cycle surge in LH and FSH secretion is attributed to the positive feedback effect of an increased, critical concentration of oestradiol for a sufficient length of time during the latter part of the follicular phase (Fig. 12.23). This stimulatory effect of oestradiol on gonadotrophin secretion has not been demonstrated in prepubertal or early pubertal girls; it is a later

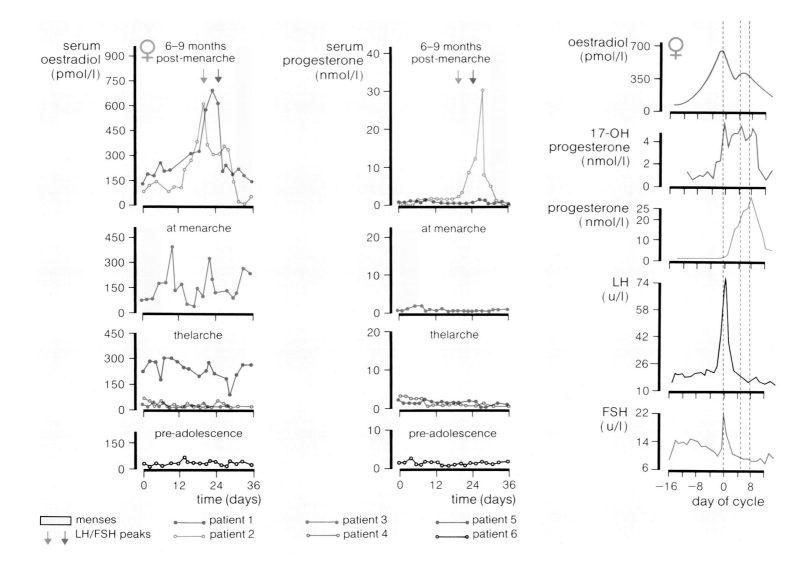

Fig. 12.22 Changes in steroid concentrations in serial samples obtained from six perimenarchal girls. The increment of serum progesterone in one of the two post-menarchal girls suggests that she had had an ovulatory cycle. Redrawn from Winter and Faiman (1973), by courtesy of the publishers, Williams and Wilkins Company.

Fig. 12.23 Graphs of serum gonado-trophin and steroid levels during the menstrual cycle of normal women.

maturational event and does not occur before mid-puberty (Fig. 12.24). In these two mid-pubertal girls, oestradiol was administered on five successive days. This was followed, when oestrogen levels were elevated, by LH spikes (in one instance to a level comparable to that seen later in an unstimulated LH burst). It appears that the development of the positive feedback action of oestradiol requires: (i) ovarian follicles primed by FSH to secrete sufficient oestradiol to reach and maintain a critical level in the

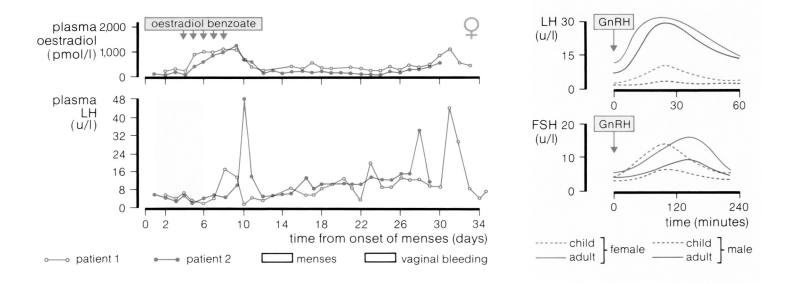

Fig. 12.24 Graph demonstrating the induction of LH secretion by exogenous oestradiol benzoate administration. Such an increment of LH is only seen in girls who are in mid-puberty or later. This represents a positive feedback mechanism.

Fig. 12.25 Graph showing the response of pituitary gonadotrophs to exogenous administration of GnRH. The maturity-related increment of LH is seen from prepubertal to pubertal levels, with a further rise during adulthood. The sex differences in GnRH-induced FSH release are also demonstrated.

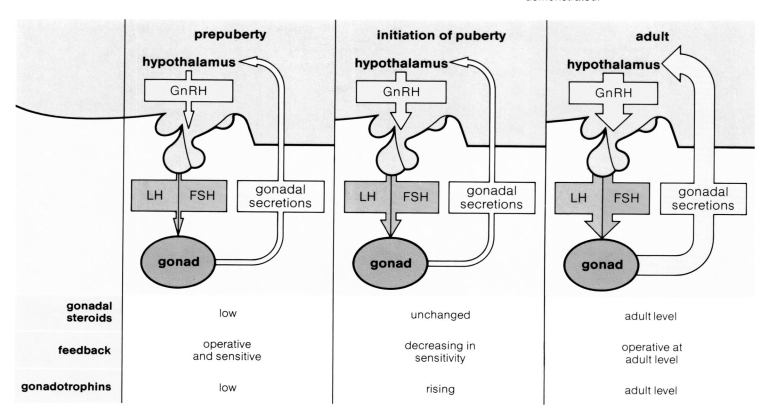

Fig. 12.26 Diagram showing the changing sensitivity to negative feedback at puberty.

12.12

circulation; (ii) a pituitary gland that is sensitised by oestrogen to amplify and augment the effect of GnRH, and which also contains a large enough pool of releasable LH to provide an LH surge and (iii) in addition to the usual adult pattern of pulsatile GnRH secretion, a sufficiently large readily-releasable pool of GnRH for the GnRH neurosecretory neurons to respond to the oestradiol stimulation with an acute increase in GnRH release.

Despite gonadotrophin cyclicity and oestrogen-induced positive feedback, by mid-puberty and prior to menarche, the positive feedback loop does not appear to be complete at that time, with consequent irregularity of ovulatory cycles. Indeed, the modulating action of the pubertal ovary and its output of oestradiol on the hypothalamo-pituitary-gonadotrophin axis appears insufficient to induce an ovulatory LH surge, even when there are adequate pituitary stores of readily-releasable LH and FSH. The ovary (from lack of sufficient gonadotrophin stimulation or decreased responsiveness) does not secrete oestradiol in a sufficient amount or duration to induce the ovulatory LH surge. Thus, during the first two years of post-menarche, as many as fifty to ninety per cent of the cycles are anovulatory, decreasing to less than twenty per cent of cycles by five years post-menarche.

Interaction of Synthetic GnRH with Gonadotrophin Secretion

If increased secretion of gonadotrophins with the approach of puberty is a consequence of a change in neural and hormonal modulation of synthesis and pulsatile secretion of GnRH, increased GnRH secretion should be followed by augmented pituitary gonadotrophin synthesis and secretion. Since GnRH secretion is not easily measured directly in humans, endogenous release can be assessed indirectly and qualitatively by the

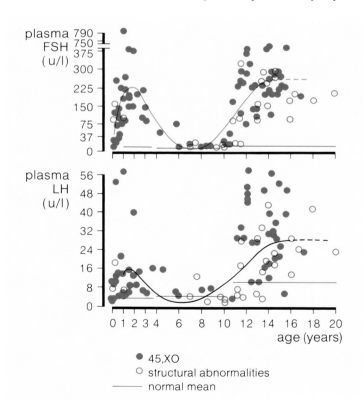

Fig. 12.27 **Graph demonstrating the diphasic pattern of LH and FSH levels in patients with gonadal dysgenesis.** The curve is a polynomial regression plot of the data. The qualitative data shown in the normal subjects are similar to that in patients with agonadism. Redrawn from Conte et al. (1975), by courtesy of the publishers, Williams and Wilkins Company.

gonadotrophin response to exogenous GnRH (Fig. 12.25). With the availability of synthetic GnRH, the pituitary sensitivity to GnRH and the dynamic reserve of pituitary gonadotrophins has been examined during different stages of pubertal maturation and in many disorders involving the hypothalamo-pituitary-gonadal axis.

The results support the concept that the prepubertal state is characterised by functional GnRH insufficiency. The release of LH following administration of GnRH is minimal in prepubertal children beyond infancy, increases strikingly during puberty and is still greater in adult males and females. Changes in maturity-related patterns of FSH release after administration of GnRH are quite different from that of LH, and result in a striking reversal of the FSH:LH ratio of gonadotrophin release. Prepubertal and pubertal females release much more FSH than males at all stages of sexual maturation. Prepubertal females have a larger dynamic reserve pool of pituitary FSH than either pubertal females or peripubertal males. Since basal levels of serum FSH and LH are similar in prepubertal children, the dramatic difference in secretion of FSH and LH evoked by GnRH administration is similar except for the heightened LH release during mid-cycle and in the luteal phase of females.

Regulation of the Onset of Puberty

In both humans and primates the increased LH and FSH secretion in the fetus and in early infancy is followed by a long period (approximately one decade) in which the reproductive endocrine system is suppressed. The factors involved in inhibiting the onset of puberty are not well understood. Two mechanisms have been invoked to explain prepubertal restraint of gonadotrophin secretion by the central nervous system: one is a sex steroid dependent mechanism, whilst the other is independent of sex steroids. The sex steroid dependent mechanism is a highly-sensitive hypothalamo-pituitary-gonadal negative feedback system (Fig. 12.26). The inhibition of hypothalamic GnRH release and lowered pituitary gonadotrophin secretion after fetal life appear to be consequences of the increasing sensitivity of the hypothalamic 'gonadostat' (probably the arcuate GnRH neurosecretory neurons) to inhibitory effects of concentrations of sex steroid. During childhood, this tonic control mechanism is exquisitely sensitive to the suppressive effects of the low levels of circulating sex steroids present in normal children. Coincident with the onset of puberty, the hypothalamic gonadostat (and possibly the pituitary gland) becomes progressively less sensitive to the inhibitory effects of sex steroids upon GnRH release. This results in the increased release of GnRH, in a pulsatile manner, and also elevated secretion of gonadotrophins. In adults, the hypothalamo-pituitary negative feedback mechanism is even less sensitive to feedback by sex steroids. There is considerable evidence for a highly-sensitive negative feedback mechanism in prepubertal children, primarily the rapid cessation of even the low level of gonadotrophin secretion in childhood upon administration of tiny amounts of sex steroids.

The sex steroid independent mechanism is ascribed to 'intrinsic' CNS inhibitory influences. Experimental data supporting such an additional mechanism are derived from studies of gonadotrophin secretion reserve in agonadal children. The diphasic pattern of basal FSH and LH secretion from infancy to adulthood (i.e. higher in the first year of life than in the next eight to ten years) is qualitatively similar in normal individuals to those in patients without gonads. In agonadal patients, however, gonadotrophin levels are much higher except during the mid-childhood nadir (Fig. 12.27). The striking fall in gonadotrophin secretion and reserve in this period indicates that CNS inhibitory influences independent of gonadal sex steroid secretion are present, and that these restrain gonadotrophin production and delay the onset of puberty. Such a pattern cannot be explained by gonadal sex steroid feedback (since functional gonads are lacking) nor by increased secretion of adrenal sex steroids (since concentrations are low and dexamethasone suppression of the adrenal does not augment serum gonadotrophin levels). The nature of this postulated intrinsic CNS inhibitory system during infancy and childhood (Fig. 12.28) is uncertain. Suppression of this neural inhibitory mechanism may lead to re-activation of gonadotrophin secretion at puberty. In patients with true precocious puberty due to hypothalamic lesions, the intrinsic CNS inhibitory system is impaired resulting in the premature appearance of the augmented, pulsatile gonadotrophin secretion characteristic of puberty.

Adrenarche or Control of Adrenal Androgenesis

The role of the adrenal component of adolescent maturation, with its characteristic prepubertal increase in adrenal androgen secretion, is not clearly understood.

A significant increment in adrenal androgen secretion by eight years of age is found in both boys and girls (see Fig. 12.19). In contrast, a progressive rise in plasma concentrations of adrenal androgens occurs during late childhood and adolescence. This correlates with the development and growth of the zona reticularis of the adrenal cortex, reaching adult levels in late adolescence (Fig. 12.29). Gonadotrophin and gonadal steroid concentrations do not begin to increase until ten to twelve years of age or approximately two years after the adrenarche. Thus, it appears that activation of the adrenal androgen secreting system (adrenarche) normally precedes activation of a hypothalamo-

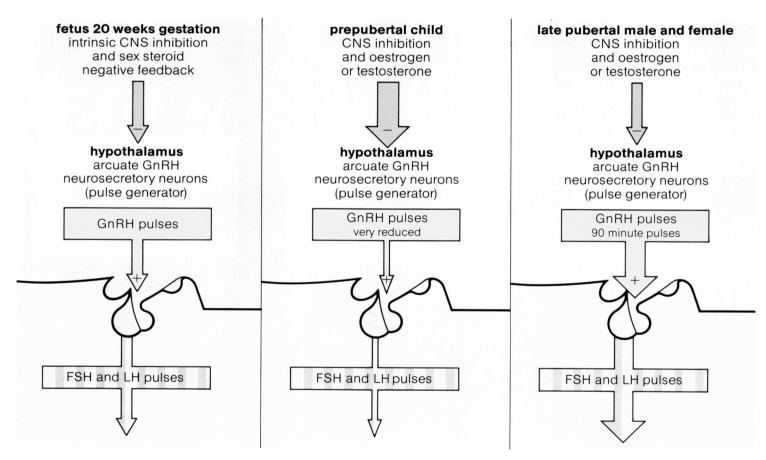

Fig. 12.28 Diagram of the ontogeny of changes in the arcuate nucleus GnRH pulse generator activity. This diagram demonstrates the hypothesis that functional GnRH insufficiency in the prepubertal child is a consequence of CNS restraint by sex steroid dependent and sex steroid independent mechanisms.

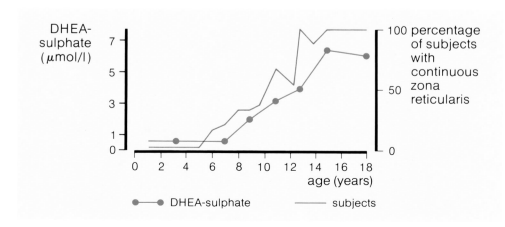

Fig. 12.29 Graph showing the change in serum DHEA-sulphate with age compared with the growth of the adrenal zona reticularis. Redrawn from Grumbach et al. (1978), by courtesy of the publishers, Academic Press Inc.

pituitary-gonadotrophin-gonadal axis (gonadarche). This temporal relationship between the adrenarche and maturation of gonadal function suggests that adrenal androgens may play an important role in regulating the onset of the gonadarche.

However, there are substantial data to indicate that the adrenarche and gonadarche are independent events, apparently controlled by separate mechanisms, and that the adrenarche is not essential for the onset of gonadarche (Fig. 12.30). The early production of adrenal androgens (as in precocious adrenarche) together with the occurrence of prepubertal children who have chronic adrenal insufficiency with deficient adrenal androgenesis, which does not interfere with the normal onset and progression of puberty, support this hypothesis. In patients with idiopathic precocious puberty, functional agonadism (e.g. gonadal dysgenesis) or isolated gonadotrophin deficiency, the

dissociation between adrenarche and gonadarche is quite apparent and further suggests the separate modulation of adrenal androgen secretion. At least three different explanations for the independence of adrenarche and gonadarche have been made: (i) intrinsic alteration in the activities of the enzymes involved in adrenal androgenesis; (ii) the secretion of an extra-pituitary stimulatory factor, such as oestrogen, and (iii) the presence of a pituitary adrenal androgen stimulating hormone, as yet uncharacterised.

The elusive adrenal androgen stimulating hormone (AASH), in the presence of adrenocorticotrophic hormone (ACTH), may induce differentiation of the zona reticularis and also synthesis and secretion of adrenal androgens and thus adrenarche, an event occurring independently of activation of the hypothalamo-pituitary-gonadal axis.

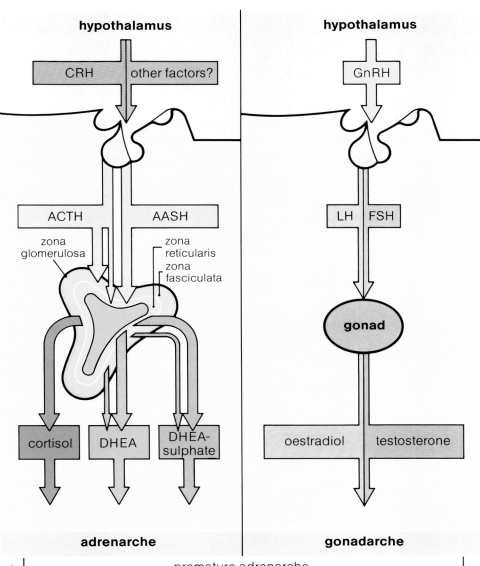

Fig. 12.30   Relationship between the adrenarche and gonadarche. Although temporally associated processes, adrenarche and gonadarche are controlled by different mechanisms with no apparent interaction. Redrawn from Grumbach (1980), by courtesy of the publishers, Hospital Practice Publishing Company Inc.

adrenarche		gonadarche
+	premature adrenarche	−
−	primary adrenal insufficiency	+
−	idiopathic precocious puberty (onset <6 years)	+
+	idiopathic precocious puberty (onset >6 years)	+
+	gonadal dysgenesis syndrome	−
+	isolated gonadotrophin deficiency	−
−	constitutional delayed adolescence	−

DISORDERS OF PUBERTAL MATURATION

Delayed adolescence occurs in twenty-five per thousand children and is thus a problem of considerable frequency. In 2.5 per cent of normal males, the onset of sexual development is delayed more than two years after the usual age of initiation, and in 0.1 per cent the delay is more than three years. Clinical experience suggests a higher incidence of delayed sexual maturation in boys than in girls. Boys should be evaluated if no sign of sexual development (testicular enlargement) has occurred by the age of fourteen years; girls should be evaluated if there is absence of breast budding at thirteen years of age.

There are many causes of delayed adolescence (Fig. 12.31). Constitutional delay in growth and development is, however, by far the most common form of delayed adolescent growth and maturation encountered. Delayed pubertal development may be associated with abnormalities of the central nervous system or those associated with the gonads. Central nervous system abnormalities lead directly or indirectly to a deficiency of GnRH production and consequently delayed production of pituitary gonadotrophins; whereas gonadal problems lead to diminished production of sex steroids.

Constitutional Delayed Adolescence

Constitutional delayed adolescence or the syndrome of familial slow growth and delayed maturation (Fig. 12.32) occurs frequently in males in whom there is a family history of delayed pubertal maturation. Such individuals may be seen either as patients being assessed for short stature during mid-childhood or for delayed sexual development in early adolescent years. Skeletal maturation is delayed, with progression through puberty slow but eventually successful. The ultimate height attained by those with constitutional delayed adolescence is normal for their family.

The clinical appearance of two brothers with constitutional delayed adolescence is shown in Figure 12.33. Both boys had significant delayed maturation and showed an extremely immature habitus. They subsequently achieved an adolescent growth spurt, reaching adult height normal for their family at the ages of twenty-three and twenty-two years.

The typical growth pattern for children with constitutional delay in growth and pubertal maturation is shown in Figure 12.34. Height is usually just below the normal range throughout most of the childhood years and a normal rate of growth is present.

The growth velocity of a child with constitutional delay either will not change at the time that his peers are having an adolescent growth spurt, or will decrease (pre-adolescent growth dip). Finally, however, the patient begins to have an increment in height at approximately fifteen years of age and, after 20cm of growth over a three-year period, has achieved a normal height of approximately 167.5cm (5'7"). The endocrinological concomitants

Causes of Delayed Adolescence

systemic disease	central nervous system	gonadal
gastrointestinal	constitutional delay	Noonan's syndrome
genitourinary	congenital anomalies e.g. craniopharyngioma	gonadal dysgenesis
cardiorespiratory	inflammatory diseases	trauma
endocrine	neoplasm	neoplasm
malnutrition	trauma	orchitis, vanishing testis syndrome
	gonadotrophin deficiency	
collagen-vascular	panhypopituitarism	errors of testosterone biosynthesis

Fig. 12.31 The differential diagnosis of the syndrome of delayed adolescence.

Characteristics of Constitutional Delayed Adolescence

familial late maturation (usually short male)
delayed bone age
slow progression through puberty
ultimate height normal for family

Fig. 12.32 Definition of the syndrome of constitutional delayed adolescence.

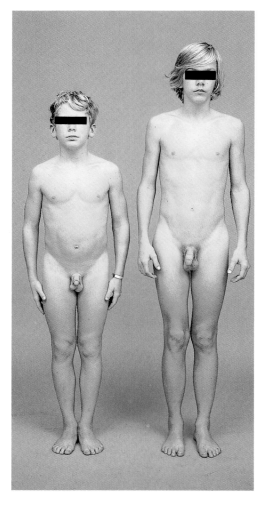

Fig. 12.33 Photograph of brothers with constitutional delayed adolescence. The brothers have chronological ages of 17 and 20 and bone ages of 13 and 15 respectively.

of this rather striking growth curve are being re-evaluated. Some children examined in mid-childhood years, have been considered to have subtle abnormalities of growth hormone (GH) secretion and have been treated with GH despite the absence of classical GH insufficiency. Whether such GH therapy will lead to a greater final adult height is unknown, but it does permit a patient to attain his adult height at a much earlier time and thus avoid many of the psychological and behavioural stresses which are faced during early teenage years.

Hypogonadotrophic Hypogonadism

Diseases which delay sexual maturation by involving the hypothalamo-pituitary axis are associated with decreased secretion of LH and FSH (i.e. hypogonadotrophic hypogonadism). Hypothalamic abnormalities may result from congenital factors (e.g. absence of GnRH, malformations, intra-uterine infections and perinatal hypoxia) or from acquired abnormalities (e.g. encephalitis, meningitis, head trauma or neoplasms). In these individuals (see Fig. 12.35) there is inadequate production and release of GnRH, leading to impaired synthesis and secretion of pituitary gonadotrophins.

In those patients in whom no obvious structural or acquired abnormality of the brain is found, the syndrome of isolated gonadotrophin deficiency, often associated with anosmia or hyposmia (Kallman's syndrome), may be present. This syndrome appears to be inherited as an autosomal dominant disorder, in which there is variable penetrance. Patients are generally tall with small testes, have minimal sexual development and exhibit a eunuchoid habitus. A large number of congenital anomalies may be associated with Kallmann's syndrome and include cleft lip and cleft palate, cryptorchidism, various skeletal defects and congenital deafness. Treatment for isolated hypogonadotrophic hypogonadism, which appears to result from a deficiency of GnRH secretion, has included the administration of testosterone, chorionic gonadotrophin and, more recently (and perhaps more logically), chronic intermittent administration of synthetic GnRH (see Chapter 10).

Noonan's Syndrome (Pseudo-Turner Syndrome)

The major clinical characteristics of Noonan's syndrome (Fig. 12.36) include short stature, a webbed neck, ptosis, delayed puberty with cryptorchidism, an abnormal facial appearance and many other features similar to those seen in patients with Turner's syndrome. Childhood Noonan's syndrome occurs with equal frequency in males and females and is an autosomal dominant inheritance. In contrast to girls with Turner's syndrome, however, cardiac abnormalities tend to be right-sided, the chest deformity is often pectus excavatum, mental retardation is frequent and the karyotype is normal.

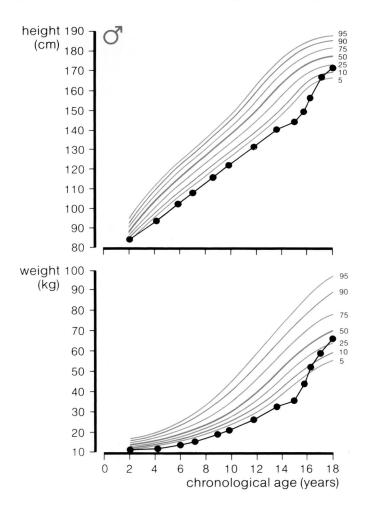

Fig. 12.34 Typical growth curve of a patient with constitutional delayed adolescence. The slow linear growth velocity in early teenage years is followed by the delayed growth spurt, thus normal adult height is finally attained, but later than normal.

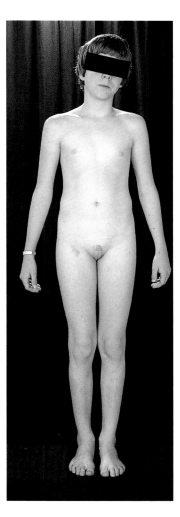

Fig. 12.35 Photograph of an adolescent male with hypogonadotrophic hypogonadism.

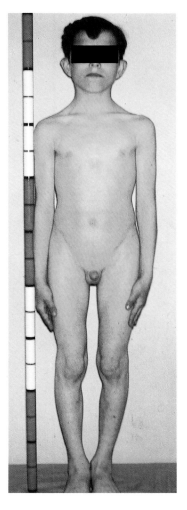

Fig. 12.36 Photograph of an adolescent male with Noonan's syndrome. The habitus resembles Turner's syndrome, with the presence of a webbed neck and short stature.

12.17

Hypopituitarism and Delayed Development

In patients with GH deficiency, there may frequently be delayed pubertal maturation (Fig. 12.37), although full pubertal development will eventually be attained without exogenous sex steroid therapy. In males, external genitalia may be remarkably small. Patients with isolated GH deficiency usually have pituitary LH and FSH secretion within the normal range when given exogenous GnRH.

Prader-Willi Syndrome

Another example of a syndrome with hypothalamic dysfunction and hypogonadotrophic hypogonadism is the Prader-Willi syndrome (Fig. 12.38). This condition is characterised by infantile hypotonia and poor fetal activity; it is often associated with neonatal failure to thrive, but with episodes of massive obesity throughout childhood. Severe mental retardation, impaired psychological maturation and characteristic facies, with almond-shaped eyes and poor dentition are often present. In addition, there may be primary failure of gonadal development.

Anorexia Nervosa

The syndrome of anorexia nervosa (Fig. 12.39) which may be a life-threatening psychiatric condition, results from major disturbances of body image and an almost incurable fear of gaining weight. The syndrome rarely occurs in males, almost always affecting adolescent and young adult women. Amenorrhoea is a uniform finding, often preceding major weight loss. In severe anorexia with starvation and hypothalamic dysfunction, life-threatening autonomic nervous system abnormalities may occur. In terms of endocrine disorders, tonic LH secretion is diminished, pulsatile LH bursts are infrequent and GnRH-induced LH release is in the hypogonadotrophic range. The aetiology of anorexia nervosa remains obscure.

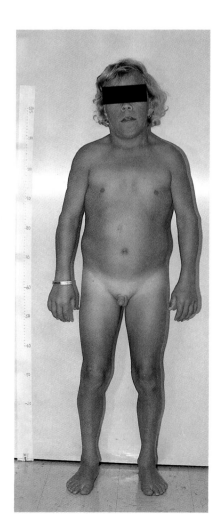

Fig. 12.37 Delayed development in a patient with growth hormone deficiency.

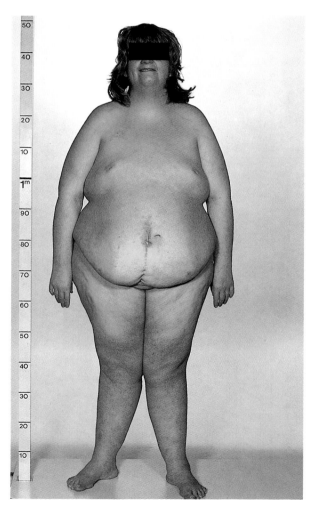

Fig. 12.38 Photograph of a patient with the Prader-Willi syndrome. Massive obesity is present.

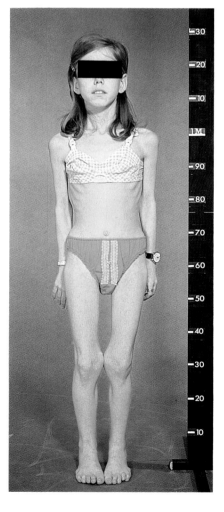

Fig. 12.39 Photograph of an adolescent female with anorexia nervosa. This life-threatening condition is commonest in young girls. By courtesy of Dr. D. Grant.

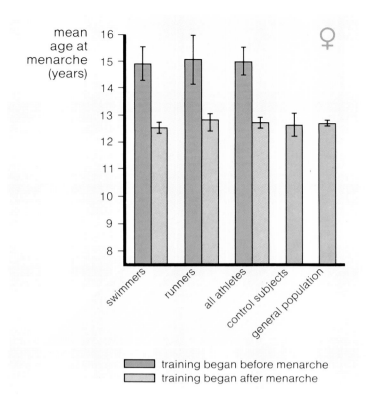

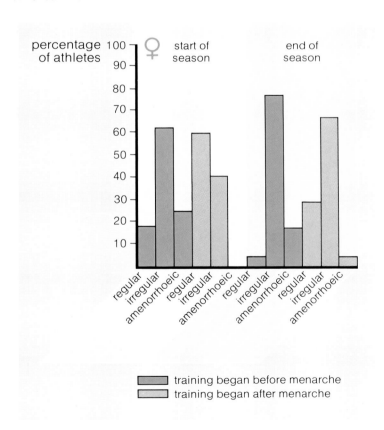

training began before menarche
training began after menarche

Fig. 12.40 Graph showing the mean menarchal age of swimmers and runners in whom training began either prior to or after menarche. These data are compared with a control population, as well as the general population. Standard errors are shown. Redrawn from Frisch et al. (1981), by courtesy of the publishers, the American Medical Association.

Menstrual Abnormalities and Excessive Energy Utilisation

Routine strenuous exercise is one of many factors which can interfere with normal human menstrual cycles. A complex relationship exists between energy utilisation, total body weight loss, diminished total body fat and menstrual dysfunction with associated reversible hypogonadotrophic hypogonadism. Frisch and her co-workers (1981) demonstrated that female athletes who had begun extensive physical training prior to menarche had a mean menarchal age of 15.1 years, contrasting with control subjects who had a menarche at 12.7 years and with a group of athletes trained after the menarche with a mean menarchal age of 12.8 years (Fig. 12.40). Menarche was delayed approximately five months for each year of training prior to menarche. At the start of the season of extensive training, only sixteen per cent of the group of athletes trained before the menarche had regular menstrual cycles, contrasting with sixty per cent of athletes trained following menarche (Fig. 12.41). Nonetheless, during the athletic season, both athletes trained before and after the menarche had an increased incidence of oligomenorrhoea or amenorrhoea. In all the female athletes there was a raised lean/fat ratio compared with normals, while their body weights were normal or increased, presumably because of a greater amount of muscle and less adipose tissue for the same amount of weight than in non-athletic women. Such data suggest the importance of body fat in affecting the hypothalamo-pituitary-gonadal axis, but does not exclude the influence of the tension and stress of training and competition.

The association of physical activity with the age of menarche extends beyond instances of women who are involved in the endurance training found in sports. As shown in Figure 12.42, menarche was remarkably delayed in young ballet dancers, occurring at a mean age of 15.4 years, significantly older than in a

training began before menarche
training began after menarche

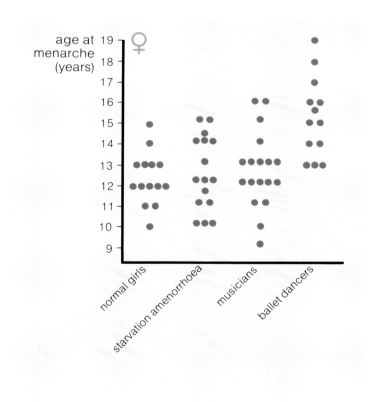

Fig. 12.41 Graph showing the influence of physical training on menstruation. The percentage of athletes with menstrual cycle disorders at the start and end of the season, with training beginning before or after menarche, is shown. Redrawn from Frisch et al. (1981), by courtesy of the American Medical Association.

Fig. 12.42 Graph showing the age of menarche in ballet dancers. The age of menarche in normal girls, in those with secondary amenorrhoea due to starvation and in a group of musicians is also shown. Redrawn from Warren (1980), by courtesy of the publishers, Williams and Wilkins Company.

group of age-matched controls, women with starvation amenorrhoea, and in a group of music students (and very similar to the athletes trained before menarche). This group of ballet dancers had a mean weight of 48 kg and were well within the range expected at menarche in normal girls. Warren suggests that these dancers, although achieving appropriate weight and body composition for several months prior to menarche, were still delayed. Factors causing the delay might include significant energy drain with concomitant tenuous nutrition occurring early in pubertal development. It is suggested that such an energy drain (in association with a diminished percentage of body fat) may have an important modulatory effect on the hypothalamo-pituitary 'set

point' at puberty, and may thus prolong the prepubertal state and delay menarche. When these same ballet dancers were examined periodically, the progress of pubertal development was significantly affected by the intensity of exercise. In the lower panel of Figure 12.43, the number of dancers with amenorrhoea was related to the amount of body fat as well as the hours of exercise per week. As can be seen, amenorrhoea increased in frequency as the hours of exercise became greater, with exaggeration in those dancers who had diminished body fat. In the upper panel, pubertal progression was markedly decreased with increase in physical exercise; when individual dancers were assessed, the progression of puberty, the onset of regular menses and the reversion of secondary amenor-

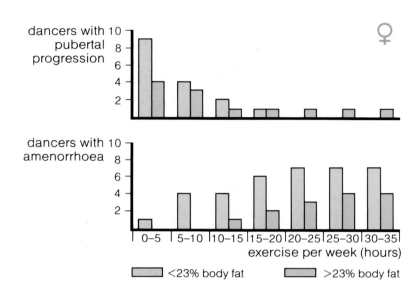

Fig. 12.43   Graph showing the relationship of exercise to pubertal progression and frequency of amenorrhoea in ballet dancers. Redrawn from Warren (1980), by courtesy of the publishers, Williams and Wilkins Company.

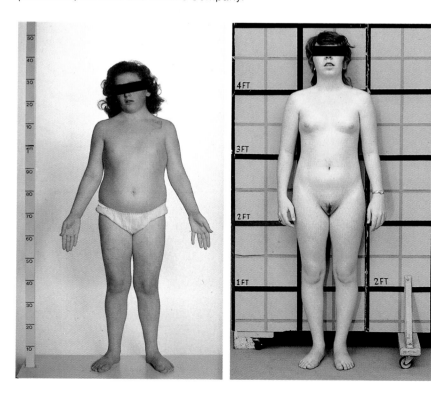

Fig. 12.44   Photographs of typical adolescent females with Turner's syndrome.

Characteristics of Turner's Syndrome

short stature
less than five feet
normal GH levels
poor response to GH therapy
intra-uterine growth retardation

sexual infantilism
dysgenetic streak-like gonads
fibrous whorls, no ova, epithelioid
  hilar cells
low oestrogen; high FSH, LH
hyper-responsive to GnRH

somatic stigmata

FACIES:
micrognathia
epicanthal folds
prominent ears
fish-like mouth
ptosis

CHEST:
broad shield-like

NECK:
short, webbed, low hairline

CARDIOVASCULAR:
coarctation of aorta
aortic valve disease
hypertension

RENAL:
rotation of kidney
horseshoe kidney
duplication/hydronephrosis

SKIN:
naevi
keloids
hypoplastic nails
lymphoedema

SKELETAL:
cubitus valgus
short 4th metacarpal/tarsal
sloping medial tibial plateau
osteoporosis
high arched palate

Fig. 12.45   Table summarising the features of the syndrome of gonadal dysgenesis (Turner's syndrome).

rhoea were frequently related to a discontinuation of energy drain – especially in dancers who had lower body fat. Weight gain alone also appeared to reverse amenorrhoea. It would appear that both total body fat and energy utilisation have significant effects upon hypothalamic production of GnRH.

Gonadal Dysgenesis: Turner's Syndrome and its Variants

Monosomy or partial monosomy of the X chromosome leads to classical Turner's syndrome, as well as to clinical variants of that syndrome. The typical subject with XO gonadal dysgenesis (Fig. 12.44) has short stature, sexual infantilism at puberty, varied somatic stigmata, streak gonads and hypergonadotrophic

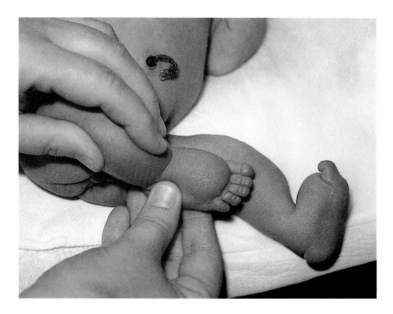

Fig. 12.46 Photograph of lymphoedema in a neonate with Turner's syndrome. This is the so-called Bonnevie-Ullrich syndrome which is most characterised by striking lymphoedema of the distal extremities.

hypogonadism. Short stature occurs invariably in patients with a 45 XO karyotype with a mean height of 142cm. Intra-uterine growth retardation is frequent and linear growth velocity is generally slow; by five years of age the patients are more than 2.5 standard deviations below the mean height for their age. The aetiology of the growth retardation is unknown.

Multiple somatic stigmata in patients with Turner's syndrome are listed in Figure 12.45. In infants, a striking phenotypic appearance of lymphoedema of the distal extremities (Fig. 12.46) and loose folds of skin over the back of the neck have been described. There is striking puffiness of the dorsum of the hands and feet, and a characteristic tightening of skin over the joints. There are multiple skeletal abnormalities, including shortening of the metacarpals, an osteoporosis similar to that seen in post-menopausal women and a wide carrying angle at the elbows.

The typical patient with Turner's syndrome has hypergonado-trophic hypogonadism. The ovaries (Fig. 12.47) are streak-like with fibrous stroma arranged in whorls, but lacking primordial follicles. Primordial follicles are present in gonads of embryos studied after spontaneous abortion. These primordial germ cells appear to degenerate in an accelerated fashion with any surviving oöcytes undergoing accelerated atresia. In longitudinal studies of patients with gonadal dysgenesis (see Fig. 12.27) extremely high gonadotrophin levels are found prior to three years of age and after eleven years of age. There is also a hyper-responsivity to GnRH administration.

In patients with partial sex chromosome monosomy (e.g. in individuals with XO/XX mosaicism), deletion of one or both arms of the X chromosome, or combinations of these, will give varied quantities of the clinical manifestations of Turner's syndrome, with variable degrees of somatic anomalies, shortness of stature and sexual infantilism.

Growth in patients with Turner's syndrome is slow and below the fifth percentile. Ultimate adult height may be variable, depending upon the chromosomal constitution, but does not exceed 153cm in those with a 45/XO karyotype. Varied

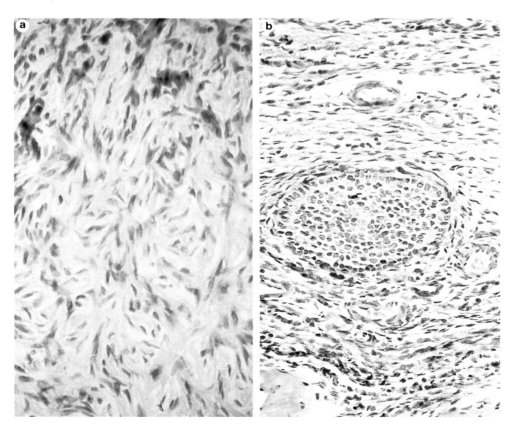

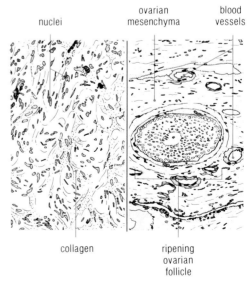

Fig. 12.47 Histological appearance of a streak gonad (a) compared with that of a normal ovary (b).

nuclei   ovarian mesenchyma   blood vessels

collagen   ripening ovarian follicle

therapeutic trials have been attempted in such patients, including the administration of androgens, GH and oestrogens. Androgen therapy does not affect the final adult height. Effects of GH treatment are not yet clear; initial trials suggest a positive response, but treatment with higher dosage and greater frequency may be needed to significantly augment final height. Finally, low-dose, early oestrogen treatment has been utilised (Fig. 12.48); the dosage of 100 ng/kg ethinyloestradiol and also a comparable dose of conjugated oestrogens have been tried. Final heights are not significantly altered. Whether low-dose oestrogen therapy together with GH therapy will be of value remains to be assessed. Breast development usually occurs immediately following oestrogen therapy; but it does not often result in substantial growth. Withdrawal bleeding usually begins within one year after the start of oestrogen therapy. Osteoporosis may be delayed or prevented. After withdrawal bleeding has occurred, medroxyprogesterone acetate (Provera) is administered between the twelfth and twenty-first day of the month to yield a physiological menstrual flow and possibly prevent endometrial hyperplasia or dysplastic changes.

Diagnostic Approach to a Patient with Delayed Puberty

Failure of pubertal development at the age of thirteen years in girls and fourteen years in boys is an indication for further assessment (Fig. 12.49). The initial history, physical examination and laboratory studies will identify patients with some form of systemic illness (e.g. malnourishment or chronic illness). Measurement of the gonadotrophins LH and FSH will differentiate between those with hypergonadotrophic hypogonadism (e.g. dysgenetic gonads, syndromes of pseudohermaphroditism, damaged gonads and inborn errors of sex steroid production) and those with hypogonadotrophic hypogonadism. CT scanning may be needed to delineate structural abnormalities. Differentiating between hypogonadotrophic hypogonadism and constitutionally delayed sexual maturation in early adolescence can be extremely difficult. Although the diagnosis will become apparent with time, this form of diagnosis is not generally acceptable. Administration of GnRH has been used in an attempt to separate the two entities in clinical trials (Fig. 12.50). However, when GnRH is administered in a single bolus, there is substantial overlap between results seen in prepubertal children and those seen in pubertal subjects and adults. Patients who have low levels of serum gonadotrophins are more difficult to assess.

GnRH-induced Gonadotrophin Release

When exogenous GnRH is administered, the readily-releasable pool of pituitary gonadotrophins may be determined (see Fig. 12.50). Prepubertal children show a small amount of LH release following GnRH treatment, with greater release in pubertal subjects and much greater secretion in adults. Large numbers of patients have been assessed and mean data in the three maturational groups differ significantly; however, the releasable gonadotrophin pools are comparable in some circumstances, thus making interpretation of a test in a specific patient occasionally difficult.

GnRH test results have been interpreted in different ways. Early suggestions were that patients with hypogonadotrophic hypogonadism with little or no responses had primary pituitary disease, while others with more LH release had hypothalamic dysfunction. More recent interpretations of the data suggest that all patients without obvious neoplasms or developmental hypoplasia of the pituitary have variable deficiencies of hypothalamic GnRH. The degree of deficiency of GnRH is reflected in the synthesis and secretion of gonadotrophins by the pituitary.

Patients with minimal to moderate GnRH deficiency demonstrate a dissociation between basal gonadotrophin secretion and that which is evoked by GnRH administration. In patients with large deficits of GnRH production, pituitary gonadotroph storage of gonadotrophins is also minimal, so the GnRH-induced releasable pool of gonadotrophins will be low or absent.

A diagrammatic representation of higher centre restraints on pubertal maturation relating to delayed adolescence is shown in Figure 12.51 (cf. Fig. 12.28). Central nervous system inhibition is exaggerated and leads to a relative or complete insufficiency of production of GnRH. Thus, gonadotrophin synthesis and secretion, gonadal development and hormone production are all diminished. In constitutional delay the central nervous inhibition is eventually decreased to a normal pubertal level, thus permitting the patient to attain normal sexual maturation.

In true, sustained hypogonadotrophic hypogonadism, either the central nervous system inhibition does not disappear or there is an intrinsic abnormality of the hypothalamic arcuate nucleus which is associated with a permanent failure to produce GnRH.

Treatment of Diminished Gonadal Function

In patients with hypergonadotrophic hypogonadism, no therapy other than sex steroid replacement is available (Fig. 12.52). This is administered either as cyclic oestrogen/progesterone treatment in females or as parenteral testosterone in males. In patients with hypogonadotrophic hypogonadism, the same sex steroid therapy may be used. A more physiological therapy for such patients would be intermittent pulsatile administration of GnRH (see Chapter 10). This is not yet used widely because of the need for pump administration. The appropriate therapy for patients with constitutional delayed adolescence is under much debate. There are significant psychosocial effects on adolescents who differ substantially from their peer group in growth and development.

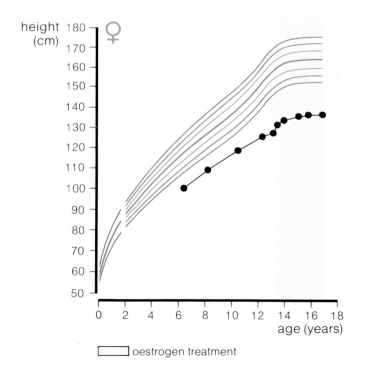

Fig. 12.48 Graph showing the response of a patient with gonadal dysgenesis to treatment with exogenous oestrogen. A slight increment in growth occurs after initiation of therapy, but this 'tails off' when a height of 140cm is reached.

Accordingly, the administration of low-dose sex steroid therapy to initiate development of secondary sexual characteristics should be considered.

In some early adolescents in whom skeletal maturation is substantially delayed, GH treatment may be reasonable. Although there is little longitudinal information on the value of GH administration to individuals who do not have classical GH insufficiency, the rapid growth which can frequently occur in such children when treated with GH may be of considerable psychological benefit to the delayed adolescent.

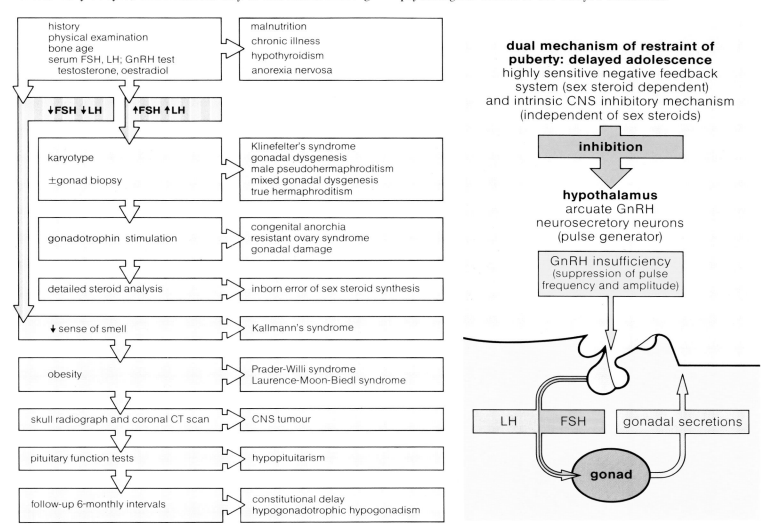

Fig. 12.49 Flow-chart of the assessment of a patient with delayed sexual maturation. The initial assessment will distinguish between patients who have systemic disorders, those with hypogonadotrophic hypogonadism and those with hypergonadotrophic hypogonadism.

Fig. 12.51 Diagram of the dual mechanism of restraint in puberty in delayed adolescence. Inhibition is great and the amount of GnRH production is small; a state of GnRH insufficiency is therefore present.

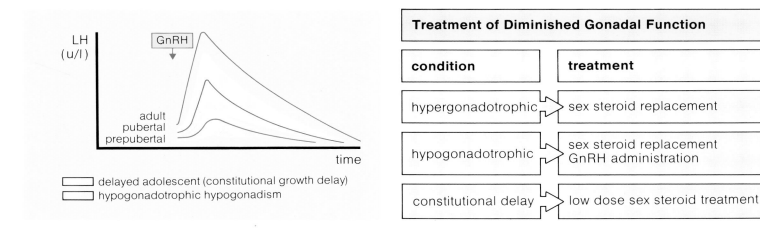

Fig. 12.50 Graph showing the response of pituitary gonadotrophs to exogenous GnRH. Patients with constitutional delayed adolescence, and those with hypogonadotrophic hypogonadism are compared with normal subjects. A substantial degree of overlap occurs between the groups.

Fig. 12.52 Flow-chart showing the treatment of hypogonadism and constitutional delayed puberty.

12.23

True Isosexual Precocious Puberty

The age at which a child is considered to have precocious puberty (in girls and in boys) has been defined as the mean pubertal age minus 2.5 standard deviations from the mean. It is based upon the appearance of testicular enlargement or pubic hair growth in the male, or breast growth or pubic hair growth in the female. This is a somewhat arbitrary definition as the incidence of 'precocious puberty' increases gradually after six years of age in both sexes. By our definition, 0.6 per cent of normal children will have evidence of pubertal development before the stated ages, thus forming a group of individuals with 'constitutional precocious puberty' which presumably has a similar mechanism to normal puberty although it occurs at an earlier age.

The differential diagnosis of isosexual precocious puberty (i.e. those in whom the development is consonant with their sex) is shown in Figure 12.53. Heterosexual precocious puberty will not be considered in this chapter. In so-called complete or true precocious puberty, there is early initiation of GnRH production by the arcuate nucleus of the hypothalamus. This is most commonly idiopathic, but can be associated with central nervous system disorders of a structural or physiological type, hypothalamic neoplasms (some of which may produce human chorionic gonadotrophin-HCG), various congenital anomalies or cysts, or brain dysfunction following infection or trauma. Incomplete precocious puberty, though yielding a result consonant with the sex of the individual, does not involve premature activation of the hypothalamo-pituitary system. Of considerable interest are the two syndromes in which it appears that intragonadal regulation of sex steroid production has become abnormal. In the male, there is a syndrome of Leydig cell hyperfunction ('testitoxicosis') and, in the female, the development of ovarian cysts which, when associated with dermatological and skeletal abnormalities, is referred to as the McCune-Albright syndrome. In addition, there are variants such as premature breast development (thelarche) and pubarche (adrenarche or premature sex hair growth) in which there is neither progression of complete sexual development, nor of any activation of the hypothalamo-pituitary-gonadal axis.

Causes of Isosexual Precocious Puberty

complete or 'true'

idiopathic: possibly raised GnRH production by the brain

structural CNS disorders

  neoplasms: possibly HCG-producing

  congenital anomalies

  cysts

  post-infection

  post-trauma

incomplete

HCG-producing neoplasms

sex-steroid producing tumours of the adrenal, ovary and testis

extragonadal androgen: congenital adrenal hyperplasia

loss of 'intragonadal regulators' leading to: Leydig cell hyperfunction ('testitoxicosis'), ovarian cysts and McCune-Albright syndrome

exogenous sex steroids

variants

precocious thelarche

precocious pubarche (adrenarche)

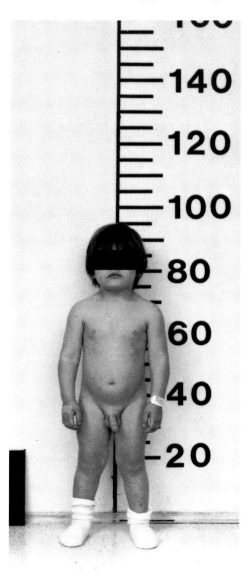

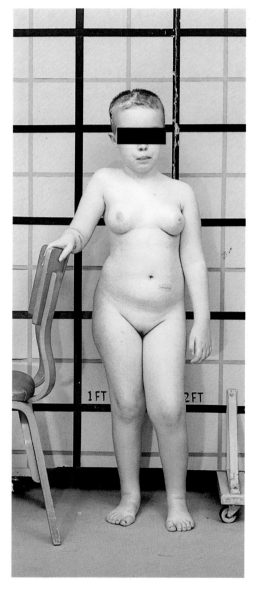

Fig. 12.53 Differential diagnosis of isosexual precocious puberty. If the sex-steroid producing tumours of the adrenal produced oestrogens in males or androgens in females, heterosexual precocity would ensue.

Fig. 12.54 Photograph of a boy with idiopathic precocious puberty. This child is four years of age.

Fig. 12.55 Photograph of a girl with precocious puberty. This premature development was caused by an intracranial cyst within the third ventricle.

A young male with idiopathic precocious puberty is shown in Figure 12.54. The accelerated height and muscle growth, the increased phallic and testicular size and the development of pubic hair and body odour are all striking and could be associated with substantial embarrassment, social difficulty and parental anxiety. Similarly, the girl with precocious puberty associated with an intracranial cyst shown in Figure 12.55, has accelerated height growth, increased skeletal maturation, adult size breast development, pubic and axillary hair growth, but is only six years of age.

The McCune-Albright syndrome (Fig. 12.56), a sporadic disorder more common in females than males, does not have any known aetiology. It is characterised by precocious puberty, large café au lait spots, and polyostotic fibrous dysplasia. The precocious puberty is associated with ovarian cysts and excessive oestrogen production. The size and function of these ovarian cysts varies considerably during the course of the disease. Of interest, is the finding that menarche may precede the appearance of all other sexual development in such patients.

In the syndrome of neurofibromatosis, tumours such as optic and hypothalamic gliomas lead, by unknown mechanisms, to increased production of hypothalamic GnRH and progressive true sexual precocity (Fig. 12.57).

In isosexual precocious puberty, activation of the hypothalamo-pituitary-gonadal axis is similar to that described for normal puberty, but occurs at a much earlier age. The dynamic status of the reproductive endocrine system in prepubertal children is demonstrated in Figures 12.58 and 12.59, showing small amounts of GnRH production, low levels of gonadotrophin secretion and small amounts of sex steroid production (cf. Fig. 12.26). In contrast, patients with precocious puberty have pubertal levels of sex steroid production, normal circulating gonadotrophin concentrations (with pubertal basal levels, episodic pulses and cyclicity), normal GnRH-induced LH release and normal pubertal results for dynamic tests of negative and positive feedback.

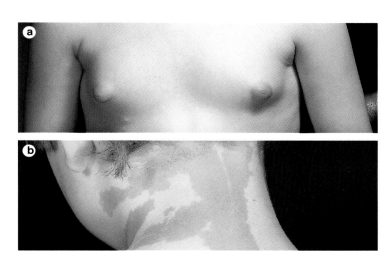

Fig. 12.56 Photographs of a girl with the McCune-Albright syndrome. Characteristic breast enlargement (a) and skin pigmentation over the neck (b) can be seen. Courtesy of Dr. P.H.W. Rayner.

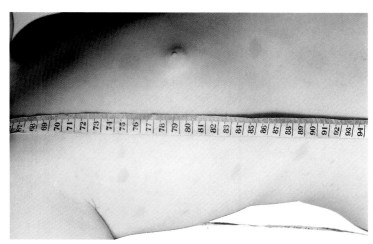

Fig. 12.57 Photograph of a girl with neurofibromatosis. Typical café au lait spots and breast enlargement are shown. Courtesy of Dr. P.H.W. Rayner.

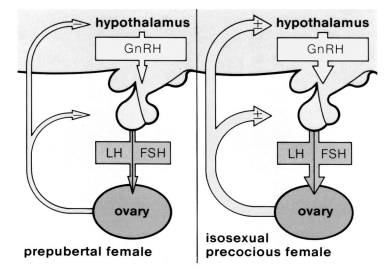

Fig. 12.58 Diagram of the hypothalamo-pituitary-gonadal axis in true precocious puberty in females.

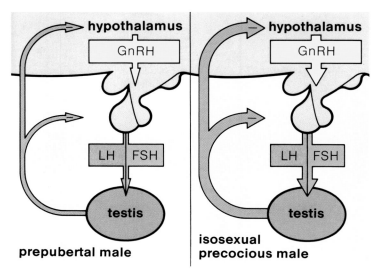

Fig. 12.59 Diagram of the hypothalamo-pituitary-gonadal axis in true precocious puberty in males.

A dual mechanism of restraint of puberty was described for normal pubertal development earlier in the chapter (see Fig. 12.28). In individuals with prepubertal chronological age, who have true sexual precocity, the negative feedback system is less sensitive than that in normal prepubertal children and approaches the pubertal level (Fig. 12.60). The intrinsic CNS inhibitory mechanisms are also diminished. The CNS restraint is therefore markedly decreased, thus permitting the arcuate nucleus of the hypothalamus to begin to synthesise and secrete hypothalamic GnRH, with increasing pulse frequency and amplitude. This then leads to the cascade of events resulting in normal, though extremely early, pubertal maturation.

Diagnosis of Precocious Puberty

A flow-chart of the diagnostic approach to the child with precocious puberty is shown in Figure 12.61. The initial history, physical examination and laboratory studies lead to clear diagnostic separations. It is of considerable importance to exclude the possibility of gonadal or adrenal neoplasms, or HCG-secreting tumours. When these possibilities have been eliminated, information is of paramount importance. If progression has been slow, there should be follow-up after several months to estimate the rate of change. Absence of progression suggests the presence of incomplete syndromes of sexual development (such as thelarche or adrenarche) whereas steady progression indicates true idiopathic precocious puberty. Diagnosis is confirmed by a pubertal response to GnRH administration and rising sex steroid levels. A CT-scan with coronal sections through the hypothalamo-pituitary area is necessary, as hypothalamic hamartomas are being found with increasing frequency. In some circumstances, these may be surgically removed.

Treatment of Precocious Puberty

The treatment of precocious puberty is varied depending upon the cause (Fig. 12.62). In those unusual patients who have gonadal or adrenal neoplasms, the treatment of sexual precocity is straight-forward (i.e. removal of the neoplasm). In circumstances in which central nervous system lesions may be treated surgically, a neurosurgeon with considerable experience should be consulted in view of potential morbidity. In patients with hypothalamic dys-germinomas (midline tumours of germ cell origin, causing precocious puberty in boys) or in individuals with optic or hypothalamic gliomas, CNS irradiation may have considerable value. The treatment of true precocious puberty without obvious

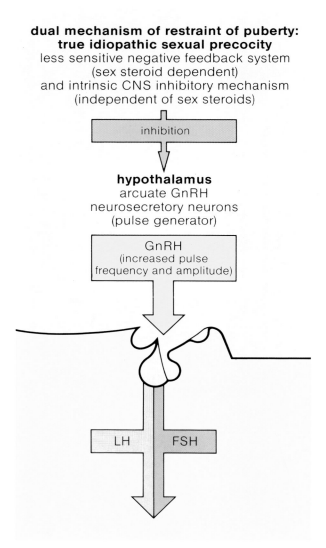

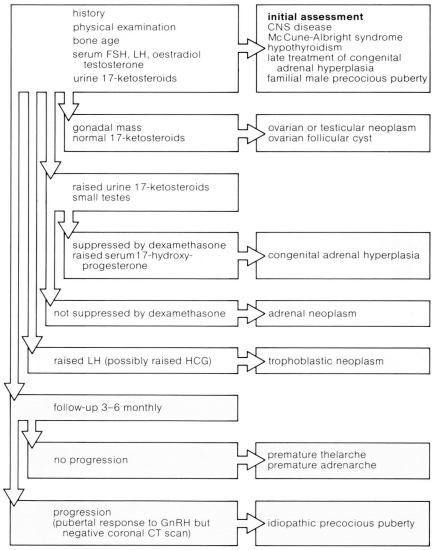

Fig. 12.60 The dual mechanism of restraint of puberty in true isosexual precocious puberty. Inhibition is diminished and GnRH production is increased.

Fig. 12.61 The differential diagnosis and assessment of children with sexual precocity. Historical data and physical examination, in conjunction with screening laboratory studies, will discriminate between steroid-producing neoplasms, other tumours, syndromes of premature thelarche and premature adrenarche and idiopathic precocious puberty.

neoplasms is aimed at suppression of gonadotrophin secretion. The most common treatment for idiopathic precocious puberty is the administration of medroxyprogesterone acetate (Provera). It is given in weekly or twice-monthly intramuscular doses of 100–200mg/m² per day. Cyproterone acetate therapy is rather more effective and works in a similar manner, but is not available in all countries. Treatment reduces basal gonadotrophin secretion as well as diminishing the readily-releasable pool of GnRH-induced gonadotrophin secretion. This gives rise to the suppression of menses and diminished breast growth in girls, and reduced testicular size and frequency of erections in boys. Improvement of facial acne and, occasionally, decreased pubic hair growth may be seen in boys. The rate of bone age maturation and rate of increased linear growth velocity are affected to varying degrees. In view of the inadequacy of standard treatments in some patients, a new agent has been used to achieve gonadotrophin suppression. Highly potent analogues of GnRH have been developed; these lower LH and FSH synthesis and secretion (Fig. 12.63). This leads to the subsequent decrease in sex steroid production and prevents accelerated epiphyseal closure, leading to diminished final adult height. The use of these potent GnRH agonist analogues was suggested after findings that continuous administration of GnRH and intermittent administration of potent agonists initially stimulate, but later diminish the release of gonadotrophins. 'Down regulation' of pituitary GnRH receptors with decreased synthesis and secretion of pituitary gonadotrophins may explain the initial stimulation and later inhibition of gonadotrophin secretion.

The effects of GnRH analogues on gonadotrophin secretion are shown in Figure 12.63. Basal LH and FSH levels are measured at twenty-minute intervals at two different four-hourly periods. The peak values are the highest gonadotrophin concentrations following a standard GnRH test in patients with idiopathic precocious puberty. Both basal and GnRH-induced LH secretion were markedly suppressed during treatment with the GnRH analogue. Currently, although long-term efficacy and risk are not clearly delineated, GnRH agonist treatment of precocious puberty would appear to be the most adequate pharmacological means of completely suppressing the hypothalamo-pituitary-gonadal axis, with concomitant slowing of skeletal maturation and growth and presumed increase in final adult height.

Fig. 12.62 Flow-chart of the treatment of various forms of precocious puberty.

Treatment of Precocious Puberty

surgical treatment for adrenal, ovarian, testicular neoplasms

CNS surgery for cysts and operable lesions

CNS irradiation for hypothalamic tumours

administration of medroxyprogesterone acetate (MPA) or a GnRH analogue to suppress LH and FSH release

Fig. 12.63 Graph showing the effects of GnRH analogue therapy upon children with precocious puberty. The basal and GnRH-induced peak LH and FSH levels prior to, during and after therapy with the GnRH analogue are shown. Redrawn from Comite (1981), by courtesy of the publishers, the New England Journal of Medicine.

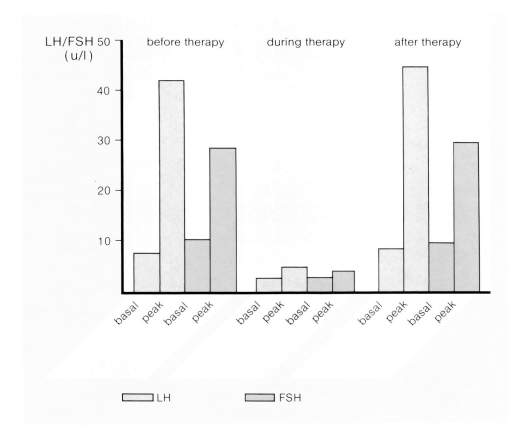

Precocious Thelarche

Premature breast development, without any other subsequent evidence of precocious sexual maturation, is referred to as precocious thelarche. The patient is typically a female infant, during her first eighteen months of life, in whom some breast tissue may have been palpable from birth. Although the disorder is self-limiting, palpable breast tissue may persist into mid-childhood, and occasionally until the process of puberty is re-initiated at the normal age. There is no acceleration of growth or bone maturation and other signs of precocious development (i.e. sexual hair or menses) do not appear. In nearly ninety per cent of such patients, precocious thelarche begins during the first year of life. In one-third of the children, breast tissue disappears by two years after onset; however, in the other two-thirds there is persistence or even further growth of breast tissue. The differential diagnosis of precocious thelarche (Fig. 12.64) mainly includes true sexual precocity, small ovarian cysts, or a large ovarian cyst or tumour. A rectal examination may reveal the presence of a large pelvic mass. Skeletal age is advanced in true sexual precocity, but not in the other entities.

Basal serum oestradiol levels will be normal or only minimally elevated in the child with premature thelarche; a finding similar to that in a child with a small ovarian cyst. Basal levels of gonadotrophins will be in the prepubertal range, other than in true sexual precocity. GnRH-induced LH secretion will also be in the prepubertal range in the patient with premature thelarche.

There is no treatment necessary for this entity and calm reassurance is most useful.

Precocious Pubarche or Adrenarche

The appearance of pubic and axillary hair prior to eight years of age in girls or nine years of age in boys without any other evidence of premature sexual development has been referred to as premature pubarche or adrenarche. It is most common in girls, particularly in the two years prior to onset of normal puberty. Otherwise, adolescent development is completely normal since the adrenarche is physiologically separable from the gonadarche.

A differential diagnosis of the syndrome of precocious adrenarche includes the true sexual precocity, congenital adrenal hyperplasia (CAH) and adrenal neoplasia (Fig. 12.65). Concentrations of DHEA-sulphate are dramatically increased in adrenal carcinoma, but only modestly in the other entities. Testosterone levels are normal in precocious adrenarche and variably elevated in congenital adrenal hyperplasia or adrenal cancer. 17-hydroxy-progesterone is most clearly elevated in congenital adrenal hyperplasia due to 21-hydroxylase deficiency. Dexamethasone suppression immediately lowers adrenal steroidogenesis in precocious adrenarche. Gonadotrophins and GnRH-induced LH release are in the prepubertal range in precocious adrenarche, strongly suggesting that there has been no activation of the hypothalamo-pituitary-gonadal axis.

	true sexual precocity	small ovarian cyst	large ovarian cyst or tumour	premature thelarche
rectal examination	negative	negative	mass	negative
bone age	advanced	normal	normal	normal
oestradiol	pubertal	slightly raised	raised	slightly raised
LH, FSH	pubertal	prepubertal	prepubertal	prepubertal
GnRH test	pubertal	prepubertal	prepubertal	prepubertal

Fig. 12.64   Table showing the differential diagnosis of the causes of premature thelarche.

	true sexual precocity	CAH	adrenal cancer	precocious adrenarche
DHEA-sulphate	slightly raised	slightly raised	raised	raised
testosterone	normal	raised	slightly raised	normal
17-hydroxyprogesterone	normal	raised	raised or slightly raised	normal
dexamethasone suppression	yes	yes	no	yes
LH, FSH	pubertal	variable	variable	prepubertal
GnRH test	pubertal	variable	variable	prepubertal

Fig. 12.65   Table showing the differential diagnosis of the causes of premature adrenarche (sex hair growth).

13 Thyroid Physiology and Hypothyroidism

W Michael G Tunbridge, MD, FRCP

The thyroid gland produces two major active thyroid hormones, thyroxine (T_4) and tri-iodothyronine (T_3). The production of these hormones within the thyroid is regulated by thyrotrophin (thyroid stimulating hormone, TSH), a glycoprotein secreted by the anterior pituitary (Fig. 13.1). In turn, the production and release of TSH is controlled by thyrotrophin releasing hormone (TRH), a tripeptide synthesised and released from the hypothalamus. Higher cerebral centres are also known to influence hypothalamic function. Circulating levels of T_4 and T_3 exert a negative feedback effect on TSH secretion via the pituitary and possibly also the hypothalamus, whereby high levels of T_4 or T_3 suppress TSH and low levels of T_4 or T_3 stimulate TSH secretion.

EMBRYOLOGICAL DEVELOPMENT OF THE THYROID GLAND

The thyroid gland develops as a pouch in the midline of the ventral aspect of the pharynx between the first and second pharyngeal pouches, towards the end of the fourth week of fetal development (Fig. 13.2). The pouch rapidly becomes bilobular, connected by a narrow hollow neck – the thyroglossal duct. The neck gradually becomes a solid stalk then atrophies, but its pharyngeal connection remains as a pit, the foramen caecum, towards the back of the tongue in adults. In contrast, the parathyroid glands develop from the third and fourth pharyngeal pouches, then move towards the posterolateral aspect of the thyroid where they are situated in adult life.

By the seventh week of fetal development the thyroid is located at the level of the developing trachea as the pharynx grows anteriorly (Fig. 13.3). The gland now has two lateral lobes connected by a narrow isthmus. Thyroid follicles develop at this stage. Cells of the ultimobranchial body are incorporated into the developing thyroid and give rise to the parafollicular or C-cells which then produce calcitonin.

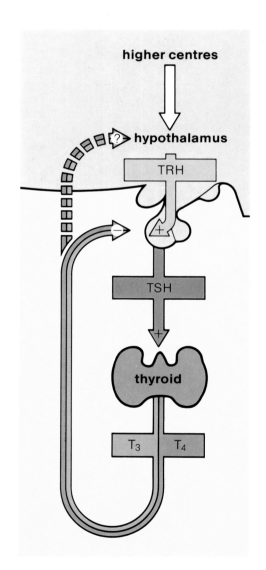

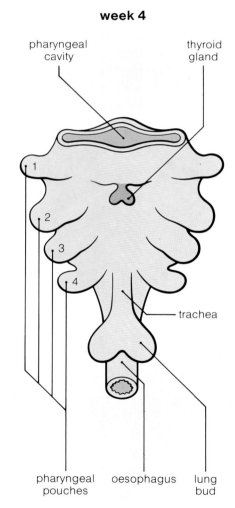

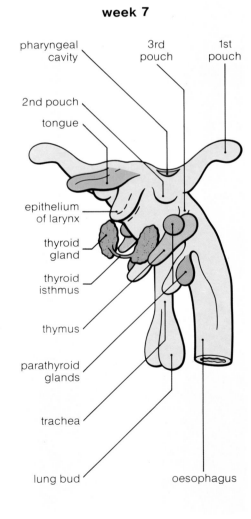

Fig. 13.1 Schematic representation of the hypothalamo-pituitary-thyroid axis. Circulating thyroid hormones exert a negative feedback effect predominantly at the pituitary level.

Fig. 13.2 Ventral aspect of the pharynx in the fourth week of fetal development. The thyroid gland develops as a pouch in the midline of the ventral aspect of the pharynx between the first and second pharyngeal pouches, towards the end of the fourth week of development.

Fig. 13.3 Representation of the developing thyroid at the seventh week of fetal life. The thyroid is recognisable at this stage as a bilobular organ connected by an isthmus.

FETAL: MATERNAL THYROID RELATIONSHIPS AT BIRTH

Between the eighth and twelfth weeks of fetal development, the thyroid and the pituitary differentiate histologically and functionally. Serum T_4 and thyroxine binding globulin (TBG) levels rise rapidly, in parallel, to plateau at term levels by the end of the second trimester. Serum T_3 levels are low, but detectable, in the third trimester and remain lower than maternal levels even at term (Fig. 13.4), probably resulting from a low peripheral conversion of T_4 to T_3. TSH is detectable at the same gestational age as circulating T_4. Levels of TSH approach term values by sixteen weeks and are higher in the fetus than in normal childhood or in maternal serum, possibly due to the low T_3 level.

CHANGES IN THYROID HORMONE LEVELS FOLLOWING BIRTH

TSH, T_4 and T_3 levels change following birth (Fig. 13.5) with a sharp rise in serum TSH, commencing with delivery, which peaks approximately thirty minutes after birth. This decreases rapidly after four hours, then more slowly over the next forty-eight hours to reach normal levels within a week of birth. Persistently high TSH values (> 50 mu/1) occur five days after birth in congenital hypothyroidism (cf. Fig. 13.21).

T_4 levels rise rapidly during the first forty-eight hours after birth with values reaching the hyperthyroid range. Levels peak between twenty-four and forty-eight hours and fall back into the normal adult range within two weeks.

T_3 levels are low at delivery and rise rapidly due to increased peripheral conversion of T_4 to T_3. Peak values occur approximately twenty-four hours after birth and then fall to normal levels over succeeding days.

THE ADULT THYROID GLAND

The normal thyroid gland in the adult consists of two conical lateral lobes joined by an isthmus which lies over the second and third tracheal rings opposite the fifth, sixth and seventh cervical vertebrae (Fig. 13.6). Ectopic thyroid tissue may be found anywhere along the line of the obliterated thyroglossal duct. Remnants of the duct may persist as isolated nests of functioning thyroid tissue, for example as a lingual thyroid, as a pyramidal lobe adjacent to the normal gland, or as non-functioning cysts.

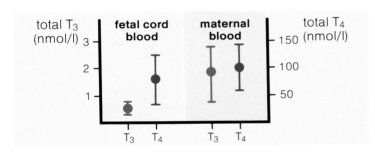

Fig. 13.4 Serum total T_3 and T_4 levels in the fetus at birth compared with maternal levels. Fetal T_3 levels tend to be low; this is probably the result of poor peripheral T_4 to T_3 conversion

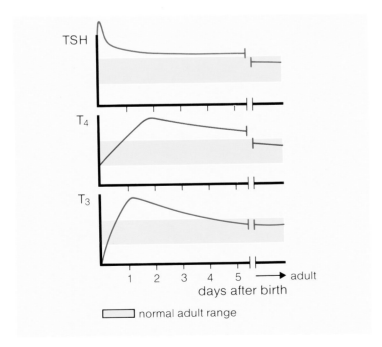

Fig. 13.5 Changes in fetal serum TSH, T_4 and T_3 levels following birth. TSH levels rise sharply at delivery to peak at thirty minutes after birth. TSH then gradually declines to reach normal values within one week of birth.

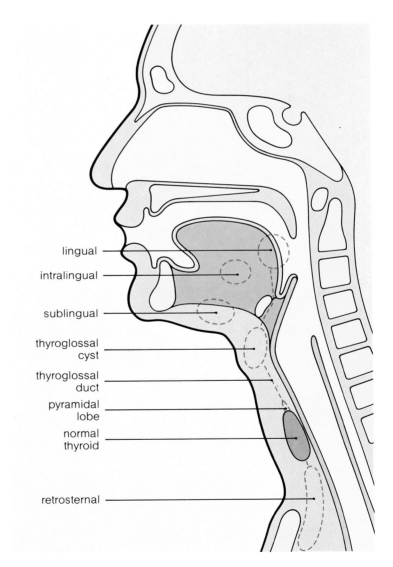

Fig. 13.6 Sites of normal and ectopic thyroid tissue along the line of the thyroglossal duct. Remnants of the duct may persist as isolated nests of functioning thyroid tissue, for example as a lingual thyroid, a pyramidal lobe or as simple thyroglossal cysts.

The thyroid gland itself consists of numerous functional units or follicles of varying size separated by connective tissue (Fig. 13.7). Each follicle is spherical and lined by epithelial cells surrounding a central colloid space. The base of each cell is adjacent to a capillary and the apex consists of microvilli pointing into the colloid.

The parafollicular or C-cells of ultimobranchial body origin secrete calcitonin. These cells are buried within the connective tissue of the gland.

THYROID HORMONE SYNTHESIS AND RELEASE

The two major active hormones produced by the thyroid are T_3 and T_4. These are synthesised from tyrosine residues in the thyroid follicles in a series of discrete steps (Fig. 13.8). They are subsequently stored in the colloid, bound to thyroglobulin, and later released from the follicular cells into the circulation.

The steps involved in thyroid hormone synthesis are: (i) iodine transport, (ii) oxidation, (iii) coupling, (iv) colloid resorption, (v) proteolysis and (vi) deiodination.

Dietary iodine is wholly absorbed from the gut and 100-200 μg are required daily. Inorganic iodide is concentrated in the follicles by active transport across the cell membrane and then rapidly transferred across the cell into the colloid lumen. During this process iodide is oxidised to iodine by peroxidase and linked to tyrosine molecules to form mono-iodotyrosines (MIT) and di-iodotyrosines (DIT) – neither of which is metabolically active.

The iodotyrosines form a large part of the thyroglobulin molecules (which are synthesised by the follicular cells and secreted into the lumen). Mono- and di-iodotyrosines linked to thyroglobulin are then coupled by further enzyme action to form the metabolically active T_3 and T_4 (Fig. 13.9) which are still linked with thyroglobulin and stored in the colloid.

The thyroglobulin-linked T_4 and T_3 are then resorbed into the follicular cells as colloid drops by the process of endocytosis.

T_4 and T_3 are subsequently separated, by proteolysis, from the thyroglobulin by lysosomes rich in proteases and peptidases.

Uncoupled mono- and di-iodotyrosines are further deiodinated to release tyrosine and iodide which may be available for recycling. Finally, T_4 and T_3 are secreted into the circulation.

Whilst T_4 is produced entirely by the thyroid, T_3 is also produced by peripheral conversion from T_4 in cells of the kidney, liver, heart, anterior pituitary and other tissues. T_4 is reduced either to the active metabolite T_3 or to a biologically inactive metabolite called reverse T_3 (Fig. 13.10). The mechanisms controlling these conversions are unclear. In healthy individuals T_4 is chiefly converted to T_3, but in severely ill people suffering from a variety of acute and chronic non-thyroid illnesses, less T_3 and more reverse T_3 is produced. T_3 and reverse T_3 are subsequently further deiodinated or conjugated into metabolically inactive compounds.

THYROID HORMONE TRANSPORT

T_4 and T_3 are largely bound to plasma proteins in the circulation. TBG has the greatest affinity for T_4 and T_3, although a small proportion of these hormones also binds to pre-albumin and to a lesser extent to albumin. Albumin has a low affinity but a large capacity for T_4 and T_3.

Measurement of circulating total thyroid hormone concentrations includes both protein-bound and free fractions of the hormones (Fig. 13.11), although the free fractions represent a tiny proportion of the total. The normal concentration of the free fraction of T_4 lies between 9–24pmol/l (0.7–1.9ng/100ml), whereas the total T_4 concentration lies between 50–140nmol/l (4–11μg/100ml). The normal concentration of free T_3 lies between 5–10pmol/l (0.33–0.65ng/100ml) and that of total T_3 between 1–3nmol/l (65–195ng/ml).

The level of free hormones governs the patient's metabolic state and thyroid status.

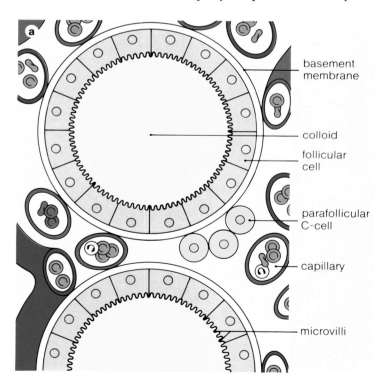

basement membrane

colloid

follicular cell

parafollicular C-cell

capillary

microvilli

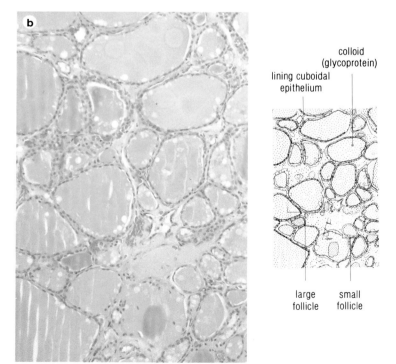

colloid (glycoprotein)

lining cuboidal epithelium

large follicle

small follicle

Fig. 13.7 Structure of the thyroid follicle. View (a) is a schematic representation of a high power view of thyroid follicles, showing their relationship with capillaries and parafollicular C-cells. The histology of normal thyroid tissue is shown in view (b). Thyroid follicles of variable sizes can be seen. They contain colloid and are lined by cuboidal epithelium. Haematoxylin and eosin stain, magnification X 120. By courtesy of Prof. I Doniach.

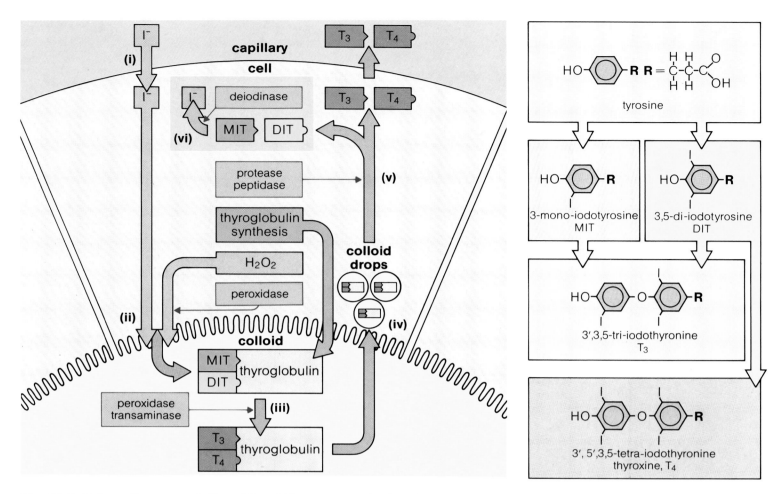

Fig. 13.8 Schematic representation of thyroid hormone synthesis and release in a single cell of a thyroid follicle. The six major stages in the biosynthesis and release of thyroid hormones, namely (i) iodine transport, (ii) oxidation, (iii) coupling, (iv) colloid resorption, (v) proteolysis and (vi) deiodination are shown.

Fig. 13.9 Biosynthesis of iodotyrosines and iodothyronines from tyrosine.

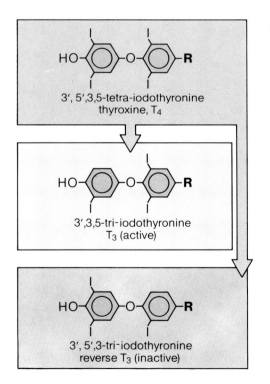

Fig. 13.10 Reduction of thyroxine to tri-iodothyronine (T₃) or its inactive metabolite reverse T₃ (rT₃). The conversion of T₄ to rT₃ occurs during acute or chronic illness such as severe infection and starvation.

Thyroid Hormone Transport

	percentage distribution		plasma concentration	
	T₄	**T₃**	**T₄**	**T₃**
free hormone	0.015	0.5	9–24 pmol/l	5–10 pmol/l
thyroxine binding globulin (TBG)	70	77	–	–
thyroxine binding pre-albumin (TBPA)	10	8	–	–
albumin	20	15	–	–
total hormone	100	100	50–140 nmol/l	1–3 nmol/l

Fig. 13.11 Thyroid hormone transport. Nearly all T₄ and T₃ (>99%) is transported in a bound state – predominantly bound to TBG, but to a lesser extent to TBPA and albumin.

MEASUREMENT OF THYROID HORMONES

Direct Methods

Direct assays of free T_4 and of free T_3 are now available (Fig. 13.12) and are useful in the assessment of a patient's thyroid status. Free thyroid hormone levels should not be affected by the concentration of normal thyroid hormone binding proteins.

Assays of total T_4 and total T_3 concentrations are widely used in clinical practice. They are a valid reflection of a patient's thyroid status in most cases, but are influenced by thyroid hormone binding protein concentrations which may lead to anomalous results.

Protein bound iodine (PBI) reflects that part of total serum iodine which is precipitated with serum proteins. Most of the organic iodine is in the form of T_4. Abnormal iodoproteins and large quantities of inorganic iodide will lead to artifically high PBI values. For these reasons the measurement of PBI, although simple, cheap and accurate, has largely been superseded.

Direct measurement of TBG enables altered TBG states to be identified. Anomalous total T_4 levels may be 'corrected' by deriving a T_4:TBG ratio.

Indirect Methods

Indirect methods of thyroid hormone estimations are also used (Fig. 13.13). In thyroid hormone binding tests, the patient's serum is incubated with an excess of ^{125}I-labelled T_3 which occupies binding sites on the thyroid hormone binding proteins, mainly TBG not already occupied by T_4, whilst the remainder is left in solution. The bound and free fractions are separated by addition of a resin or Sephadex. The proportion of free to bound ^{125}I-T_3 is determined by the residual binding capacity of thyroid hormone binding proteins and is inversely related to the total T_4 concentration. The results are related to a standard reference serum and are reported as a ratio.

Some methods, indeed most resin uptake tests, are a measure of the radioactivity in the free fraction, whereas others reflect the protein bound radioactivity (e.g. the Sephadex uptake test). Thus confusion can occur if the method used is not clearly stated. If the free fraction is measured, the ratio of the radioactivity in the test serum to that in the control is increased in hyperthyroidism and decreased in hypothyroidism. If the bound fraction is measured, the ratio is decreased in hyperthyroidism and increased in hypothyroidism.

Thyroid hormone binding tests are often wrongly and misleadingly referred to as 'T_3 tests'. They utilise ^{125}I-T_3 but are not a measure of total or free T_3. They are an indirect measure of TBG capacity and allow adjustment of total T_4 concentrations in altered TBG status.

The free thyroxine index (FTI) is calculated from the results of a total T_4 estimation and a thyroid hormone binding test. Depending upon the method used for the thyroid hormone binding test, the calculation is as shown in Figure 13.13.

The FTI gives a value for T_4 which is corrected for alterations in TBG capacity and is of particular value in subjects taking oral contraceptive therapy, in pregnancy and in hypoproteinaemic states. The FTI is widely used for these reasons, but it involves the use of two tests and therefore may be superseded by the advent of a direct free thyroid hormone assay.

A summary of thyroid hormone concentrations and distribution is shown in Figures 13.14 and 13.15.

Changes in the concentration of binding proteins will therefore have dramatic effects on the total T_4 levels. The effect of increased and decreased TBG concentration on the total T_4 levels is shown in Figure 13.15. Drugs may also bind onto thyroid hormone binding proteins and may interfere with the estimation of thyroid function. The causes of increased and decreased TBG capacity are summarised in Figure 13.16. It should be noted that, although alteration in the concentration of serum proteins or in their residual binding capacity will affect total thyroid hormone levels (e.g. by competitive binding from drugs such as phenytoin), free hormone levels are not usually affected.

Increased TBG capacity will produce falsely elevated total T_4 and T_3 levels in euthyroid patients. Decreased TBG capacity will produce false low T_4 and T_3 levels in euthyroid patients. These may be corrected by using the T_4:TBG ratio or by deriving the FTI.

Measurement of Thyroid Hormones

direct methods

circulating levels of free hormones

free thyroxine (fT_4)

free tri-iodothyronine (fT_3)

circulating levels of total hormones

total thyroxine (T_4)

total tri-iodothyronine (T_3)

protein bound iodine (PBI)

thyroid hormone binding proteins

thyroxine binding globulin (TBG)

Fig. 13.12 Table of the direct methods of measurement of thyroid hormones.

Measurement of Thyroid Hormones

indirect methods

thyroid hormone binding tests

free thyroxine index (FTI)

$$FTI = \frac{T_4 \times \text{resin uptake ratio}}{100}$$

or

$$FTI = \frac{T_4 \times 100}{\text{Sephadex uptake ratio}}$$

Fig. 13.13 Table of the indirect methods of measurement of thyroid hormones.

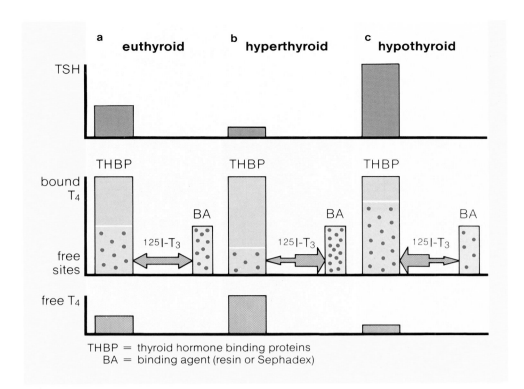

a **euthyroid** b **hyperthyroid** c **hypothyroid**

THBP = thyroid hormone binding proteins
BA = binding agent (resin or Sephadex)

Fig. 13.14 Thyroid function tests in various states. The distribution of isotope between binding agents (resin or Sephadex) and the free sites on thyroid hormone binding proteins is shown.
(a) In the euthyroid state, levels of free T_4, total T_4 and TSH are within the normal range. Using indirect testing, ^{125}I-T_3 attached to a binding agent (BA), normally resin or Sephadex, competes for free binding sites on the thyroid hormone binding proteins (THBP), mainly TBG, and competition between BA and THBP is approximately even.
(b) In the hyperthyroid state, levels of free T_4 and total T_4 are increased but TSH levels are suppressed. On indirect testing, few binding sites are unoccupied on THBP and most ^{125}I-T_3 remains attached to the binding agent.
(c) In primary hypothyroidism, levels of free T_4 and total T_4 are low but TSH is increased. On indirect testing, many binding sites are unoccupied on THBP and will therefore take up ^{125}I-T_3 leaving only a small quantity on the BA.

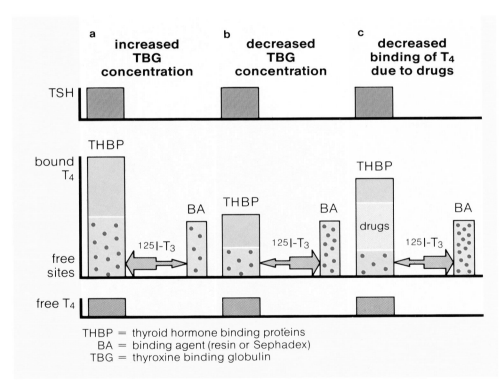

a **increased TBG concentration** b **decreased TBG concentration** c **decreased binding of T_4 due to drugs**

THBP = thyroid hormone binding proteins
BA = binding agent (resin or Sephadex)
TBG = thyroxine binding globulin

Fig. 13.15 Thyroid function tests: the effects of alteration to binding proteins. The distribution of isotope between binding agents (resin or Sephadex) and free sites on thyroid hormone binding proteins is shown. In the euthyroid state free T_4 and TSH levels are normal, but alterations in TBG concentration or capacity will affect total T_4 levels.
(a) Increased TBG concentration increases total T_4 levels. The number of free binding sites is also increased and these avidly take up ^{125}I-T_3 (as in hypothyroidism).
(b) Decreased TBG concentration decreases total T_4 levels. There are also fewer free binding sites so most ^{125}I-T_3 remains attached to the binding agent (as in hyperthyroidism).
(c) Drugs (e.g. phenytoin) compete for binding sites on THBP, thus levels of total T_4 are low. There are also only a few free binding sites on THBP so ^{125}I-T_3 remains mainly attached to the BA (as in hyperthyroidism).

Causes of Altered TBG Capacity

Fig. 13.16 Table of the causes of altered TBG capacity. Several factors can both increase or decrease TBG levels.

increased
pregnancy
oestrogens
oral contraceptives
myxoedema
genetic TBG excess
drugs e.g. phenothiazines,
  clofibrate

decreased
severe hypoproteinaemia
  e.g. nephrotic syndrome
malnutrition
severe illness
thyrotoxicosis
genetic TBG deficiency
drugs e.g. anabolic steroids,
  phenytoin, phenylbutazone

DYNAMIC TESTS OF THYROID FUNCTION

One dynamic test of thyroid function in clinical practice is that of radionuclide uptake using ^{123}I, or ^{99m}Tc (see Fig. 13.17). The proportion of a known tracer dose of such radionuclides present in the thyroid after a given time can be used as a marker test of thyroid function. The uptake is affected by the patient's iodine state and by disorders of iodide trapping. Radioiodine uptake is increased in hyperthyroidism and decreased in hypothyroidism, but discrimination between normal and mildly disturbed thyroid function is poor. ^{123}I has a shorter half life than ^{131}I and permits less exposure to radioactivity; the test is also quicker. Technetium is trapped but not organified by the thyroid and is therefore often used instead of radioiodine to provide a rapid assessment of thyroid function in suspected hyperthyroidism. It has no value, however, in discriminating between hypothyroid and normal thyroid states.

Radioiodine uptake tests have been largely superseded by more precise direct hormone assays; however, they are still used in combination with thyroid scanners to provide a map of the thyroid. Scans are particularly useful when delineating areas of active and inactive tissue in the investigation of nodular goitre.

The T$_3$ suppression test has been used to demonstrate thyroid autonomy. A radioiodine uptake test is repeated after the patient has taken a suppressive dose of T$_3$ (at least $20\,\mu$g three times daily for a week). In normal individuals radioiodine uptake is suppressed to at least fifty per cent of the pretreatment value. Failure of suppression occurs in thyrotoxicosis and patients with autonomous 'hot' nodules. The test is seldom necessary and the addition of T$_3$ can be dangerous to patients who are already hyperthyroid. The TSH stimulation test involves the administration of pharmacological doses of TSH (10 iu intramuscularly, daily for three days) followed by a radioiodine uptake test. This test is also seldom necessary as it has been superseded by more sensitive direct measures of thyroid failure such as TSH estimation. However, it may occasionally be useful for demonstrating the presence of suppressed thyroid tissue.

TESTS OF THE THYROID-PITUITARY AXIS

There are currently two tests of the thyroid-pituitary axis in use. One is the measurement of basal serum TSH levels, the other is a measure of the serum TSH response to exogenous TRH. A summary graph of basal TSH values and the TSH response to TRH is shown in Figure 13.18.

Basal TSH Estimation

The lower limit of detection of serum TSH in most radioimmunoassays is 0.5 mu/l. The range of basal TSH in the normal healthy population is 0 – 6 mu/l with a median of approximately 2 mu/l. Basal TSH is usually suppressed in hyperthyroidism but poor assay discrimination in conventional TSH radioimmunoassay between low normal and subnormal values means that there is little value in estimating serum TSH in suspected hyperthyroidism. New highly-sensitive TSH assays may, however, allow discrimination between suppressed and normal values, since TSH is a sensitive indicator of primary thyroid failure. Values above 6 mu/l are indicative of some degree of thyroid failure and in severe hypothyroidism values may be in the range 10–100 mu/l or higher. A normal TSH value excludes primary hypothyroidism provided that the hypothalamo-pituitary axis is intact.

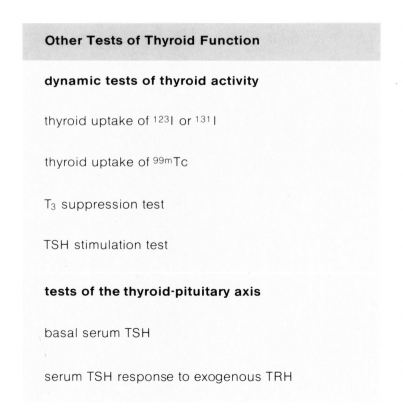

Other Tests of Thyroid Function

dynamic tests of thyroid activity

thyroid uptake of ^{123}I or ^{131}I

thyroid uptake of ^{99m}Tc

T$_3$ suppression test

TSH stimulation test

tests of the thyroid-pituitary axis

basal serum TSH

serum TSH response to exogenous TRH

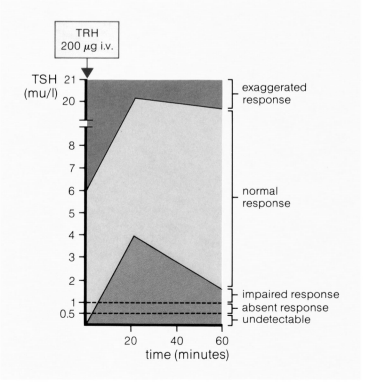

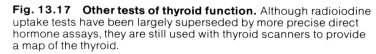

Fig. 13.17 Other tests of thyroid function. Although radioiodine uptake tests have been largely superseded by more precise direct hormone assays, they are still used with thyroid scanners to provide a map of the thyroid.

Fig. 13.18 The TSH response to TRH. An impaired TSH response to TRH is found in hyperthyroidism, whilst in hypothyroidism an exaggerated response to TRH is characteristic.

The TRH Test

Exogenous TRH, given intravenously in a pharmacological dose of 200 μg, induces a rise in TSH which peaks approximately twenty minutes later then declines, but not to basal levels, by sixty minutes in normal subjects.

The peak TSH response to TRH is proportional to basal TSH. In hypothyroid subjects the basal TSH is elevated and the TSH response is exaggerated. However, it is seldom necessary to perform a TRH test in the diagnosis of hypothyroidism.

In hyperthyroidism the TSH response to TRH is suppressed. Absent response to TRH may also be found in certain patients with nodular goitre who are otherwise euthyroid and in patients with ophthalmic Graves' disease who are not toxic. An absent TSH response is thus consistent with, but not diagnostic of, hyperthyroidism. A normal TSH response to TRH excludes hyperthyroidism and this is the main value of the test. Thyroid autonomy may result in a flat TSH response to TRH but the correlation with the T_3 suppression test is not so close as might be expected, perhaps because the two tests measure different aspects of the thyroid-pituitary axis.

CAUSES OF HYPOTHYROIDISM

Iodine deficiency is the commonest cause of hypothyroidism and goitre worldwide. However, in non iodine-deficient areas auto-immunity is the commonest cause of hypothyroidism (Fig 13.19), but destructive therapy by surgery or radioiodine for thyrotoxicosis accounts for approximately one third of all cases. Excessive iodine (e.g. as a result of chronic ingestion of proprietary cough medicines) may also cause hypothyroidism. Primary hypo-thyroidism due to failure of the thyroid gland itself is much more common than failure secondary to pituitary or tertiary hypo-thyroidism due to hypothalamic disease. The effects of iodine on the thyroid gland are multiple and complex (Fig. 13.20).

Chronic iodine deficiency, caused by reduction of dietary iodine intake below the minimum daily requirement, leads to a reduced thyroid hormone production and a compensatory increase in TSH secretion. There is preferential secretion of T_3 rather than T_4. The frequency of goitre and severity of hypothyroidism is related to the degree of iodine deficiency. In moderate endemic areas with urinary iodide excretion between 25–50 μg/g creatinine, the prevalence of goitre is twenty to fifty per cent. In areas with urinary iodide less than 25 μg/g creatinine, goitre prevalence may be greater than fifty per cent, but not all individuals in such communities are necessarily hypothyroid.

In excess iodine exposure, an acute increase in intracellular iodine concentration in normal glands interferes with iodination and temporarily inhibits thyroid hormone synthesis and release. The gland subsequently escapes from this effect, perhaps by a reduction in the affinity of the iodide trap. Use has been made of this effect in preparing thyrotoxic patients for surgery by administration of iodide solution for several days prior to operation.

The introduction of iodine therapy in areas of iodine deficiency has led to an increase in the frequency of thyrotoxicosis (Jod-Basedow phenomenon) perhaps by unmasking thyroid abnormalities previously protected from exposure by iodine deficiency. The phenomenon has also been reported to occur sporadically in patients given large doses of iodine (e.g. radiographic contrast media) in non-endemic areas.

Prolonged iodide ingestion (e.g. from proprietary cough medicines containing iodine) may lead to goitre formation and hypothyroidism in individuals with an underlying abnormality of thyroid hormone synthesis. Congenital goitre and hypothyroidism may also be produced by maternal ingestion of excess iodides.

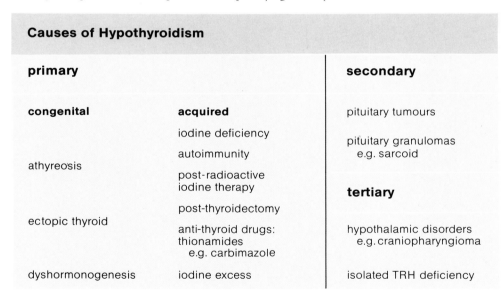

Causes of Hypothyroidism

primary		secondary
congenital	**acquired**	pituitary tumours
	iodine deficiency	pituitary granulomas
	autoimmunity	e.g. sarcoid
athyreosis	post-radioactive iodine therapy	**tertiary**
	post-thyroidectomy	
ectopic thyroid	anti-thyroid drugs: thionamides e.g. carbimazole	hypothalamic disorders e.g. craniopharyngioma
dyshormonogenesis	iodine excess	isolated TRH deficiency

Fig. 13.19 Causes of hypothyroidism. These can be broadly classified into 'congenital' and 'acquired' categories.

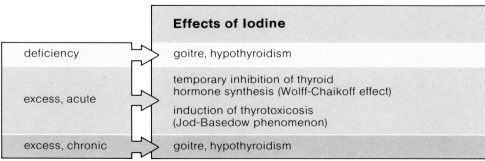

Effects of Iodine

deficiency	goitre, hypothyroidism
excess, acute	temporary inhibition of thyroid hormone synthesis (Wolff-Chaikoff effect)
	induction of thyrotoxicosis (Jod-Basedow phenomenon)
excess, chronic	goitre, hypothyroidism

Fig. 13.20 Various effects of iodine on thyroid function. Whereas iodine deficiency will lead to goitre formation and hypo-thyroidism, iodine excess can temporarily inhibit thyroid hormone synthesis (Wolff-Chaikoff effect) or induce thyrotoxicosis (Jod-Basedow phenomenon). Chronic iodine excess can also cause goitre formation and hypothyroidism.

13.9

CONGENITAL HYPOTHYROIDISM

The incidence of congenital hypothyroidism in non iodine-deficient areas in Europe and North America is approximately 1 in 4,000 live births. The condition usually results from absence of the thyroid or an ectopic thyroid, but is not widely recognisable clinically at birth. If not recognised and treated in the early stages, it leads to retarded physical and mental development.

Congenital hypothyroidism may be detected biochemically by screening all neonates five days after birth (Fig. 13.21). Persistent elevation of serum TSH at this stage will reveal hypothyroidism due to primary thyroid failure, but measurement of TSH will not detect the rare patient with hypothyroidism secondary to pituitary-hypothalamic disease. Low T_4 levels at this stage will also reveal secondary hypothyroidism, but false low T_4 levels may be found in premature infants and misleading normal T_4 levels may occur with ectopic thyroids. Replacement thyroxine therapy should be commenced as soon as high TSH levels are detected.

ACQUIRED HYPOTHYROIDISM

In non iodine-deficient communities primary hypothyroidism is ten times more common in women than in men. The prevalence in women of all ages is two per cent of the population (with one third of these cases presenting with iatrogenic hypothyroidism). The annual incidence of primary hypothyroidism in women of all ages is two per thousand population. It is most common in middle-aged women, but can occur at any age.

The incidence of hypothyroidism following radioiodine therapy is highest during the first year after treatment, regardless of the dose of ^{131}I, but continues to accumulate slowly and may reach fifty per cent after ten years (Fig. 13.22). The incidence of hypothyroidism after partial thyroidectomy, whilst less than that after radioiodine treatment, is also cumulative and may reach twenty-five to thirty-five per cent after ten years. Hypothyroidism secondary to destructive therapy to the thyroid accounts for approximately one third of all cases of hypothyroidism in the general population.

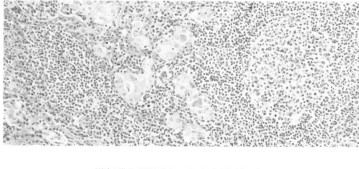

Congenital Hypothyroidism		
TSH screening	1: ≃ 4,000 live births	
T_4 screening	1: ≃ 8,000 live births	
	T_4	**TSH**
false positive	prematurity low TBG laboratory error	laboratory error
false negative	ectopic thyroid laboratory error	hypopituitarism laboratory error
recall rate	>1%	≃0.1%

Fig. 13.21 Incidence of congenital hypothyroidism using TSH or T₄ for screening. Neonates are screened five days after birth.

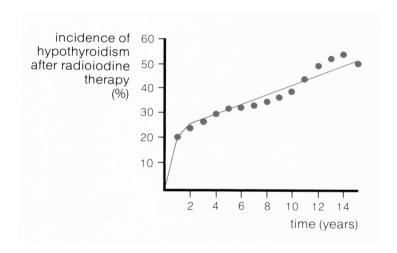

Fig. 13.22 Cumulative incidence of hypothyroidism after radioiodine therapy for thyrotoxicosis.

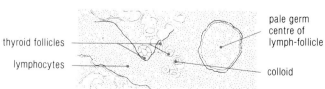

thyroid follicles
lymphocytes
pale germ centre of lymph-follicle
colloid

Fig. 13.23 Histological appearance of the thyroid in a patient with Hashimoto's thyroiditis. The parenchyma (comprising colloid-containing follicles) is almost totally replaced by oxyphil cells (Askenazy cell change). On the right of the field shown, a lymph-follicle containing a large, pale, germ centre can be seen. Haematoxylin and eosin stain, magnification X 80.

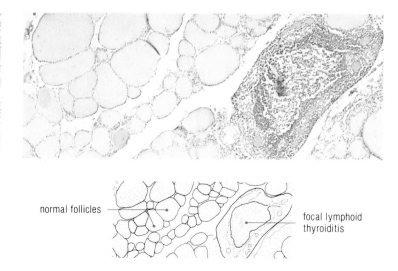

normal follicles
focal lymphoid thyroiditis

Fig. 13.24 Focal lymphoid thyroiditis. In this condition most of the thyroid follicles are normal, but focal lymphoid infiltration is seen. The follicles lie separately in a diffuse mass. Haematoxylin and eosin stain, magnification X 30.

AUTOIMMUNE THYROID DISEASE AND HASHIMOTO'S THYROIDITIS

The term 'Hashimoto's thyroiditis' is probably best reserved for the patient with a large multinodular goitre and evidence of an autoimmune process. Circulating thyroid auto-antibodies are strongly positive. Histological examination of the thyroid shows diffuse lymphocytic infiltration, lymphoid follicles with germinal centres, and Askenazy cell change in the remnants of thyroid follicles (Fig. 13.23).

Focal lymphoid thyroiditis (Fig. 13.24) with normal follicles is a common finding at autopsy in patients without evidence of clinical thyroid disease during life. Such histological changes have been shown to correlate with the presence of thyroid antibodies in the circulation. Many patients with thyroid antibodies, whilst asymptomatic, can be shown to have minor biochemical disturbances of thyroid function characterised by mild or moderately elevated TSH levels, whilst the serum T4 is in the normal range. This is called subclinical hypothyroidism.

Thyroid microsomal and thyroglobulin antibodies are more common in women than in men at all ages and are most common in postmenopausal women (Fig. 13.25). Raised TSH values show a similar age and sex distribution and there is a close correlation with thyroid antibodies.

Patients with thyroid antibodies may maintain normal thyroid function for their lifetime. However, approximately fifty per cent of people with thyroid antibodies also have raised TSH levels and such patients progress to overt hypothyroidism at the rate of approximately five per cent per annum. Prophylactic thyroxine replacement therapy merits consideration in individuals with evidence of underlying autoimmune thyroiditis and subclinical hypothyroidism.

SEVERE HYPOTHYROIDISM

In severe primary hypothyroidism patients have thickened, dry, flaking skin – termed myxoedema (Fig. 13.26). The histology of the thyroid in a patient with severe myxoedema is shown in Figure 13.27. The thyroid is replaced with fibrous tissue, there is minimal lymphocytic infiltration and few follicles remain. This process is believed to be the end result of an autoimmune destructive process in most cases.

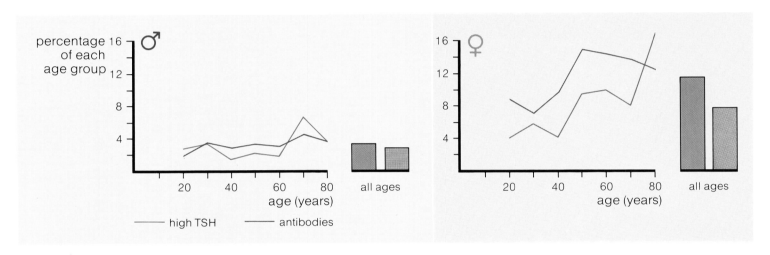

Fig. 13.25 Prevalence of thyroid antibodies and raised TSH in a cross-section of a population in North East England.

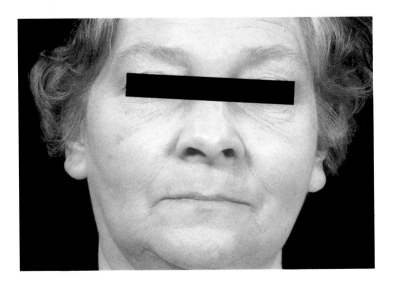

Fig. 13.26 Photograph of a patient with myxoedema. A 'puffy' face, dry skin, diffuse capital hair loss and skin pallor are characteristic of this condition.

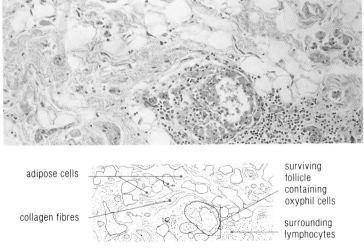

Fig. 13.27 Histology of the thyroid in a patient with severe myxoedema. There is severe destruction of the normal thyroid architecture with much fibrous replacement. Some surviving parenchyma is present and many lymphocytes can also be seen. Haematoxylin and eosin stain, magnification X120. By courtesy of Prof. I. Doniach.

CLINICAL FEATURES IN HYPOTHYROIDISM

The symptoms of hypothyroidism (Fig. 13.28) are non-specific and may be attributed by both patient and doctor to ageing; the onset usually being insidious. The diagnosis of hypothyroidism should be considered in the absence of other obvious explanations, particularly in older women with any of the above symptoms. These symptoms may be even less apparent in secondary hypothyroidism, depending upon the degree of failure of other pituitary hormones. Overt hypothyroidism with thickened dry flaking skin, which led to the term myxoedema, is usually well-advanced before it is recognised clinically.

The signs of hypothyroidism (Fig. 13.29) are non-specific and are easily overlooked, especially if mild. These signs are usually even less apparent in secondary hypothyroidism when features of other pituitary hormone deficiencies tend to predominate.

THE CHANGES IN THE HYPOTHALAMO-PITUITARY-THYROID AXIS IN HYPOTHYROIDISM

In primary thyroid failure the low circulating thyroid hormone levels stimulate the pituitary to increase TSH output (Fig. 13.30). The combination of low T_4 and a high basal TSH is therefore diagnostic of primary hypothyroidism. A normal basal TSH thus excludes primary hypothyroidism. The TSH response to TRH is typically exaggerated but the rise in TSH is proportional to the basal level and the TRH test is seldom necessary except to clarify borderline elevated basal TSH values. Serum T_3 levels may be normal even though T_4 levels are low and TSH is raised. The preservation of normal T_3 levels may be interpreted as a compensatory mechanism of thyroid hormone

production; the measurement of T_3 levels is thus a poor diagnostic test of hypothyroidism.

In secondary hypothyroidism, low circulating thyroid hormone levels are due to failure of TSH output as a result of pituitary disease (Fig. 13.31). The T_4 levels are low, but so are the basal TSH levels. There is no TSH response to exogenous TRH in severe pituitary failure but a blunted TSH response may still occur in less severe pituitary disease. The T_3 levels may be normal despite low T_4, as in primary hypothyroidism, therefore the measurement of T_3 is not a good diagnostic test for hypothyroidism of any origin.

Hypothalamic disease is a rare cause of thyroid failure. In such instances, circulating T_4 levels are low, T_3 may be normal or low and basal TSH is normal or low (Fig. 13.32). The pituitary TSH response to exogenous TRH is usually sluggish and delayed, and values at sixty minutes are higher than at twenty minutes after TRH administration.

A summary of the diagnostic tests for hypothyroidism is shown in Figure 13.33. Whilst a low T_4 is common to all causes of hypothyroidism, it is not absolutely diagnostic. This is because a variety of severe acute and chronic illnesses, together with interference of drugs in thyroid function tests, may also cause low T_4 values (Fig. 13.34). Thus low TBG levels or competitive binding by drugs alter the binding capacity and total T_4 levels are reduced, but free T_4 levels are usually normal. Even when TBG levels are not affected, severe illness may alter T_4 production and T_4 to T_3 conversion. Reverse T_3 levels are usually increased and TSH levels are normal. In asymptomatic autoimmune thyroiditis, total T_4 levels may be towards the lower limit of normal but TSH levels are often mildly elevated.

Symptoms of Hypothyroidism	
usual	**rare**
lethargy	
constipation	deafness
weight gain	
cold intolerance	psychosis
facial puffiness	
dry skin	cerebellar disturbance
hair loss	
hoarseness	myotonia
acroparaesthesiae	

Fig. 13.28   Symptoms of hypothyroidism.

Physical Signs of Hypothyroidism
change in appearance
periorbital oedema
dry, flaking, yellowish skin
diffuse hair loss
bradycardia
signs of median nerve compression (carpal tunnel syndrome)
effusions in body cavities e.g. ascites, pericardial effusion
delayed relaxation of reflexes
croaky voice
goitre

Fig. 13.29   Common physical signs in hypothyroidism.

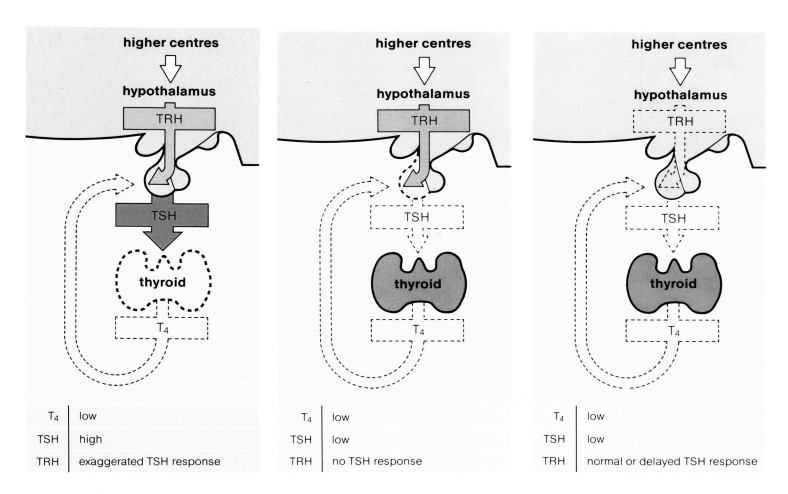

T$_4$	low	T$_4$	low	T$_4$	low
TSH	high	TSH	low	TSH	low
TRH	exaggerated TSH response	TRH	no TSH response	TRH	normal or delayed TSH response

Fig. 13.30 Schematic representation of the changes in the hypothalamo-pituitary-thyroid axis in primary hypothyroidism. The TSH response is typically exaggerated.

Fig. 13.31 Schematic representation of the changes in the hypothalamo-pituitary-thyroid axis in secondary hypothyroidism. In this situation, there is an absent TSH response to TRH because of pituitary disease.

Fig. 13.32 Schematic representation of the changes in the hypothalamo-pituitary-thyroid axis in hypothalamic hypo-thyroidism. In this form of 'tertiary' hypothyroidism, the sixty-minute TSH response in the TRH test is greater than the twenty-minute response.

Hypothyroidism – Summary of Diagnostic Tests

	T$_4$	basal TSH	TRH response
primary hypothyroidism	low	raised	exaggerated
secondary hypothyroidism (pituitary)	low	low or normal	absent
tertiary hypothyroidism (hypothalamic)	low	low or normal	normal or delayed
non-thyroid illness	low	normal	normal

Fig. 13.33 Summary of diagnostic tests for hypothyroidism.

Causes of a Low Serum T$_4$ in Clinically Euthyroid Patients

low TBG / normal TSH	hypoproteinaemia / drugs / hereditary
normal TBG / normal TSH	acute non-thyroid illness / chronic non-thyroid illness
normal TBG / raised T$_3$ / raised TSH / antibody +ve	autoimmune thyroiditis 'subclinical hypothyroid' or 'compensated euthyroid'

Fig. 13.34 Causes of low serum T$_4$ concentrations in clinically euthyroid patients.

TREATMENT

Hypothyroidism is treated with replacement thyroxine therapy (Fig. 13.35). Replacement doses usually start at 50 μg T_4 daily, being increased in a stepwise fashion at two-weekly intervals to 150 μg daily, and the response is assessed clinically and biochemically. When the patient is euthyroid, the TSH should be suppressed into the normal range and the T_4 levels also returned to normal. Maintenance therapy should be continued for life and the patient should be rechecked annually. Some patients may only require 100 μg T_4 daily and others 200 μg T_4 daily for full replacement therapy.

In patients with ischaemic heart disease, replacement therapy should be introduced cautiously, perhaps with starting doses of 25 μg per day. Increments should also be small. If an exacerbation of angina occurs, the dose of T_4 may need to be reduced and the patient also given a beta-blocking agent (i.e. propranolol).

Myxoedema coma is a rare complication of severe hypothyroidism but carries a mortality rate of over fifty per cent. It may be difficult to distinguish from hypothermia *per se*. Treatment is empirical and the optimum form of management remains to be defined. One method is outlined in Figure 13.36. As recovery proceeds the dose of T_3 can be increased over succeeding days to 20μg eight-hourly then eventually changed to T_4 maintenance therapy. The dose of steroids can be reduced stepwise and 'tailed' off.

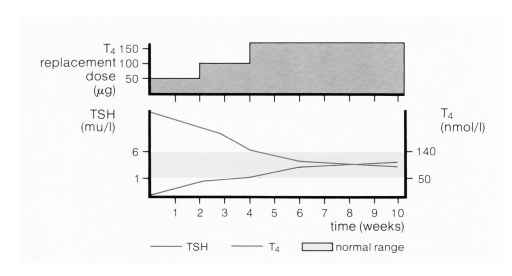

Fig. 13.35 Changes in serum TSH and T_4 with thyroxine replacement therapy. With the gradual increase in T_4, the TSH slowly descends to the normal range.

Fig. 13.36 A suggested plan for the management of myxoedema coma.

Protocol for the Management of Myxoedema Coma

1 take blood for diagnostic tests: T_4, TSH and plasma cortisol

2 maintain adequate ventilation

3 treat hypothermia with gradual rewarming using a space blanket

4 give i.m. hydrocortisone 100mg immediately and repeat 6-hourly

5 give T_3 5–10μg i.m. or by nasogastric tube 12-hourly

6 treat any heart failure with diuretics

7 correct any electrolyte disturbance

14 Carcinoma of the Thyroid

Israel Doniach, MD, FRCPath, FRCP

Carcinoma of the thyroid is a rare cause of fatal malignant disease accounting for only 400 deaths each year in England and Wales, compared with 35,000 from carcinoma of the lung and 12,000 from carcinoma of the breast. The number of newly diagnosed cases reported annually averages 750, the majority presenting as a solitary thyroid nodule which proves to be well differentiated and carries a good prognosis. Solitary nodules are comparatively common and must be investigated further since approximately twelve per cent that are 'cold' on radioactive iodine or pertechnetate scan (i.e. take up less radioactivity than the surrounding normal thyroid) prove to be malignant. This percentage is higher still in children and young adults. Anaplastic thyroid carcinoma is rapidly fatal, but is much rarer and occurs mostly in the elderly. A histopathological classification of thyroid malignancies is shown in Figure 14.1. The follicular cell differentiated carcinomas account for approximately seventy-five to eighty per cent of the total whilst the anaplastic carcinomas account for only fifteen per cent. The incidence of medullary carcinomas varies from five to

ten per cent and malignant lymphomas less than two per cent. Secondary tumours are often found at post-mortem as microscopic deposits, sometimes within benign thyroid nodules.

Carcinoma of the thyroid is nearly three times more common in females than in males (see Fig. 14.2). It occurs at all ages and the standardised incidence per 100,000 women (Fig. 14.3) rises steadily from the age of fifty-six years onwards. Although the clinical incidence in young people is high, mortality from thyroid carcinoma occurs only in the middle-aged and the elderly (Fig. 14.4). Since the majority of differentiated carcinomas are either cured or the patients live long enough to die of other causes, it follows that the prevalence far exceeds the number who die annually from this cause.

The four major types of primary thyroid carcinoma (papillary, follicular, anaplastic and medullary) are classified according to histology and clinical behaviour (Fig. 14.5). These are further divided into histopathological subtypes (Fig. 14.6) which correlate with prognosis.

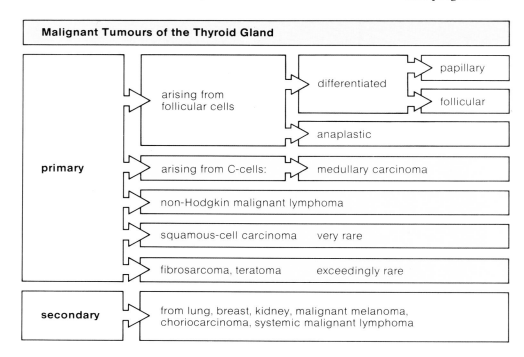

Fig. 14.1 A histopathological classification of malignant tumours of the thyroid gland.

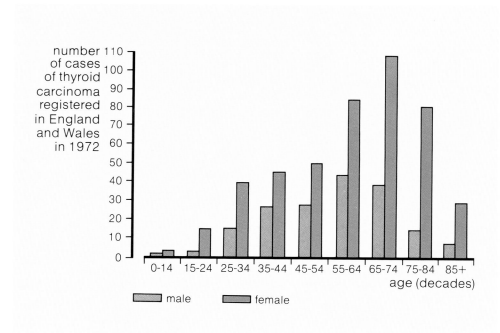

Fig. 14.2 The number of cases of thyroid carcinoma registered in England and Wales in 1972 for each age decade.

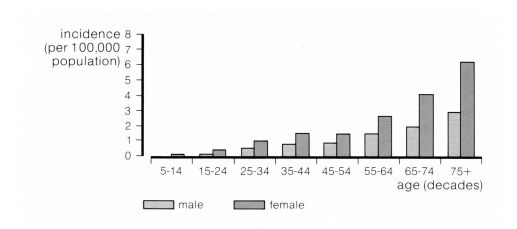

Fig. 14.3 The incidence of thyroid carcinoma per 100,000 of the population in 1972. The greater incidence of this disease in middle-aged women and in the elderly is shown.

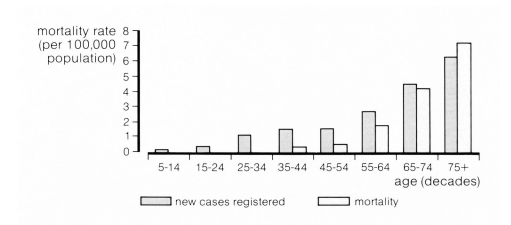

Fig. 14.4 Mortality attributed to thyroid carcinoma per 100,000 of the population. There is negligible mortality in the younger age groups.

Distribution of Clinicopathological Types	Subtypes	Prognosis: Deaths Within 10-20 Years
papillary 60-70%	microcarcinoma:	less than 1%
	intrathyroid:	less than 5%
	extrathyroid:	more than 50%
follicular 15-20%	microangioinvasive	less than 5%
	angioinvasive:	more than 50%
anaplastic 10-15%		100%
medullary 5-10%	confined to thyroid gland:	less than 5%
	with lymph node metastases:	more than 50%

Fig. 14.5 Distribution and prognosis of the four major clinicopathological types of primary thyroid carcinoma.

Subtypes of Differentiated Carcinomas		
papillary	microcarcinoma:	less than 1.5cm diameter, incidental finding
	intrathyroid carcinoma:	does not invade thyroid gland capsule
	extrathyroid carcinoma:	traverses thyroid gland capsule
follicular	microangioinvasive:	permeates venous sinusoids of tumour capsule
	angioinvasive:	permeates veins outside thyroid gland capsule

Fig. 14.6 The histopathological subtypes of the differentiated carcinomas of the thyroid.

14.3

PAPILLARY CARCINOMA

Papillary carcinoma is the most common type of thyroid carcinoma and occurs in all age groups. Since the majority of papillary carcinomas contain neoplastic follicles in addition to neoplastic papillae, many authors classify mixed papillary and follicular carcinomas separately from pure papillary tumours. However, there is no accepted evidence of any difference in clinical behaviour. The term 'papillary carcinoma' therefore includes all tumours that contain any neoplastic papillae. These tumours are predominantly lymphangioinvasive.

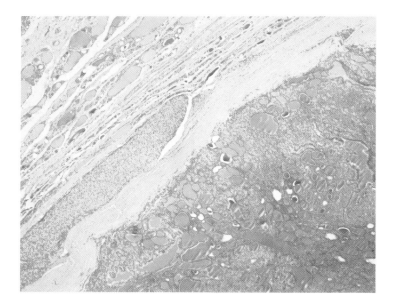

Fig. 14.7 Histology of papillary carcinoma. A typical mixture of neoplastic papillae and neoplastic colloid-containing follicles is shown. The nuclei are crowded, irregular in shape and empty-looking. Haematoxylin and eosin stain, magnification x 200.

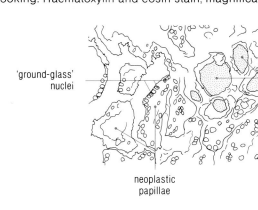

Fig. 14.8 Histology of follicular carcinoma. Follicular carcinomas consist of neoplastic colloid-containing follicles of varied sizes separated by a thick fibrous capsule from normal thyroid parenchyma. The lumen of a large venous sinusoid in the capsule is almost filled by a plug of invasive tumour. Haematoxylin and eosin stain, magnification x 20.

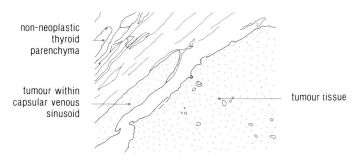

Fig. 14.9 Histology of oxyphil follicular carcinoma. Large polygonal cells with an eosinophilic granular cytoplasm (due to proliferation of mitochondria) can be seen. Haematoxylin and eosin stain, magnification x 200.

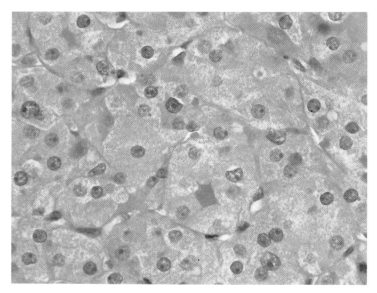

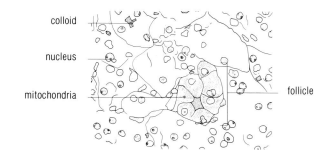

The three subtypes of papillary carcinoma are the micro-carcinomas, the intrathyroid carcinomas and the extrathyroid carcinomas. Microcarcinomas measure less than 1.5cm in diameter and are clinically occult. They are usually found unexpectedly in surgical thyroidectomy specimens, for example, in patients with Graves' disease, colloid goitre, Hashimoto's goitre or in follicular adenoma. In these circumstances follow-up has shown no evidence of either recurrence of the carcinoma or the development of metastases. Cervical lymph node metastases of papillary carcinomas are usually associated with a palpable primary tumour. Occasionally, however, an excision biopsy of a solitary enlarged cervical lymph node is found to contain a deposit of a papillary carcinoma, and the primary is subsequently demonstrated as an occult microcarcinoma of the ipsilateral lobe on thyroidectomy. Intrathyroid carcinomas present as a palpable thyroid nodule, with or without enlarged cervical lymph nodes. On section, the tumour is seen to be confined within the thyroid with no extension through the gland's capsule. Extrathyroid carcinomas are usually larger and more rapidly growing than the other subtypes of papillary carcinoma. They are more common in older patients and are found, at operation, to have penetrated the thyroid capsule and to have infiltrated adjacent tissues including the strap-muscles.

Papillary carcinomas are made up of varying quantities of neoplastic papillae and follicles (Fig. 14.7). The papillae consist of elongated, branching fibrovascular cores covered by a single layer of epithelium. The follicles, however, may contain eosinophilic colloid or appear empty. The nuclei of both papillae and follicles, in approximately sixty per cent of the tumours, are characteristically empty-looking with a prominent rim due to linear condensation of chromatin against the nuclear membrane. These nuclei are described as having a 'ground-glass' appearance, and they are large, misshapen and overlapping. Approximately fifty per cent of the tumours contain scattered, small, spherical, laminated, calcified bodies (psammoma bodies or calcospherites). These bodies are present either in the fibrovascular core of the papillae, or in the intervening connective tissue stroma, or even in the non-neoplastic thyroid stroma some distance from the tumour. In some cases there is an intense focal fibrous reaction that may be seen as thick strands within the tumour, or as a pseudo-capsule in which single or small clumps of atypical polygonal neoplastic cells lie embedded.

Occasionally, papillary carcinomas are grossly cystic – a change which can also be seen in the lymph node metastases. However, over ninety per cent of papillary carcinomas are unencapsulated, discrete and vary in degree of local infiltration. On careful microscopy other foci of tumour may be found in both thyroid lobes; however, it is not possible to determine whether these are interstitial lymph-borne metastases or whether they are separate primaries including 'harmless' microcarcinomas.

FOLLICULAR CARCINOMA

Follicular carcinomas occur more commonly in middle-aged women and are comparatively rare in children and young adults. They predominantly invade blood vessels and are divided into two subtypes, microangioinvasive and angioinvasive. Micro-angioinvasive follicular carcinomas are well differentiated encapsulated tumours whose major histological difference from adenomas is the presence of tumour tissue within the lumen of capsular venous sinusoids. The presence of bizarre giant nuclei within the tumour and also of occasional mitoses and atypical differentiation do not of themselves constitute malignancy in the absence of vascular invasion; such tumours are benign and are described as 'atypical adenomas'. Angioinvasive follicular carcinomas are less well differentiated, permeate veins outside the capsule of the thyroid gland and may infiltrate through the tumour capsule into adjacent thyroid parenchyma and extrathyroid tissues.

Follicular carcinomas consist of a mixture of variably sized colloid-containing follicles, empty acini and solid cords or alveoli of neoplastic cells (Fig. 14.8). They are surrounded by a well-defined capsule rich in arterioles, and also venous sinusoids into which there are foci of capsular invasion extending into the venous sinusoid lumen. The less well differentiated types consist predominantly of trabeculae; they also show marked infiltration of the capsule and prominent invasion not only of capsular venous sinusoids but also of veins outside the capsule of the thyroid gland. A variant follicular carcinoma is the oxyphil (Hürthle or Askenazy) tumour in which most of the neoplastic cells are large with bizarre-shaped nuclei and voluminous cytoplasm and contain abundant eosinophilic granules which are mitochondria (Fig. 14.9). Oxyphil change may also be seen in papillary carcinomas, adenomas and, focally, in non-neoplastic thyroid parenchyma – especially in autoimmune thyroiditis (see Chapter 13). The major histological characteristics of the differentiated carcinomas are summarised in Figure 14.10.

Fig. 14.10 Comparison of the histological characteristics of papillary and follicular carcinomas.

Histological Characteristics of the Differentiated Carcinomas

	papillary	follicular
capsule	−	+
papillae	+	−
follicles	+	+
'ground-glass' nuclei	+ (60%)	−
psammoma bodies	+ (50%)	−
additional tumour micro-foci	common	−
lymphatic spread	typical	rare
vascular spread	rare	typical

ANAPLASTIC CARCINOMA

Anaplastic carcinomas arise in late middle-age and in the elderly. Most tumours arise from a differentiated papillary or follicular carcinoma, sometimes with a long-standing history of goitre.

The tumours are undifferentiated (Fig. 14.11) with varying proportions of large spindle and giant cells, resembling a sarcoma. Mitoses are numerous, and many of them abnormal. Focal necrosis is often present. An undifferentiated small cell type has also been found, although current opinion is that most tumours in this group are lymphomas.

MEDULLARY CARCINOMA

Medullary carcinomas are tumours of the calcitonin-secreting parafollicular C-cells and occur in males almost as frequently as females. They represent a different entity from tumours of follicular cell origin, since the parent C-cells are derived from neural crest cells that colonise the ultimobranchial bodies which fuse in early embryonic life. The thyroid anlage is itself derived from endodermal tissue.

These tumours are discrete and non-encapsulated, and are made up of either polygonal, round or spindle-shaped cells arranged in sheets, nests or trabeculae with prominent intervening collagenous stroma (Fig. 14.12). Amyloid is present in varying amounts both within cell masses and in the stroma. The individual tumour cells show little variation in morphology with stippled nuclei of regular shape and size and finely granulated cytoplasm. In addition, surviving non-neoplastic thyroid follicles are incorporated into the periphery of the tumour.

MALIGNANT LYMPHOMA

Malignant lymphomas are characterised by the replacement of large areas of thyroid parenchyma by lymphoma cells (Fig. 14.13). In the majority of cases the lesion is high grade, often immunoblastic, and the prognosis poor. Most of the low grade lymphomas are lymphoplasmacytoid. In over half the cases, surviving non-infiltrated thyroid parenchyma shows Hashimoto's thyroiditis.

CLINICAL PRESENTATION OF MALIGNANT THYROID TUMOURS

These most commonly present as a solitary nodule in one thyroid lobe or the isthmus, often firm and indistinguishable from a colloid nodule or adenoma. The length of history is variable – in some patients the swelling is first noticed by a relative whilst others have been aware of the lump in the neck for some years. There are usually no systemic symptoms. Extrathyroid papillary carcinomas and angioinvasive follicular carcinomas present with more rapidly growing large tumours which may be associated with hoarseness, dysphagia, stridor and dyspnoea. Enlarged cervical lymph nodes due to secondary deposits are found in approximately half the cases of papillary carcinoma and much less often in follicular carcinomas.

Intrathyroid papillary carcinomas and microangioinvasive follicular carcinomas are very slow-growing tumours in patients under the age of forty years. This applies also to metastases that may not become clinically apparent until five to ten or more years after the initial thyroidectomy; such metastases tend to occur

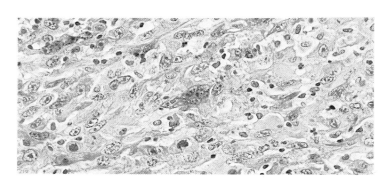

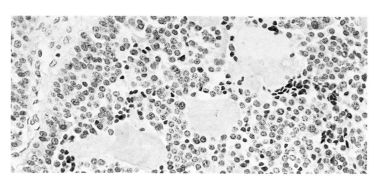

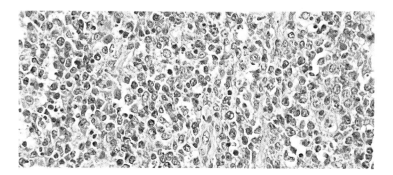

Fig. 14.11 Histology of anaplastic carcinoma. Large spindle and giant cells with bizarre-shaped nuclei are characteristic of this type of carcinoma. Haematoxylin and eosin stain, magnification x 200.

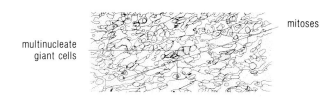

Fig. 14.12 Histology of medullary carcinoma. The tumour cells have round nuclei of regular appearance. Also present are amorphous intercellular masses of pink, congo red positively-stained amyloid deposits. Haematoxylin and congo red stain, magnification x 200.

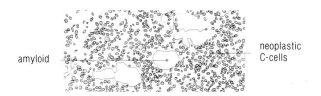

Fig. 14.13 Histology of non-Hodgkin lymphoma. This consists of a diffuse proliferation of neoplastic lymphoid cells that have replaced normal thyroid parenchyma. The lymphoid cells are mixed lymphoplasmacytoid and immunoblastic in type. Haematoxylin and eosin stain, magnification x 200.

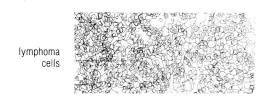

either in the lymph nodes (papillary carcinomas) or in bones (follicular carcinomas). After the age of forty years both previously diagnosed and newly diagnosed tumours show a tendency to more rapid growth and spread, usually associated with less well-differentiated histopathology.

Papillary carcinoma may prove fatal as a result of lymphatic spread to the trachea with resultant ulceration. More commonly death occurs in papillary, follicular and anaplastic carcinomas from vascular spread to the lungs, brain, liver and bones. Bone metastases usually involve the vertebrae, pelvis and ribs; however they may also occur in the long bones.

Anaplastic carcinomas give rise to a history of recent very rapid enlargement of a normal or goitrous thyroid gland with local pressure symptoms – especially that of difficulty in breathing. On examination the thyroid is markedly and asymmetrically enlarged by a large hard mass attached to adjacent structures. Vocal cord paralysis may also be present.

Malignant lymphoma of the thyroid may present as a thyroid nodule but more usually causes gross symmetrical firm enlargement of the gland, and also dysphagia and dyspnoea especially when the head is flexed. The condition may be mimicked by the fibrous variant of Hashimoto's goitre. The management, by a combination of radiotherapy and chemotherapy, is similar to that applied to lymphomas in other situations; thyroxine replacement is also indicated. The prognosis of high grade lymphomas is very poor but better in low grade tumours.

Diagnostic procedures vary between institutes. After clinical examination, thyroid function tests and radiological examination of the neck, the most commonly used next step is a radioactive iodine or pertechnetate scan to determine whether the nodule is 'cold' (Fig. 14.14). Alternatively, histology of a needle biopsy or cytology of an aspiration needle biopsy may be used in preference. Ultrasound scanning (Fig. 14.15) differentiates cysts from solid lesions; however, differentiated carcinomas are only occasionally cystic. A nodule that is 'cold' on scan may prove to be a benign cyst, a colloid nodule, an adenoma, part of an asymmetric Hashimoto's goitre, a differentiated carcinoma or a medullary carcinoma. If a solitary intrathyroid tumour is found at operation, the surgeon may either carry out a lobectomy plus isthmectomy and await the routine histology report, or he may send the lobe for frozen section diagnosis. In the latter situation, the pathologist can usually rule out non-neoplastic lesions and positively recognise papillary carcinoma, provided papillae are present in the sections taken. He is not necessarily able to distinguish adenomas from microangioinvasive follicular carcinomas but, with experience, can recognise medullary carcinomas. Routine paraffin wax embedded blocks allow much greater sampling of the tumour and more time for microscopy, and the histology of routine preparations is considerably easier to interpret than that of frozen sections. The more advanced thyroid carcinomas are usually recognisable macroscopically at operation, and are radically dealt with if operable and if the diagnosis is confirmed by routine histology.

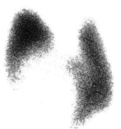

Fig. 14.14 Thyroid nodule: area of decreased uptake on isotope scan. A cold area in the lobe of the thyroid is shown. This appearance is due to a mass. Cysts, however, also show diminished uptake and an ultrasound scan is therefore needed in order to differentiate a cyst from a solid lesion.

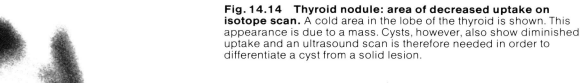

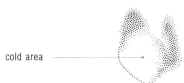

cold area

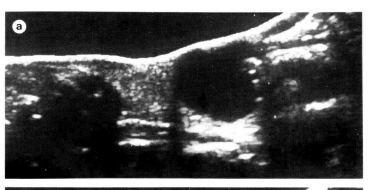

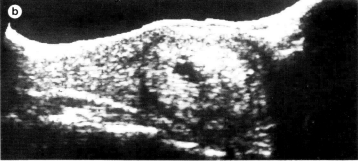

Fig. 14.15 Longitudinal ultrasound scans of thyroid lobes: (a) thyroid cyst and (b) thyroid tumour. In (a) the right lobe of the thyroid is shown. The anechoic area in the lower pole and the increased through-transmission of sound behind it are characteristic of a simple thyroid cyst. In (b) the left lobe is shown containing a solid inhomogeneous mass. The reduced echogenicity around the mass suggests the presence of a capsule. It is not possible to differentiate a benign tumour from a malignant tumour using this technique.

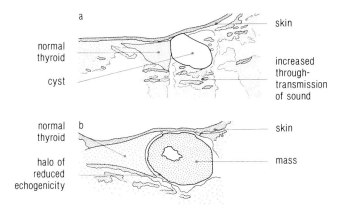

MANAGEMENT

The operation procedure varies with the surgeon's findings and predilections. In the more advanced cases, total thyroidectomy is performed with removal of macroscopically involved tissues and lymph nodes. The choice of three procedures with discrete, solitary, differentiated carcinomas is shown in Figure 14.16. Lobectomy and subtotal removal of the remaining lobe is usually advocated in order to remove occult carcinoma in the apparently normal lobe and ensure preservation of parathyroid tissue. There is also a choice of postoperative management. The scanning is first carried out at six-monthly intervals, and then at longer intervals until the patient is deemed cured but continues to attend for clinical follow-up. During the six months before each scan the patient is maintained on tri-iodothyronine (T_3). During the seven to fourteen days preceding each scan the patient stops the T_3. At other times the patient is maintained on thyroxine.

The objections raised against simple lobectomy are the possibility of the presence of occult tumour in the apparently normal lobe and the need to ablate the thyroid for follow-up scan and treatment of metastases that might arise. The arguments in favour of simple lobectomy are that recurrences or new primaries in the residual lobe do not occur after this operation in micro-angioinvasive follicular carcinoma and are very rare in intra-thyroid papillary carcinoma. If metastases are subsequently found on clinical follow-up, it is possible to ablate the residual lobe and still treat these very slow-growing tumours. The more conservative approach in young patients and the more radical approach in patients over forty years of age at the time of initial diagnosis should be favoured.

TREATMENT OF ANAPLASTIC CARCINOMA

When anaplastic carcinomas are suspected it is customary to carry out a needle biopsy for histological confirmation followed by a course of radiotherapy to the neck, even in the presence of known metastases. Untreated anaplastic carcinomas infiltrate the trachea and may ulcerate through the skin.

CLINICAL ASPECTS OF MEDULLARY CARCINOMA

Approximately eighty per cent of medullary carcinomas are sporadic and twenty per cent familial, the latter showing an autosomal dominant inheritance with strong penetrance. In sporadic cases the clinical presentation is usually that of a solitary hard thyroid nodule which is 'cold' on scan. Involvement of cervical lymph nodes at the time of presentation is observed in about fifty per cent of cases, when chest radiography may show additional involvement of the upper mediastinum.

The clinical symptoms that may be associated both with sporadic and familial cases are summarised in Figures 14.17 and

14.18. The diarrhoea is severe and watery in type due to a combination of intestinal hurry and excessive secretion. It is relieved by removal of the tumour and recurs with metastases. The cause of the secretion has not been identified but calcitonin, a bradykinin-producing kallikrein, prostaglandins and vasoactive intestinal peptide have been suggested. The peptide hormones that have been identified in tumour tissue and in the blood are also listed (see Fig. 14.17). The basal level of calcitonin is high and rises greatly after a provocative infusion of ionised calcium or alcohol by mouth. In all of the familial syndromes leading to medullary carcinomas (see Fig. 14.18) the thyroid shows marked hyperplasia of C-cells plus two or more medullary carcinomas. In types 2 and 3 the adrenals show bilateral medullary hyperplasia and multiple phaeochromocytomas. These might present clinically before or after the thyroid tumours. In type 3 the mucosal neuromas are present on the eyelids, lips and tongue (see Chapter 9), and there may be ganglioneuromatosis of the small and large intestines. These patients have thick blubbery lips, marfanoid habitus, high arched palate and pes cavus. In all types, relatives of clinically diagnosed patients must be screened routinely for the presence of raised calcitonin and, in 2 and 3, for raised catecholamine secretions.

Both sporadic and medullary carcinomas vary in their degree of malignancy. In some, the condition is cured by thyroidectomy. In others, especially in patients who present initially with lymph node metastases, the tumour may metastasise widely within one or two years, to mediastinal nodes, lungs, bones and liver.

EPIDEMIOLOGY

The incidence of reported new cases of thyroid carcinomas shows considerable geographical variation (Fig. 14.19) from less than 1 per 100,000 women in Hamburg to 9 per 100,000 in Hawaii. This is thought to result from both ethnic and environmental factors. Geographical variation is also seen in the distribution of histological types associated with iodine content of the diet (Fig. 14.20). In areas of iodine deficiency (present or past) follicular carcinomas are more predominant than papillary carcinomas, and the converse is true where iodine is readily available. Reports from Switzerland have shown a decrease in percentage of follicular carcinomas and an increase in papillary carcinomas since the iodization of salt. In Iceland, where the dietary intake of iodine is unusually large, the high incidence of thyroid malignancy is due mainly to papillary carcinomas. An interesting finding has been the variation in geographical incidence of microcarcinomas in step-sectioned post-mortem glands in women from seven per cent in Colombia to twenty-eight per cent in Japanese residents in Hawaii. The equivalent figures for men were five per cent and twenty per cent.

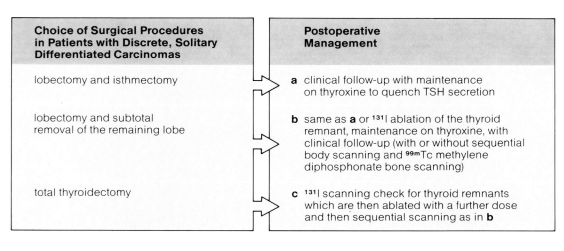

Choice of Surgical Procedures in Patients with Discrete, Solitary Differentiated Carcinomas	Postoperative Management
lobectomy and isthmectomy	**a** clinical follow-up with maintenance on thyroxine to quench TSH secretion
lobectomy and subtotal removal of the remaining lobe	**b** same as **a** or ^{131}I ablation of the thyroid remnant, maintenance on thyroxine, with clinical follow-up (with or without sequential body scanning and ^{99m}Tc methylene diphosphonate bone scanning)
total thyroidectomy	**c** ^{131}I scanning check for thyroid remnants which are then ablated with a further dose and then sequential scanning as in **b**

Fig. 14.16 Choice of procedures for surgery and postoperative management of discrete, solitary, differentiated carcinomas.

Medullary Carcinoma

associated clinical syndromes		peptide hormones secreted	
intractable diarrhoea	in 20% of cases	calcitonin	always
		somatostatin	common
		carcinoembryonic antigen	common
		gastrin releasing peptide (bombesin)	common
carcinoid syndrome	rare	histaminase	common
		serotonin	rare
		ACTH	rare
		corticotrophin releasing activity	very rare
		prolactin stimulating activity	very rare
Cushing's syndrome	very rare	nerve growth factor	very rare

Fig. 14.17   The associated clinical syndromes and peptide hormones secreted by medullary carcinomas.

Types of Familial Inheritance

1 medullary carcinoma alone

2 medullary carcinoma and phaeochromocytoma

3 medullary carcinoma, phaeochromocytoma and mucosal neuromas

hyperparathyroidism due to parathyroid adenoma or hyperplasia may be associated with any of the three types, especially 2

Fig. 14.18   Types of familial inheritance of medullary carcinoma.

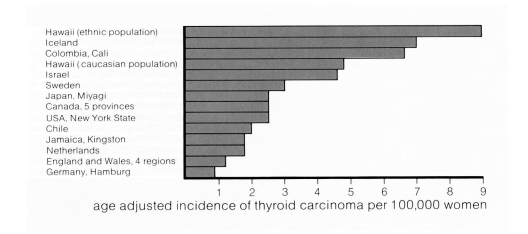

Hawaii (ethnic population)
Iceland
Colombia, Cali
Hawaii (caucasian population)
Israel
Sweden
Japan, Miyagi
Canada, 5 provinces
USA, New York State
Chile
Jamaica, Kingston
Netherlands
England and Wales, 4 regions
Germany, Hamburg

1 2 3 4 5 6 7 8 9
age adjusted incidence of thyroid carcinoma per 100,000 women

Fig. 14.19   Chart showing differing incidence of thyroid carcinoma with geographical location.

	Ratio of Papillary to Follicular Thyroid Carcinoma in Various Series			
	author	number of cases	papillary/ follicular ratio	country
		papillary	follicular	
normal dietary iodine	Woolner 1968	736	208	3.5:1	USA, Mayo clinic
	Russell 1973	552	124	4.5:1	USA, Texas
	Lindsay 1960	178	76	2.3:1	USA, San Francisco
low dietary iodine	Correa 1969	105	169	0.6:1	Colombia, Cali
	Silink 1966	43	81	0.5:1	Czechoslovakia
	Heitz 1976	145	225	0.6:1	Switzerland, Basel

Fig. 14.20   The incidence of papillary carcinoma compared with follicular carcinoma. This rises with an increase in dietary iodine and varies geographically.

AETIOLOGICAL CONSIDERATIONS

The possible aetiological factors associated with thyroid carcinoma are listed in Figure 14.21. In the past, the two major aetiological factors were thought to be iodine deficiency with its accompanying maintained TSH stimulation, and malignant change in a long-standing adenoma. Epidemiological surveys have not confirmed any excess incidence of thyroid malignancy in iodine deficient areas. Current opinion is that malignant change in an adenoma must be a rare event since adenomas are common and follicular carcinomas rare.

A major and definite aetiological factor which has been demonstrated is ionising radiation to the thyroid gland, given, in the past in some centres, in non-sterilizing dosage to infants and children. Doses reported to have induced thyroid carcinoma vary from a few rads (cGy) given to epilate the scalp in the treatment of ringworm to 1500 rads for the treatment of tuberculous glands in the neck. Other conditions include prophylactic irradiation of the thymus in infants and therapeutic irradiation of acne, enlarged tonsils, skin tumours of the head and neck, and Hodgkin and non-Hodgkin lymphomas of the cervical lymph nodes. The carcinogenic risk factor has been calculated to be one per cent per 100 rads in twenty years. The latent period is approximately ten to twenty years, or even longer. Occasional cases have been reported in irradiated adults. Therapeutic sterilizing doses of radiation to the thyroid, for example radiological treatment of laryngeal carcinoma or ^{131}I treatment of Graves' disease, are not associated with cancer induction; in fact the patients are liable to develop hypothyroidism.

Histology of the thyroid parenchyma in papillary carcinoma shows an increased incidence of focal lymphocytic thyroiditis usually considered to be an effect rather than a cause. In view of the frequency of occult papillary microcarcinomas suggested that these might be *in situ* carcinomas that are sometimes promoted to invasive tumours either by unknown endogenous or environmental factors, or both.

Fig. 14.21 The possible aetiological factors in thyroid carcinoma. Ionising radiation is a major cause.

Possible Aetiological Factors in Thyroid Carcinoma	
iodine deficiency goitre	no clear evidence
precursor adenoma	possibly, rarely
precursor occult papillary microcarcinoma	possibly
ionising radiation	yes
dyshormonogenesis	yes, rarely
autoimmune thyroiditis	no
excessive iodine consumption	possibly
genetic	familial medullary carcinoma

15 Hyperthyroidism and Graves' Disease

Reginald Hall, BSc, MD, MB BS, FRCP

Hyperthyroidism is the clinical condition which results from increased circulating levels of thyroid hormones. It occurs in about 1.8 per cent of the adult population, but is much rarer in childhood. Women are affected more often than men (ratio about 10:1) and the mean age at diagnosis is forty-eight years.

AETIOLOGY

The causes of hyperthyroidism are shown in Figure 15.1. In most countries, Graves's disease is the commonest cause of hyperthyroidism, followed (in Europe) by toxic nodular goitre and then toxic adenoma. In North America, viral thyroiditis (de Quervain's disease) and silent thyroiditis are much more common than in Europe.

Graves' disease (Fig. 15.2) is a useful omnibus term used to describe a combination of eye signs, goitre and hyperthyroidism and, more rarely, of localised myxoedema, thyroid acropachy and other associated features. Partial forms of Graves' disease can occur, e.g. ophthalmic Graves' disease (Fig. 15.3) where the eye signs occur in the absence of hyperthyroidism in a patient who has never been hyperthyroid. In some patients a goitre is absent, in others the goitre may precede the development of hyperthyroidism.

Neonatal hyperthyroidism (Fig. 15.4) occurs at, or shortly after, birth and is due to the transplacental passage of thyroid-stimulating antibodies (TSAb).

PATHOGENESIS OF GRAVES' DISEASE

Graves' disease is one of the group of autoimmune thyroid (AIT) diseases (Fig. 15.5) which includes myxoedema (Fig. 15.6) and Hashimoto's disease. All of the AIT diseases are characterised by lymphocytic infiltration of the thyroid gland and the presence of circulating thyroid antibodies. The hyperthyroidism of Graves' disease results from the action of TSAb which are antibodies to the thyrotrophin receptor on the surface of the thyroid cell (Fig. 15.7), which bind to the receptor and activate the enzyme adenylate cyclase in the same manner as thyroid stimulating hormone (TSH). In some patients, antibodies may bind to the TSH receptor but fail to activate it. These blocking antibodies may contribute to the development of hypothyroidism in some patients.

Graves' disease is often familial and genetic factors are involved in its development. There is an association of Graves' disease with human leucocyte antigens HLA A1, B8, DW3 (Fig. 15.8), and genes at the D locus are thought to be responsible for the coding of antigens involved in the abnormal immune response.

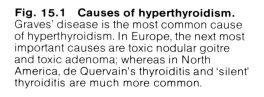

Causes of Hyperthyroidism

main causes

Graves' disease and variants

toxic multinodular goitre

toxic nodule

rarer causes

Jod-Basedow

disseminated thyroid autonomy

thyroiditis:
  de Quervain's
  silent

factitious

hypothalamic – pituitary:
  with or without a
  pituitary tumour

post-partum:
  probably variant
  of silent

molar pregnancy

choriocarcinoma

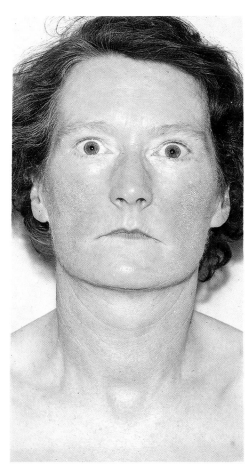

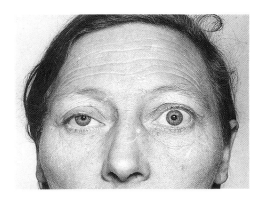

Fig. 15.3 Ophthalmic Graves' disease. The eye signs of Graves' disease, which may be asymmetrical, can occur (as here) in a euthyroid patient with no history of hyperthyroidism.

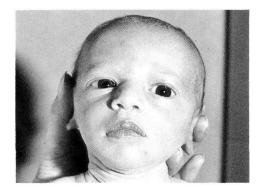

Fig. 15.1 Causes of hyperthyroidism. Graves' disease is the most common cause of hyperthyroidism. In Europe, the next most important causes are toxic nodular goitre and toxic adenoma; whereas in North America, de Quervain's thyroiditis and 'silent' thyroiditis are much more common.

Fig. 15.2 Typical facial appearance in Graves' disease. This patient has a goitre and lid retraction causing an enlarged palpebral fissure with sclera visible above the superior margin of the limbus.

Fig. 15.4 Neonatal hyperthyroidism. Hyperthyroidism in the new-born results from transplacental passage of thyroid stimulating antibodies (TSAb) into the foetal circulation. A goitre is normally present. This baby has minimal exophthalmos.

Organ-Specific Autoimmune Diseases

chronic hepatitis	hypoparathyroidism (some forms)
Hashimoto's disease	
myxoedema	diabetes mellitus (some forms)
lymphocytic thyroiditis	vitiligo
Graves' disease	
	premature ovarian failure
pernicious anaemia	
Addison's disease	allergic alveolitis

Fig. 15.5 Table of the organ-specific autoimmune diseases. All of these disorders are characterised by the presence of circulating antibodies and lymphocytic infiltration of the gland or tissue.

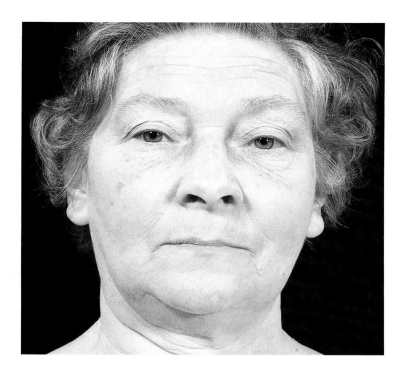

Fig. 15.6 Typical facial appearance in myxoedema. The skin is dry, coarse, and usually cold. Pallor is common, as is a yellowish tinge of the skin caused by hypercarotinaemia. The hair is thinned, coarse and brittle.

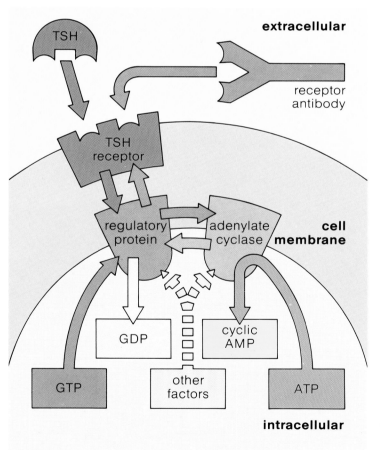

Fig. 15.7 Possible mechanism of action of stimulating thyroid antibodies. The antibody occupies the TSH receptor and can therefore activate adenylate cyclase.

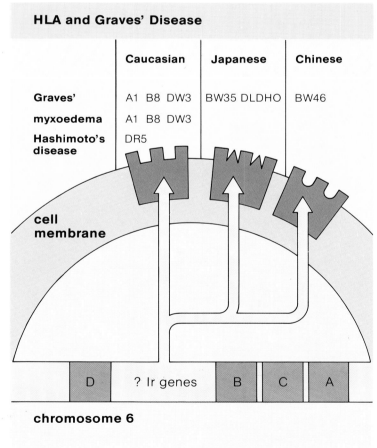

HLA and Graves' Disease

	Caucasian	Japanese	Chinese
Graves'	A1 B8 DW3	BW35 DLDHO	BW46
myxoedema	A1 B8 DW3		
Hashimoto's disease	DR5		

cell membrane

D	? Ir genes	B	C	A

chromosome 6

Fig. 15.8 Human leucocyte antigen (HLA) associations of autoimmune thyroid disease in three ethnic groups.

DIAGNOSIS

The diagnosis of hyperthyroidism consists of demonstrating increased circulating levels of thyroxine (T_4) or tri-iodothyronine (T_3) (Fig. 15.9) and then determining the cause of the hyperthyroidism (Fig. 15.10). The cause of the dysfunction may be clinically apparent, (e.g. the eye signs in a patient with Graves' disease). Serological tests, for example, the demonstration of microsomal or receptor antibodies, may be required before AIT disease can be confirmed (Fig. 15.10).

The most sensitive test to exclude hyperthyroidism is the thyrotrophin releasing hormone (TRH) test. A normal response to TRH excludes hyperthyroidism. Most patients with hyperthyroidism have raised serum T_3 levels, unless there is some illness or drug impairing conversion of T_4 to T_3. In overt hyperthyroidism, routine tests usually suffice to confirm the diagnosis (e.g. serum T_4 measured by RIA). Thyroid hormone binding tests, thyroid hormone uptake tests or direct thyroxine-binding globulin (TBG) estimations may be required to correct the T_4 for alterations in binding proteins. Assay of free-T_4 is now being adopted as a useful test unaffected by changes in binding proteins. Free T_3 estimations are now proving helpful in diagnosis, particularly when TBG levels are altered.

CLINICAL FEATURES
Hyperthyroidism

The symptoms of hyperthyroidism are relatively non-specific, but weight loss combined with an increased appetite is a useful diagnostic combination. A fine tremor of the outstretched fingers (Fig. 15.11) warm moist skin, tachycardia, atrial fibrillation with a hyperdynamic circulation and systolic hypertension are the major signs of hyperthyroidism. Onycholysis, the recession of the nails from the nail beds (the so-called 'Plummer's nails'), may cause difficulty in keeping the nails clean. Erythema of the fingers and palms may be apparent (Fig. 15.12).

Thyroid Function Tests

mild hyperthyroidism

thyrotrophin releasing hormone test

serum T_3

overt hyperthyroidism

T_4-radioimmunoassay
T_3-radioimmunoassay
thyroid hormone binding/uptake tests
free T_4 index – calculated
free T_3 index – calculated
free T_4
free T_3

Diagnosis of Graves' Disease

clinical signs	laboratory tests
diffuse goitre	
eye signs	thyroid-stimulating antibodies (TSAb)
localised myxoedema	
acropachy	thyroglobulin antibodies (TgAb)
vitiligo	
family history	microsomal antibodies

Fig. 15.9   Tests used in the diagnosis of Graves' disease. For mild cases, the most sensitive test available is the thyrotrophin releasing hormone (TRH) test, a normal response to which will exclude hyperthyroidism. In overt cases, routine tests, such as T_4 measured by radioimmunoassay (RIA) will suffice to confirm the diagnosis.

Fig. 15.10   Diagnosis of Graves' disease. Diagnosis of hyperthyroidism depends upon the demonstration of increased levels of circulating T_4 or T_3, and then determining the cause of the dysfunction.

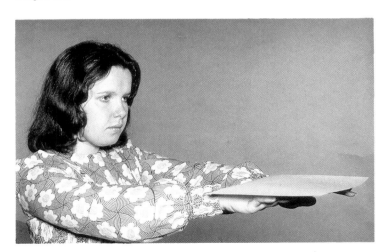

Fig. 15.11   Method of demonstrating fine tremor of the outstretched fingers.

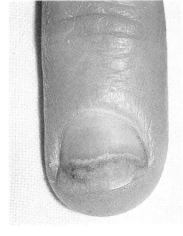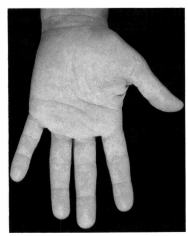

Fig. 15.12   Onycholysis (or 'Plummer's nails') and palmar erythema in thyrotoxicosis. The separation of the nails from the nail beds makes them friable and difficult to clean. Palmar and digital erythema may also be apparent.

Goitre

The goitre in Graves' disease is usually diffuse and symmetrical (Fig. 15.13), and moves readily upwards with the larynx on swallowing (Fig. 15.14). A continuous vascular murmur is almost diagnostic of hyperthyroidism (Fig. 15.15). The histological picture of the thyroid in Graves' disease consists of tall columnar epithelium, which may be unfolded, and scalloping of the colloid (Fig. 15.16) associated with varying degrees of lymphocytic infiltration.

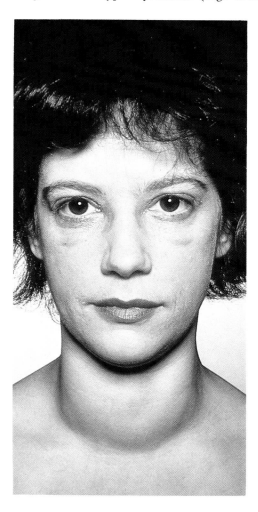

Fig. 15.13 Diffuse and symmetrical goitre of Graves' disease.

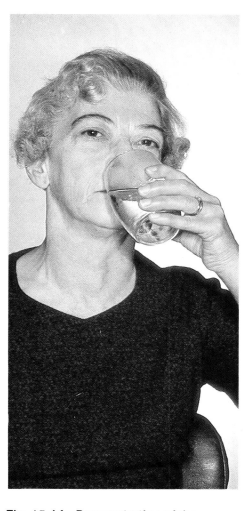

Fig. 15.14 Demonstration of the presence of a goitre. The presence of a goitre can best be shown by asking the patient to swallow, when its movement upwards with the larynx can be clearly seen.

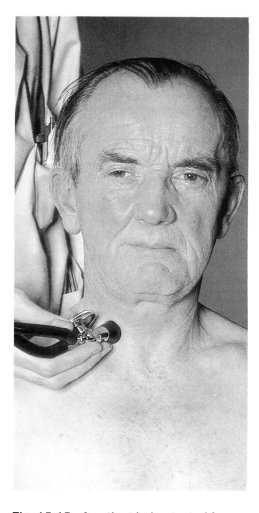

Fig. 15.15 A patient being tested for vascular murmur. Continuous vascular murmur is almost diagnostic of Graves' disease.

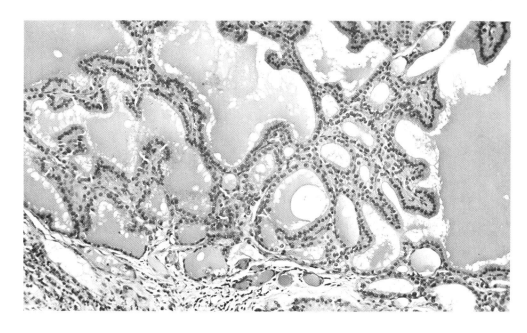

Fig. 15.16 Histology of thyroid tissue in Graves' disease. Tall unfolded columnar epithelium is present, together with scalloping of follicular colloid.

Neonatal Hyperthyroidism

This disorder is seen in children born to mothers who have, or at some time have had Graves' disease. The child usually has eye signs and a goitre as well as the peripheral features of hyperthyroidism. The mother very often has eye signs (Fig. 15.17) and localised myxoedema.

EYE SIGNS

The eye signs of Graves' disease consist of:
Exophthalmos (proptosis)
Lid elevation or retraction
Ophthalmoplegia
Periorbital swelling
Conjunctival changes including oedema and inflammation
Congestive ophthalmopathy

Exophthalmos

Protrusion of the globe from the lateral orbital margin can be measured using a Hertel exophthalmometer. The patient must be observed with the head in the vertical position and if proptosis is present, the sclera is visible between the cornea and the lower lid (Fig. 15.18). Proptosis of more than 18 mm is referred to as

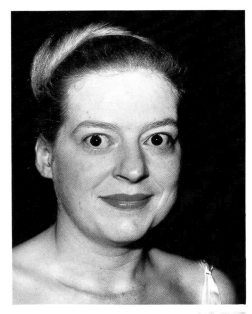

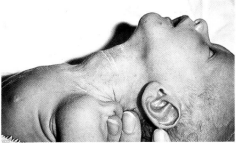

Fig. 15.17 Neonatal thyrotoxicosis.
A goitre is usually present, and this child also has eye signs. The mother shows the eye signs of Graves' disease; note the thyroidectomy scar.

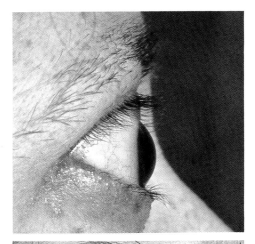

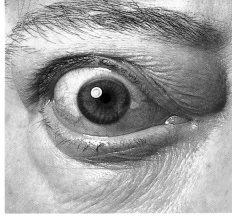

Fig. 15.18 Proptosis in Graves' disease.
The eye protrudes from the lateral orbital margin by more than 18 mm. In this case, sclera is visible both below the cornea (proptosis) and also above (lid retraction).

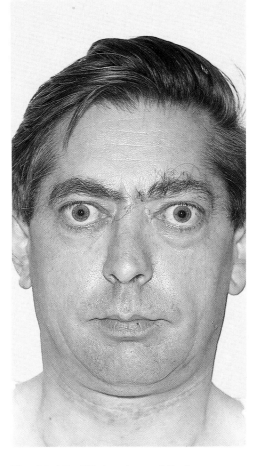

Fig. 15.19 Bilateral exophthalmos.
Exophthalmos is usually bilateral in Graves' disease, as in this instance.

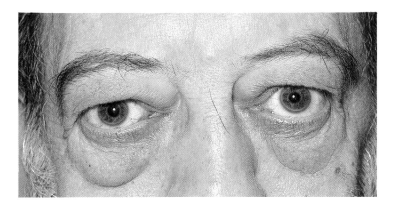

Fig. 15.20 Unilateral exophthalmos. Unilateral exophthalmos is common in ophthalmic Graves' disease.

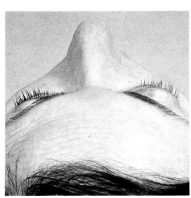

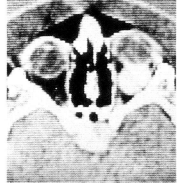

Fig. 15.21 Asymmetrical exophthalmos in excess of five mm.
This degree of asymmetry is unusual in Graves' disease, and its presence should raise the suspicion of a retro-orbital tumour.

15.6

exophthalmos which may be bilateral (commoner in Graves' disease with hyperthyroidism, Fig. 15.19) or unilateral (commoner in ophthalmic Graves' disease, Fig. 15.20). However, the asymmetry rarely exceeds 5mm in Graves' disease and any asymmetry greater than this should raise the suspicion of a space-occupying lesion in the orbit (Fig. 15.21).

Lid Retraction

In the relaxed position of forward gaze with the head vertical the upper lid should cover 3 or 4 mm of the cornea. In Graves' disease, spasm of the striated *levator palpebrae superioris* results in the upper lid becoming elevated. If the condition is sufficient to cause sclera to become visible above the cornea, lid retraction is present (Fig. 15.22). If one upper lid is merely higher than the other, giving a staring appearance, the sign is referred to as lid elevation (Fig. 15.23). Like exophthalmos, lid retraction is more often unilateral in the ophthalmic form of Graves' disease (Fig. 15.24) and bilateral in hyperthyroid Graves' (Fig. 15. 25). Lid retraction is almost diagnostic of Graves' disease but can very occasionally occur in lesions (usually vascular) affecting the upper brain stem (Fig. 15.26). Ptosis may occur in Graves' disease (Fig. 15.27) but is rare, and should always raise the suspicion of myasthenia gravis.

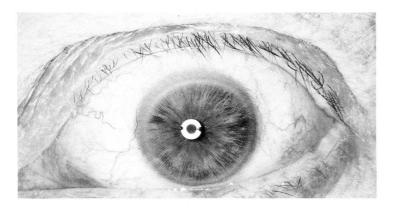

Fig. 15.22   Spasm of the levator palpebrae superioris causing lid retraction. The sclera is visible between the upper lid margin and the cornea when the head is vertical and the gaze is forward.

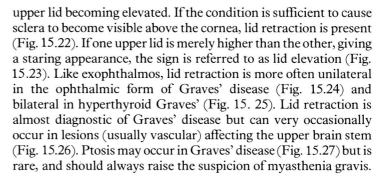

Fig. 15.23   Lid elevation giving a staring appearance.

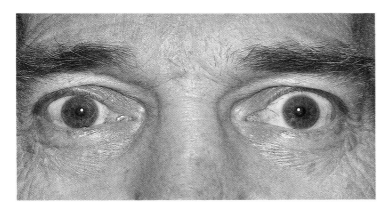

Fig. 15.24   Unilateral lid retraction. This is commonly seen in ophthalmic Graves' disease.

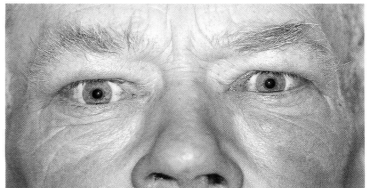

Fig. 15.25   Bilateral lid retraction in hyperthyroid Graves' disease.

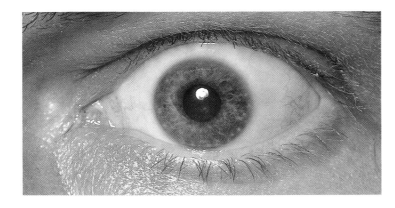

Fig. 15.26   Lid retraction. In this case, lid retraction is the result of a vascular lesion of the upper brain stem.

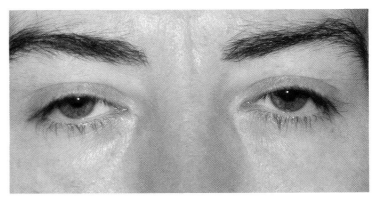

Fig. 15.27   Ptosis in Graves' disease. Ptosis is rare in Graves' disease, and care should be taken to exclude myasthenia gravis.

Ophthalmoplegia

Ophthalmoplegia in Graves' disease characteristically affects upward and outward gaze first (Fig. 15.28). Later, upward and inward gaze, lateral, medial and downward gaze are affected (in that order). The patient usually complains of diplopia in the direction of the limited ocular movement, particularly upwards (Fig. 15.29), which is mainly due to tethering of the muscles, particularly the inferior rectus below the globe. The eye may be deviated downwards due to fibrosis of the inferior rectus (Fig. 15.30).

Periorbital Swelling

Two forms of this, often associated with each other, are seen in Graves' disease. First, periorbital swelling may accompany any space-occupying lesion in the orbit which also causes exophthalmos. Second, and more characteristic of Graves' disease, is the oedematous inflammatory swelling of the lids, the upper usually being more severely affected (Fig. 15.31).

Conjunctival Changes

These consist of oedema (chemosis), inflammation, injection of the sclera over the insertion of the lateral rectus (Fig. 15.32) and swelling of the medial caruncles (Fig. 15.33). These changes are most marked in the condition of congestive ophthalmopathy.

Congestive Ophthalmopathy

This term refers to the severe, sight-threatening condition where optic nerve compression can lead to failure of vision, loss of colour vision and field defects; optic atrophy is a late sign, and conjunctival signs are prominent (Fig. 15.34), blepharospasm may be marked (Fig. 15.35) and should not be mistaken for ptosis. Corneal ulceration can occur along with the other eye signs of Graves' disease (Fig. 15.36). The term 'congestive ophthalmopathy' is preferable to 'malignant exophthalmos' since it is not malignant in the usual sense of the word and exophthalmos may not be present.

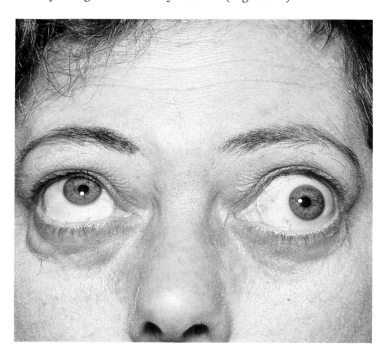

Fig. 15.28 Ophthalmoplegia in Graves' disease. Upward and outward movements are the earliest to be affected.

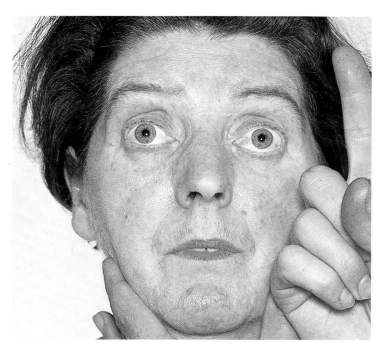

Fig. 15.29 Limitation of upward gaze. In this case, the limitation of movement is caused by tethering of the inferior rectus muscle.

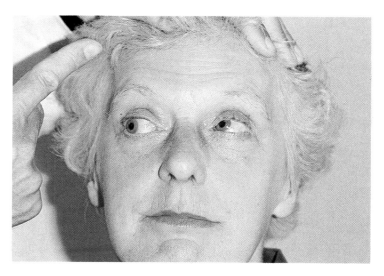

Fig. 15.30 Downward deviation of the eye, due to fibrosis of the inferior rectus muscle.

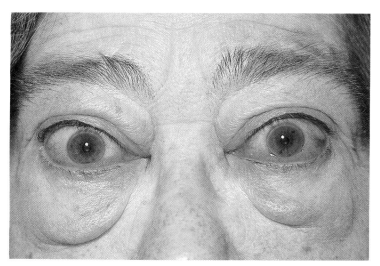

Fig. 15.31 Oedematous swelling of the eyelids in Graves' disease.

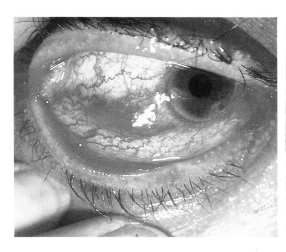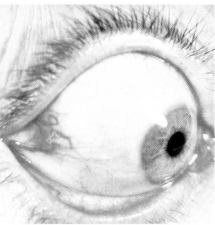

Fig. 15.32 Inflammation of the conjunctiva in Graves' disease. The right hand picture shows injection of the sclera over the insertion of the lateral rectus muscle.

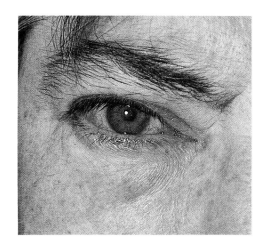

Fig. 15.33 Swelling of the medial caruncle in Graves' disease.

Fig. 15.34 Severe congestive ophthalmopathy. Optic atrophy is a late sign.

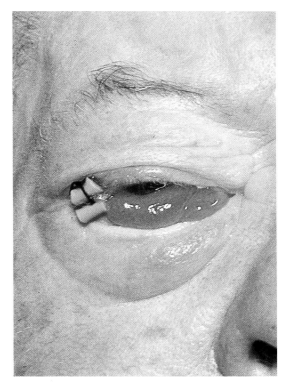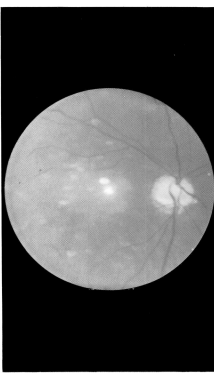

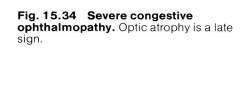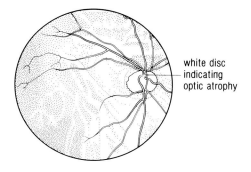

white disc indicating optic atrophy

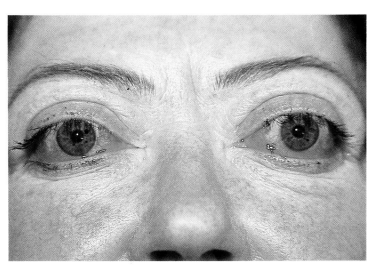

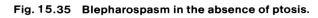

Fig. 15.35 Blepharospasm in the absence of ptosis.

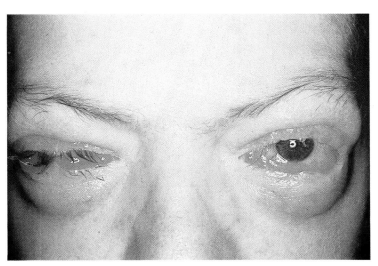

Fig. 15.36 Severe chemosis and pericorneal swelling in advanced congestive ophthalmopathy.

Localised Myxoedema

Localised myxoedema, which commonly affects the pretibial region may affect other parts of the body, determined by local pressure or trauma. It can occur in several forms (Figs. 15.37 – 15.39):

(i) A nodular form sometimes initiated by trauma which mimics erythema nodosum and may come and go.

(ii) A sheet-like form with non-pitting oedema, coarse thickening of the skin, violaceous discolouration and thickened hairs.

(iii) A horny form in which there are gross overgrowths of the skin and subcutaneous tissue on the dorsum of the feet and toes.

Thyroid Acropachy

Thyroid acropachy closely resembles clubbing of the fingers, and the curving of the nails is most apparent in the thumb and index finger (Fig. 15.40). Acropachy may be associated with patchy subperiosteal new bone formation (Fig. 15.41) and differs from hypertrophic osteoarthropathy, in which the new bone growth

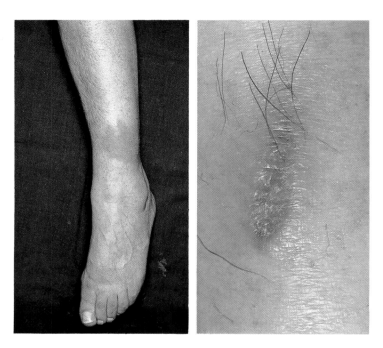

Fig. 15.37 Nodular pretibial myxoedema resembling erythema nodosum.

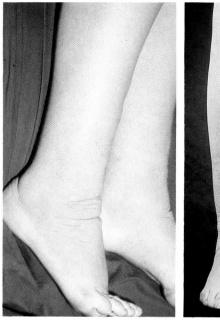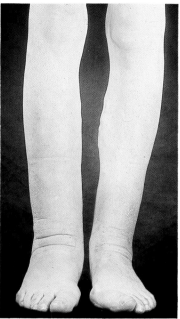

Fig. 15.38 A further variant of localised myxoedema. This type gives rise to coarse violaceous skin, thickened hair, and non-pitting oedema.

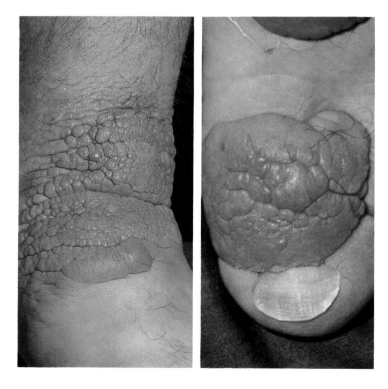

Fig. 15.39 The horny form of localised myxoedema. This type gives rise to gross papilliform overgrowth of skin and subcutaneous tissue, here involving the dorsum of the feet and toes.

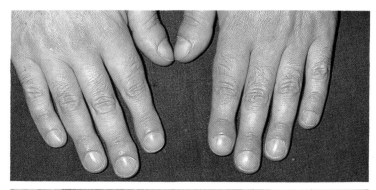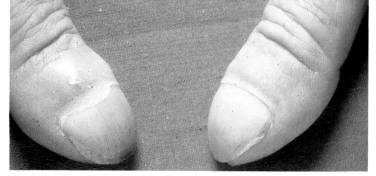

Fig. 15.40 Thyroid acropachy. Thyroid acropachy (upper) closely resembles clubbing of the fingers (lower).

develops in a linear manner. Acropachy can also affect the toes and in its gross form may cause visible swelling of the fingers and metacarpals.

Other Associated Features

Other associated features may help in the diagnosis of AIT disease. Vitiligo (Fig. 15.42) is the patchy but almost symmetrical depigmentation of the skin surrounded by increased pigmentation, which may be associated with any of the organ-specific auto-immune diseases (AIT diseases, pernicious anaemia, Type 1 insulin–dependent diabetes mellitus and Addison's disease). Premature greying of the hair and leucotrichia (Fig. 15.43) are also associated with AIT disease. Fat deposition just beyond the angle of the jaws can give an appearance of prominent jowls (Fig. 15.44) which is associated with Graves' disease, usually occurring with eye signs and localised myxoedema.

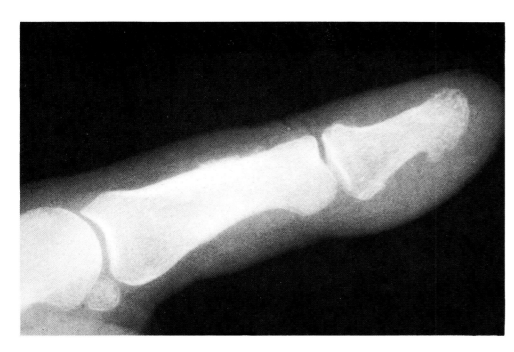

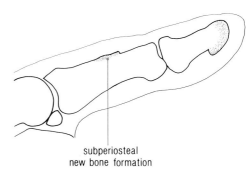

Fig. 15.41   Patchy subperiosteal new bone formation in thyroid acropachy.

subperiosteal
new bone formation

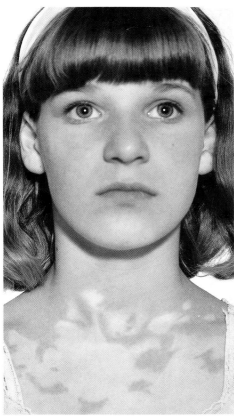

Fig. 15.42   Vitiligo. This patchy but almost symmetrical distribution of skin depigmentation may be associated with any of the organ-specific AIT diseases.

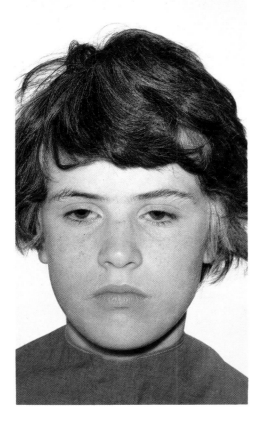

Fig. 15.43   Leucotrichia associated with autoimmune thyroiditis.

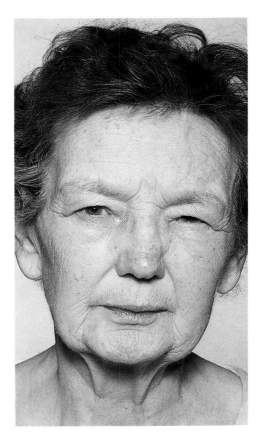

Fig. 15.44   Fat deposition beyond the angle of the jaws in Graves' disease. This problem usually occurs with eye signs and localised myxoedema.

15.11

Toxic Multinodular Goitre

This condition can be recognised clinically by the nodular and asymmetrical thyroid enlargement (Fig. 15.45) which may extend retrosternally (Fig. 15.46) and cause tracheal deviation (Fig. 15.47). Sometimes eye signs are associated with it, and it is then assumed that Graves' disease has developed in a patient with a pre-existing nodular goitre. The nodularity is best demonstrated by the patchy uptake of radioiodine in a thyroid scan (Fig. 15.48).

Toxic Adenoma

Here one, or occasionally two, thyroid nodules exhibit autonomy (Fig. 15.49). Increased levels of thyroid hormones, sometimes of tri-iodothyronine alone, may be sufficient to impair or abolish the thyrotrophin response to thyrotrophin releasing hormone without causing clinically apparent hyperthyroidism – the so-called subclinical toxic adenoma.

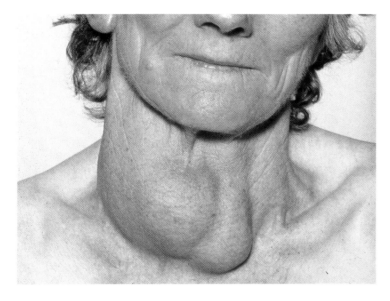

Fig. 15.45 Asymmetric, nodular thyroid enlargement.

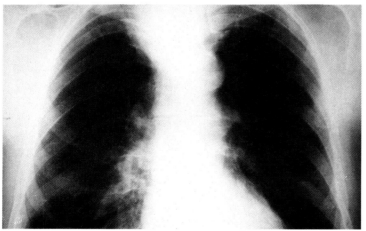

Fig. 15.46 Retrosternal extension of a goitre.

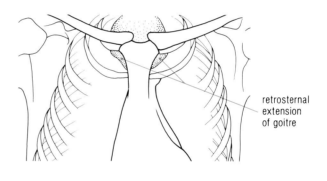

retrosternal extension of goitre

Fig. 15.47 Gross tracheal deviation caused by thyroid enlargement.

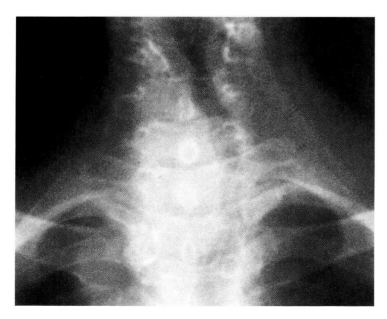

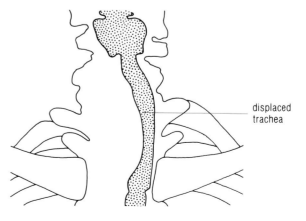

displaced trachea

TREATMENT OF HYPERTHYROIDISM

Toxic adenoma can be treated surgically (after control of hyperthyroidism by antithyroid drugs) or by radioiodine. Hypothyroidism is uncommon after the use of radioiodine, because of the suppressed uptake of isotope in the normal thyroid.

Toxic multinodular goitre can be treated in a similar fashion to toxic adenoma. In younger patients, partial thyroidectomy is preferable to radioiodine since the nodular gland is less radiosensitive and the radioiodine treatment may have to be repeated. An initial dose of 15 – 20 mCi of ^{131}I is usually given.

Graves' disease can be treated by antithyroid drugs, partial thyroidectomy or by radioiodine (Fig. 15.50).

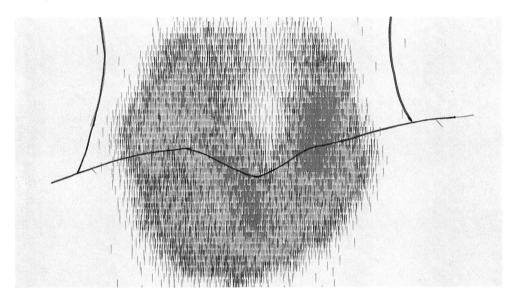

Fig. 15.48 Thyroid scan demonstrating patchy uptake of radioiodine.

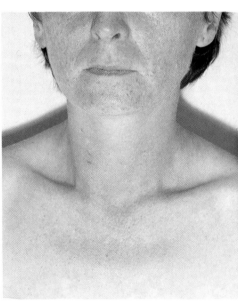
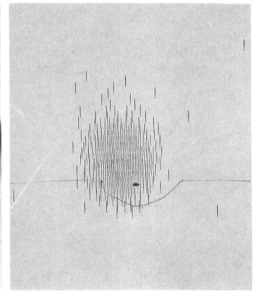

Fig. 15.49 Patient with solitary hyperactive thyroid nodule. The scintigraph scan confirms the presence of a 'hot' nodule.

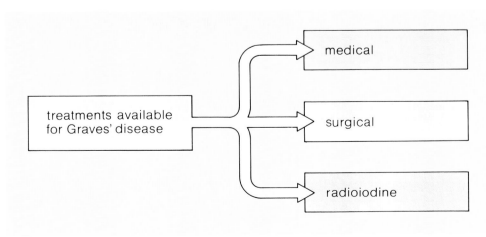

Fig. 15.50 Methods of treating Graves' disease. Graves' disease may be treated with antithyroid drugs, by partial thyroidectomy or by means of radioiodine.

Antithyroid Drugs

The indications for antithyroid therapy are shown in Fig. 15.51. There is general agreement that children with Graves' disease (Fig. 15.52) are best treated with antithyroid drugs. In the U.K. and Europe the drug of first choice is carbimazole, in an initial dose of 15 mg three times daily. When the patient is clinically euthyroid, thyroxine is added by some clinicians to the carbimazole in a dose of 0.15 mg daily in a 'blocking–replacement' regime. This allows a smooth control of circulating thyroid hormone levels without frequent hospital visits. Others do not use thyroxine and merely reduce the carbimazole alone to the level required to maintain the euthyroid state. This usually requires 10 – 15 mg carbimazole given in a single daily dose. The duration of therapy is empirical and courses vary from six months to two years. (Figure 15.53 is a table of antithyroid drugs). All patients treated with carbimazole should be warned of the risks of agranulocytosis presenting as a sore throat or ulcerated mouth. This is rare after the first three months of therapy. About sixty per cent of patients treated with a one-year course of antithyroid drugs relapse, usually within the next two years. Repeat courses may be given and occasionally patients prefer life-long carbimazole, given in a small dose once daily, to ablative therapy.

Fig. 15.54 shows the factors which may determine the results of medical treatment. Patients with severe disease and large vascular goitres who require large maintenance doses of antithyroid drugs are more likely to relapse. Relapse is more common in

Indications for Medical Treatment
patient preference
small goitre
mild disease
other diseases
children
pregnancy
ophthalmopathy
pre-operative
pre-radioiodine
thyrotoxic crisis
relapse after thyroidectomy

Fig. 15.51   Indications for medical treatment in Graves' disease.

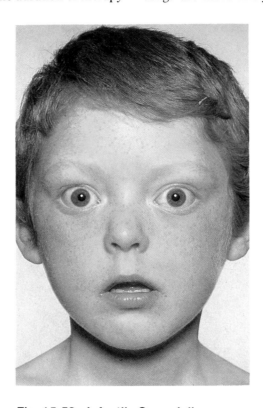

Fig. 15.52   Infantile Graves' disease. It is generally agreed that medical therapy is preferable for children with Graves' disease.

Antithyroid Drugs
carbimazole
methimazole
propylthiouracil (PTU)
potassium perchlorate
lithium
iodides
propranolol
sodium ipodate

Fig. 15.53   Table of antithyroid drugs. Carbimazole is the drug of choice in Europe. Some clinicians add thyroxine to the carbimazole in a blocking-replacement regime, once the patient is clinically euthyroid. Carbimazole is rapidly converted to methimazole (10 mg carbimazole $\equiv$ 6 mg methimazole).

Fig. 15.54   Factors determining the result of medical therapy. Patients with severe disease and large vascular goitres are more likely to relapse, as are those whose thyroidal uptake is not suppressed by T_3, and who show high initial levels of circulating thyroglobulin. HLA DR3 haplotypes are prone to relapse, along with those who have high levels of receptor antibody post-therapy. Those with high titres of microsomal antibodies are more likely to become hypothyroid after medical or surgical treatment.

Factors Determining the Results of Medical Therapy	
clinical	**laboratory**
severity of disease	T_3 suppressibility
size of goitre	TRH test
vascularity of goitre	TSAb titre
degree of goitre decrease with therapy	thyroglobulin
	HLA type
dose required for maintenance	microsomal antibody titre

patients whose thyroidal radioisotope uptake is not suppressed by T_3 and who show high initial levels of circulating thyroglobulin. An absent TSH response to TRH at the end of a course of treatment has not proved to be a consistent predictor of relapse. Patients who are HLA DR3 are more prone to relapse, as are those with high levels of receptor antibody at the end of therapy. Those with high titres of microsomal antibodies are more likely to become hypothyroid after both medical and surgical treatment. Alternative antithyroid drugs include propylthiouracil, methylthiouracil and the more recent sodium ipodate, which blocks peripheral conversion of thyroxine to tri-iodothyronine and may prove of value if rapid control of symptoms is required. The side-effects of antithyroid drugs are shown in Fig. 15.55, and other problems associated with medical therapy are shown in Fig. 15.56.

SURGERY

The indications for partial thyroidectomy are shown in Fig. 15.57. All patients should first be controlled with antithyroid drugs. The complications of operation are shown in Fig. 15.58. However, the only common complications are hypothyroidism, (occurring in about fifteen per cent) and recurrent hyperthyroidism (occurring in about five per cent). Recurrent upper pole nodules are a rare complication which may be associated with recurrent hyperthyroidism (Fig. 15.59).

Side-Effects of Antithyroid Drugs
nausea
vomiting
rashes
pruritis
leucopenia (carbimazole,PTU)
agranulocytosis (carbimazole,PTU)
aplastic anaemia (perchlorate)
drug fever

Fig. 15.55 Side-effects of antithyroid drugs. All patients treated with carbimazole should be warned of the risk of agranulocytosis presenting as a sore throat or ulcerated mouth.

Problems Associated with Drug Treatment
inconvenience to patient
high relapse rate
difficulty in predicting remission
long duration of therapy
difficulty in maintaining patient cooperation

Fig. 15.56 Other problems associated with antithyroid drugs. Drug therapy has a relatively high relapse rate, and the chance of remission is difficult to predict while the patient is undergoing treatment. Therapy may be of long duration and may involve inconvenience to the patient who may therefore find it difficult to co-operate.

Indications for Surgical Treatment
patient preference
adults up to 45 years
severe disease
large goitre
relapse after drug treatment

Fig. 15.57 Indications for surgery in Graves' disease. Partial thyroidectomy is considered by some to be the treatment of choice in adult patients up to the age of 45 years, especially in severe cases. Surgery should also be considered when a patient has relapsed after drug therapy.

Complications of Partial Thyroidectomy	
early	**late**
recurrent laryngeal nerve palsy	
superior laryngeal nerve palsy	cheloid scar
haemorrhage	
hypoparathyroidism	tethered scar
pneumothorax	
thyroid crisis	hypothyroidism
infection	
damage to thoracic duct	recurrence of hyperthyroidism
damage to carotid artery	
damage to jugular vein	recurrent upper pole nodules

Fig. 15.58 Complications of partial thyroidectomy. The only common complications are hypothyroidism and recurrent hyperthyroidism.

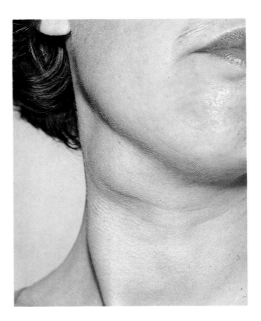

Fig. 15.59 Recurrent upper-pole nodule associated with thyrotoxicosis. This is a rare complication of surgery, which may be associated with recurrent hyperthyroidism.

15.15

Radioiodine Therapy

The indications for, and complications of radioiodine therapy are shown in Figure 15.60. There is no convincing evidence for the subsequent development of thyroid carcinoma or leukaemia. Opinions vary as to the optimum dosage schedule but the author prefers to administer a 15mCi dose to all patients, irrespective of gland size or severity of hyperthyroidism, rendering eighty-five per cent of patients hypothyroid within three months. Further doses of 15 mCi are given if required. The most common complication of radioiodine treatment is hypothyroidism, and even this should be easily controllable.

Indications for, and Complications of, Radioiodine Treatment	
indications	**complications**
patient preference	permanent hypothyroidism
patients over 45 years	transient hypothyroidism
treatment choice for recurrence after thyroidectomy	thyroiditis
severe uncontrolled disease	sialadenitis
large goitre	thyrotoxic crisis
poor patient cooperation	nodule formation
presence of other disease	malignancy (not proven)

Fig. 15.60 **Indications for radioiodine therapy and associated complications.** Radioiodine is the most effective treatment in cases of recurrence after surgery. It is suitable for older patients, in severe disease, and when patient co-operation is poor. Radioiodine is also useful in the presence of other disorders. The only problematic complication is hypothyroidism, which is relatively easy to control.

16 Growth Disorders

Charles G D Brook, MD, FRCP

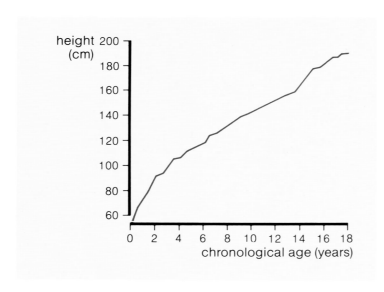

Fig. 16.1 Height distance chart showing the growth of an individual boy from birth to adulthood. All normal children follow a growth curve resembling this distance chart.

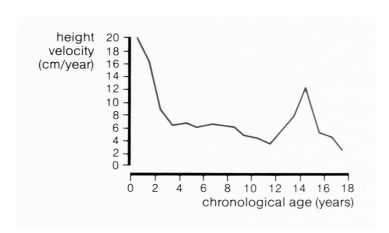

Fig. 16.2 Height velocity chart of the same boy as in Figure 16.1. To produce such a chart the annual gain in height is plotted against chronological age. The three phases of childhood growth of (i) rapid deceleration in infancy, (ii) slow deceleration in middle childhood and (iii) rapid acceleration at adolescence may be identified.

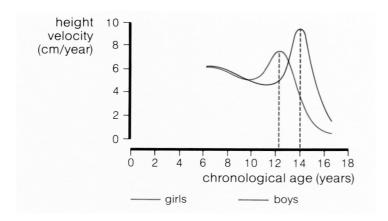

— girls   — boys

Fig. 16.3 Average height velocity chart for both males and females in the United Kingdom. The earlier onset of the adolescent growth spurt in females is shown together with the greater peak height velocity in males.

Normal growth in height and size results from the complex interplay of many intrinsic and extrinsic factors on the innate, genetically-determined capacity for growth of that individual. The ultimate height of a person is a function not only of the rate of linear growth of his bones, but also of its duration.

The growth of an individual from birth to adulthood may be pictorially represented in a height distance chart (Fig. 16.1). All normal children follow such a growth curve.

To determine the rate of growth of an individual child, a number of height measurements should be made at regular intervals, for instance, twice a year. A height velocity curve (Fig. 16.2) is obtained by plotting the height gained during each year and yields important information about the growth pattern of a child. The three phases of growth in childhood are easily recognised: there is first a period of rapid and rapidly decelerating growth in infancy, then a period of steady and slowly decelerating growth in middle childhood followed by a rapid rise and fall of growth at adolescence.

The adolescent growth spurt, which is associated with puberty in both sexes, occurs earlier in females than in males by an average of two years (see Fig. 16.3). The absence of the two years of

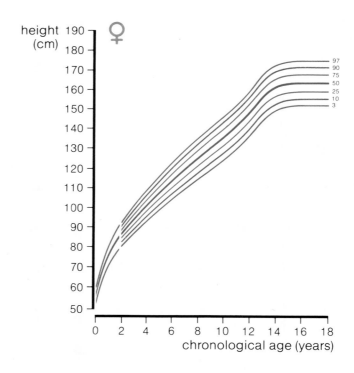

Fig. 16.4 Height distance centile chart for girls in the United Kingdom. This chart is no more than a description of the height of the female population. The fiftieth percentile is the median, so that fifty per cent of individuals are taller and fifty per cent shorter than this height.

16.2

decelerating prepubertal growth and the difference in the peak height velocity at puberty accounts for the adult height difference between men and women which is 12.6cm on average.

Height is usually plotted on a standard centile chart for distance (Fig. 16.4). This chart is no more than a description of the height in the population (in this case the population of the United Kingdom). Fifty per cent of girls aged four years have a height above 100cm, and the remaining fifty per cent have a height below 100 cm. Three per cent of all girls aged four years measure less than 92cm, and the growth of the majority of these is not abnormal. Where the height of a child lies on the centile chart at any time depends upon genetic and environmental factors, most of which are beyond the control of physicians.

Although in most children growth and developmental events follow the same orderly pattern, the pace of maturation varies widely. Thus an individual child's growth performance is better viewed in relationship to his or her stage of physical maturity than in relationship to chronological age. Using skeletal age, it is possible to predict with some degree of reliability, the final adult stature and to distinguish between children who will mature early and those in whom sexual development will be delayed. A number of systems for estimating bone age are available, but all use comparisons of the maturity of a number of epiphyseal centres with standard radiographs and, from these, derive an average maturity score. Because of the number of centres conveniently available in the hand and wrist, radiographs from these areas are usually used to make such an assessment. The hand of a girl with precocious puberty is shown in Figure 16.5. She has the maturity of a girl of ten years of age; this means that eighty-three per cent of her growth has already taken place. She now measures 128cm which is tall for her chronological age, but is short for her bone age. Her final height will be short, estimated to be approximately 154cm.

A typical problem is shown in Figure 16.6. A boy aged fourteen years is referred for evaluation of his short stature since his present height is only 140cm, which is below the third percentile. His skeletal maturity corresponds to that of a boy of eleven years of age, so his growth prognosis (170cm) is well within normal limits for the centile position of his parental heights (shown on the right of the chart). Whether he will achieve this potential, depends upon whether he is growing at a normal rate, and on how long he continues growing, which is defined by his bone age. To establish normal growth a normal growth rate must be demonstrated.

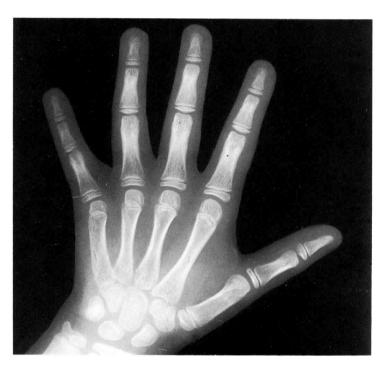

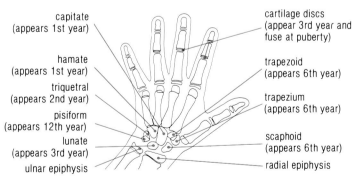

capitate
(appears 1st year)

hamate
(appears 1st year)

triquetral
(appears 2nd year)

pisiform
(appears 12th year)

lunate
(appears 3rd year)

ulnar epiphysis

cartilage discs
(appear 3rd year and
fuse at puberty)

trapezoid
(appears 6th year)

trapezium
(appears 6th year)

scaphoid
(appears 6th year)

radial epiphysis

Fig. 16.5 Radiograph of a hand used to assess skeletal maturity (bone age). The hand of a 6-year-old girl with precocious puberty is shown. Although she is tall for her chronological age, her bone age is advanced to that of a 10-year-old, which means that eighty-three per cent of her growth has taken place already. Assessment of her bone age is important since it is used to predict her final height which, in this case, will be short. The normal ages at which the bone ossification centres develop are shown in brackets.

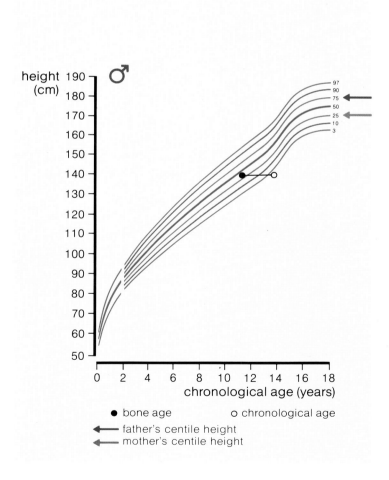

● bone age   ○ chronological age

⬅ father's centile height
⬅ mother's centile height

Fig. 16.6 Height centile graph used to evaluate growth in a short boy. Although the chronological age of this boy is 14 years his bone age is only that of an 11-year-old, suggesting that he has potential for catch-up growth.

To establish the growth rate, one measures height on two different occasions separated by a period of time. The length of time needed to establish a normal growth velocity depends upon the increment which might be expected and the accuracy of the equipment used. Instruments of the type shown in Figure 16.7 would require approximately three years to establish normality because of the high error margin when using them. When measuring the height of children, it should be remembered that all individuals shrink slightly during the day. A child must therefore be drawn out to the maximum by traction under the mastoids.

Measuring Technique

Standing height should be taken without shoes, the child standing with his heels and back in contact with an upright wall. His head is held so that he looks straight ahead with the outer canthus of the eye socket in the same horizontal plane as his external auditory meatuses, and not with his nose tipped upwards. A right angled block is then slid down the wall until the bottom surface touches the child's head and a scale (fixed to the wall) is read. During measurement, the child should be told to stretch his neck to be as tall as possible, although care must be taken to prevent his heels coming off the ground. Gentle but firm traction should be applied by the measurer under the mastoid processes to keep the child stretched. In this way, the variation in height from morning to evening is minimised.

A stadiometer, as shown in Figure 16.8, enables one to measure height on successive occasions to within a millimetre when the measurements are made with care by the same observer using the same technique. In a measurement of more than 1m, the accuracy of this instrument compares favourably with any other measurement made clinically or in the laboratory. Nevertheless, measurements made over less than three to six months may produce considerable errors and reliance should not be placed upon single estimates of height velocity made over a short period of time.

Height velocity measurements (Fig. 16.9) are converted into annual rates of growth by dividing the increment by the lapse of time. Such measurements are compared with centiles as before but, whereas a third centile position on a height distance chart may be and probably is normal, a velocity which is persistently on the third centile leads to progressive loss of height compared with children of the same age. The growth velocity of a given child must oscillate about the fiftieth percentile to maintain growth along a centile chart on a distance chart. Visual inspection on a distance chart is not a substitute for calculating the height velocity and plotting it on a centile chart.

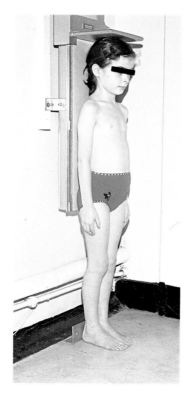

Fig. 16.7 Photograph of a stadiometer not to be recommended. This instrument should be avoided since it would take several years to produce a reliable growth curve because of the error margin involved.

Fig. 16.8 Photograph of a recommended stadiometer in use. During measurement the child should be told to stretch his neck whilst the measurer applies gentle traction under the mastoids to keep the child stretched. The outer canthus of the eye sockets of the child should be in the same horizontal plane as his external auditory meatuses, and his heels should be touching the ground.

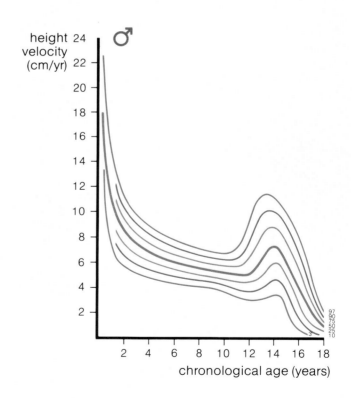

Fig. 16.9 Height velocity chart for males from birth to 18 years of age. Height velocity is the change in height over an interval of time. The length of time needed to establish a normal growth velocity depends upon the increment which might be expected and the accuracy of the equipment used. The child must maintain a height velocity at or above the fiftieth percentile to maintain growth along the centile line on a distance chart.

SHORT STATURE

Short stature is a common cause of concern amongst children, adolescents and their parents. Three per cent of the population have a height below the third percentile and will be noticeably short; however, probably fewer than one out of a hundred of these will have a primary endocrine defect. In order to detect these children, careful clinical assessment and measurements of the height velocity are needed to separate those who are small, but growing normally, from those who are failing to grow. For the latter, a diagnosis is needed in order for the appropriate treatment to be instituted without delay. The state of nutrition may help to point the diagnostic pathway but any child who is growing slowly should have diagnostic investigation to determine the cause. In assessing all short patients, a detailed history, physical examination and urine analysis are required, together with a radiograph of the non-dominant hand and wrist. The bone age can be assessed and therefore the growth potential. Short stature which is out of keeping with the family background is likely to be significant. The mid-parental height (the mean of the parental centile heights) can be calculated in order to estimate height expectation. Information should also be obtained about the growth pattern in the parents, especially concerning the time of onset of the pubertal growth spurt. Physical examination may reveal an abnormal looking child with either dysmorphic features or disproportionate short stature (short limbs or short back and limbs). The major causes of short stature in children with a normal appearance and those with disproportionate short stature are illustrated in Figures 16.10 and 16.11.

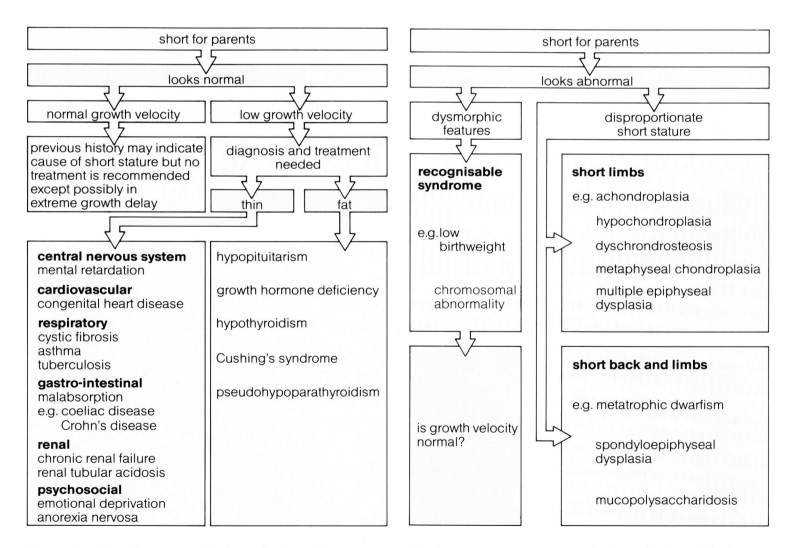

Fig. 16.10 Flow diagram used in the evaluation of short stature of patients who have a normal appearance.

Fig. 16.11 Flow diagram used in the evaluation of short stature of patients who have an abnormal phenotype.

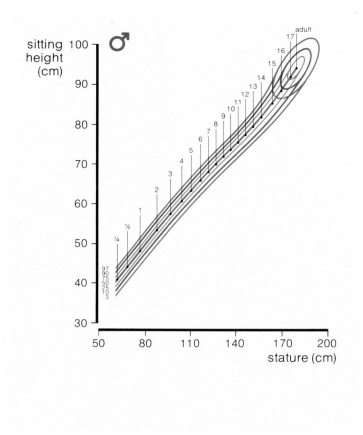

sitting height (cm)

♂

Fig. 16.12 Graph of sitting height versus stature. The measurement of body proportion is greatly facilitated in measuring sitting height and plotting the relationship of sitting height to stature.

Disproportionate Short Stature

Children who are short because they have short limbs will have plots that lie towards the upper left side of a chart of sitting height versus stature, and those with short backs the opposite (Fig. 16.12): the method of measurement of sitting height is shown in Figure 16.13. Shortness may be caused by skeletal dysplasia, for example, hypochondroplasia in which there is proportionate shortening in back and limbs which is only identifiable by clinical inspection. Where a skeletal dysplasia is suspected a full skeletal radiographic survey is needed and an experienced radiologist consulted. As few radiologists are practised in this field, only a very few know how to interpret the very subtle radiographic changes; it is a field for the super specialist.

Dysmorphic Features

Children with dysmorphic features may have a recognisable syndrome, for instance, one associated with a chromosomal abnormality, or they may have dysmorphic features resulting from low birth weight.

The dysmorphic features associated with relatively low birth weight are shown in Figure 16.14. Note the facial features, the body asymmetry and the appearance of thinness. An early history of being difficult to feed is extremely characteristic of this very common problem. Absolute low birth weight is not a prerequisite for the diagnosis. A low birth weight for the family is frequently found. If there are no obvious abnormalities on examination, and if a normal growth velocity exists, it is unlikely that there is anything amiss. However, where a low growth velocity exists, an organic cause is usually present. Short and thin children usually have a systemic cause for their short stature, whereas endocrinopathies causing short stature usually result in obesity.

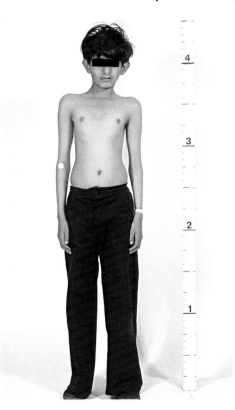

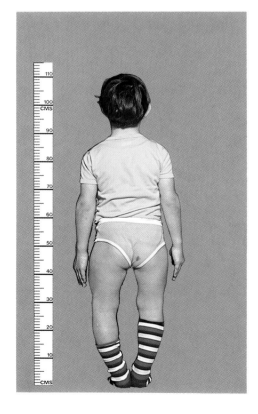

Fig. 16.13 Photograph showing the correct method of measurement of sitting height.

Fig. 16.14 Photograph of a boy showing dysmorphic features (facial asymmetry) and body thinness associated with low birth weight.

Fig. 16.15 Photograph of a child with rickets. Note the bowing of his legs which is only part of the reason for poor growth in children with rickets.

16.6

Systemic Causes of Short Stature

In systemic disease there is often delayed skeletal maturation, but the potential for catch-up growth is present if the underlying systemic disorder can be successfully treated. A child with coeliac disease, for example, will continue to have stunted growth until gluten is removed from the diet, after which rapid growth and development may occur. Other chronic disorders which may also retard growth are Crohn's disease, respiratory disease (e.g. asthma), renal disease, cardiovascular causes and nutritional causes (e.g. rickets, Fig. 16.15). In all these instances the potential for catch-up growth remains if the disease is rapidly cured.

Occult coeliac disease is a common finding amongst children growing slowly for no obvious reason. Most children with endocrine diseases are fat; therefore, in a child who is not fat, a jejunal biopsy should be performed at an early stage to exclude villous atrophy. The effect of a gluten-free diet in a late diagnosed asymptomatic coeliac patient whose only complaint was short stature is shown in Figure 16.16.

Psychosocial and Emotional Deprivation

This condition is commonly recognised in infancy and childhood. Infants suffering from maternal deprivation display behavioural abnormalities such as apathy, watchfulness and autoerotic activity as well as delayed developmental behaviour. There is often a history of maternal rejection or neglect, non-accidental injury or lack of physical handling. Emotional deprivation in childhood may lead to small stature (Figs. 16.17 and 16.18), retarded skeletal maturation and, in older children, delayed sexual maturation. Endocrine function may also be abnormal in affected patients, together with high fasting growth hormone levels and cortisol non-responsiveness with the insulin tolerance test.

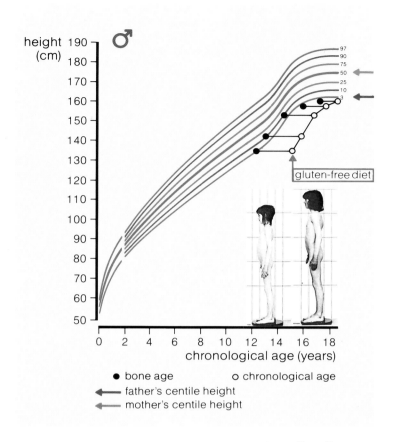

Fig. 16.16 Photograph of a child with occult coeliac disease with short stature before and after treatment. The effect of introducing a gluten-free diet on his growth is shown. Note the delayed bone age at the start of treatment.

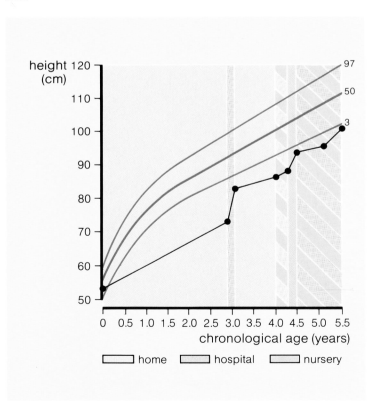

Fig. 16.17 Graph showing the effect of emotional deprivation on a child. During hospitalisation the growth rate of the child increased but 'steadied-off' during periods of emotional deprivation at home.

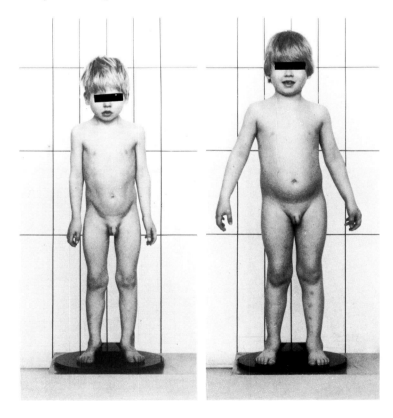

Fig. 16.18 Photograph of an emotionally-deprived 7-year-old child before treatment, and after treatment taken one year later. Note the marked short stature and the rapid growth following treatment.

16.7

Endocrine Causes of Short Stature

The important hormones concerned with growth are thyroxine, growth hormone, and sex steroids. Deficiency of any of these hormones may result in short stature.

Children with growth hormone deficiency present in two ways; either with isolated growth hormone deficiency associated with relatively straightforward management, or with a varied spectrum of additional pituitary hormone deficiences. The aetiology of isolated growth hormone deficiency (IGHD) appears to be due to pituitary somatotroph hypoplasia which may be secondary to a lack of secretion of hypothalamic growth hormone releasing hormone (a recently discovered polypeptide of forty-one to forty-four amino acid residues). Cases of growth hormone deficiency may be familial.

Birth weight is characteristically normal, and in the immediate postnatal and early life, general health is seldom a problem. Apart from short stature, a growth hormone deficient child shows features which frequently occur in this condition, but which in themselves are not unique. He has truncal obesity (Fig. 16.19) and a face young in appearance for his chronological age which is typical of many of these children. There is a tendency for crowding of the facial features to the centre of the face, suggesting maxillary hypoplasia. In males, the genitalia tend to be underdeveloped and may be of micropenis proportions. Delayed skeletal maturation is almost invariable. Body proportions tend to be normal before the normal age of puberty although IGHD children tend to have rather poor musculature. Skinfold fat is always increased. In boys delayed puberty is seen almost without exception, even in the absence of additional gonadotrophin deficiency. However, they tend to enter puberty at the normal bone age. Clearly, if they do not, concurrent gonadotrophin deficiency should be suspected.

Diagnostic investigations are an adjunct to the clinical picture. Methods of testing the hypothalamo-pituitary axis as to its ability to secrete growth hormone are legion (Fig. 16.20), suggesting that there is still none that is ideal. The investigation of immediate prepubertal children deserves special mention. Some individuals

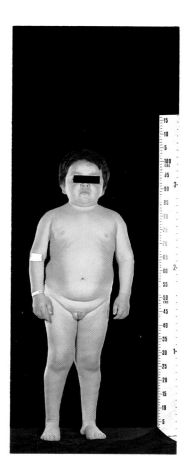

Screening Tests of Growth Hormone Reserve

exercise

sleep

Agents used in Formal Assessment of Growth Hormone Reserve

insulin tolerance test

arginine infusion

L-dopa

glucagon

clonidine

propranolol

growth hormone releasing factor

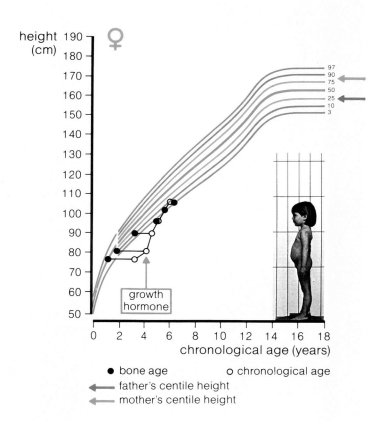

Fig. 16.19 Photograph of a boy with classical growth hormone deficiency. Such children are very small, tend to be fat and have under-developed genitalia. They have a low growth velocity and usually a retarded bone age.

Fig. 16.20 Table of commonly used screening tests for growth hormone (GH) reserve. The insulin tolerance test remains the most frequently used investigation. The GRF test is currently only a research procedure.

Fig. 16.21 Response to treatment of a girl with isolated growth hormone deficiency by injections of human growth hormone three times per week. The heights are shown as open circles and continuous lines and height plots are connected to the corresponding bone ages by solid lines.

seem to acquire a transiently impaired growth hormone response to stimuli at this stage of their development and priming with the appropriate sex steroid may be required before evaluating growth hormone reserve. This can be done by giving 100mg testosterone enanthate three days before the test in boys, or 200μg oral ethinyloestradiol daily on three consecutive days in girls. Treatment of isolated growth hormone deficiency is by injections of growth hormone three times per week. The response to a typical case receiving treatment is shown in Figure 16.21.

Laron Dwarfism

The Laron dwarf phenotype (Fig. 16.22) is identical to the growth hormone deficient child. The defect is, however, caused by somatomedin deficiency, and resting growth hormone levels are high. These patients do not respond to exogenous growth hormone.

Hypothyroidism

Hypothyroidism in children is traditionally divided into congenital hypothyroidism (cretinism, Figs. 16.23 and 16.24) and acquired hypothyroidism, although the same aetiological factors may be responsible for both.

Causes of cretinism include athyreosis, cryptothyroidism with inadequate thyroid hormone production, and dyshormonogenetic causes.

Basal thyroid function tests will reveal low levels of thyroxine together with a raised TSH. Bone age radiographs, particularly of the knees, are valuable. The distal femoral epiphyses are calcified in nearly all normal term individuals, but not in cretins.

Linear growth and skeletal maturity respond rather dramatically to thyroid hormone replacement. However, intellectual capacity in these children is inversely proportional to the age at which adequate therapy is begun. If treatment is delayed beyond the age of three to six months, the chances of attainment of normal intelligence are poor.

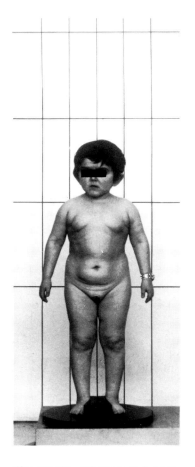

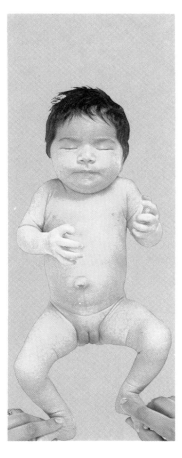

Clinical Features of Cretinism

prolonged neonatal jaundice

lethargy

feeding problems

failure to gain weight

constipation

dry skin

thick tongue

umbilical hernia

respiratory problems

goitre

mental retardation

Fig. 16.22 Photograph of a child with Laron's syndrome. The phenotype is identical to that of a growth hormone deficient child. However, since the cause is a deficiency of somatomedin, patients do not respond to exogenous growth hormones (indeed their resting growth hormone levels are high).

Fig. 16.23 Photograph of a child suffering from cretinism. Coarse features, a large tongue and an apathetic appearance are characteristic of cretinism.

Fig. 16.24 Table of the clinical features of cretinism.

Although the same aetiological causes as in cretinism may be invoked, after the age of two years, truly acquired hypothyroidism (Figs. 16.25 and 16.26) is usually caused by Hashimoto's thyroiditis or iodine deficiency. Symptoms and signs are similar to adult hypothyroidism. Short stature is very common, the bone age tends to be very retarded and children tend to maintain infantile proportions because of poor linear bone growth.

Pseudohypoparathyroidism

Pseudohypoparathyroidism (Fig. 16.27) is transmitted with an X-linked inheritance, the patients having peripheral resistance to the actions of parathyroid hormone (PTH). The typical phenotypic features include short stature, a round face, obesity, short thick neck, decreased intelligence, subcutaneous calcification as well as ossification. Shortening of the metacarpals is frequent. The diagnosis may be confirmed by the presence of low or normal serum calcium, elevated phosphate and the presence of a raised PTH level. Following PTH infusion, urinary cyclic AMP fails to rise. The condition is treated by administering high doses of vitamin D.

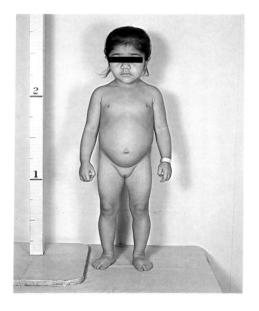
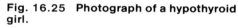

Fig. 16.25 Photograph of a hypothyroid girl.

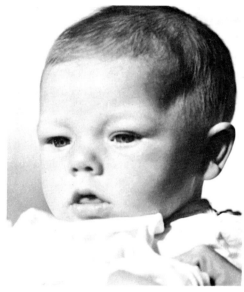
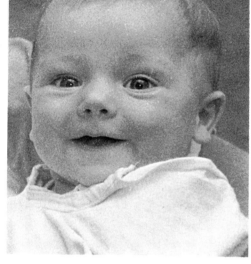

Fig. 16.26 Photograph of a hypothyroid baby before and after treatment.

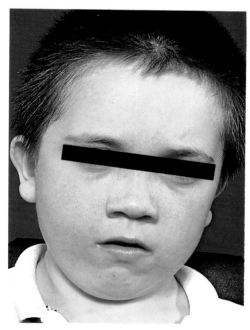
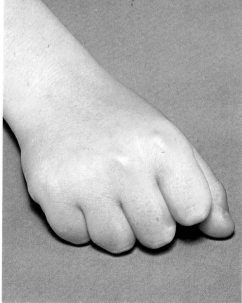

Fig. 16.27 Photograph of a boy with pseudohypoparathyroidism. Note (a) his round face and shortened neck and (b) his shortened metacarpals.

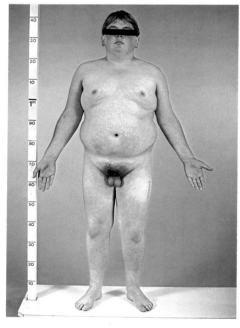

Fig. 16.28 Photograph of a patient with Cushing's syndrome. This is uncommon in childhood. Short stature is a consequence of the suppression of growth hormone secretion by corticosteroids. In addition to short stature, a plethoric 'moon' face, centripetal obesity and abdominal striae are present.

Cushing's syndrome

Except for the iatrogenic variety, Cushing's syndrome (Fig. 16.28) is unusual in infancy and childhood. Short stature results from decreased linear growth (corticosteroid suppressed growth hormone secretion). Rarely, where a preponderance of androgen secretion occurs, there may be an acceleration of growth.

Constitutional growth delay

Much the commonest cause of short stature, is constitutional growth delay with delayed puberty. The bone age is retarded, but the growth velocity is normal. A normal growth spurt in puberty can be predicted, and eventual height will be normal (Fig. 16.29).

TALL STATURE

There are relatively few pathological causes of tall stature, most children representing the upper end of normal distribution of height. Most often there is a family history of tallness in one or both parents. Ultimate height can be predicted by assessment of bone age. A diagram showing the method of evaluation of tall stature is shown in Figure 16.30. A summary of the treatment of tall stature is shown in Figure 16.31.

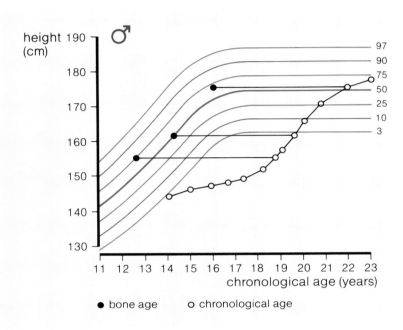

Fig. 16.29 Growth chart of a boy with constitutional growth delay. His short height during childhood would have been accompanied by a delayed bone age, and when the average boys of his age started growing rapidly in puberty this boy was left behind. Thus he was referred for short stature and delayed puberty. His pubertal stages were appropriate for his bone age and, because of the previously normal growth velocity, a normal growth spurt in puberty would be predicted and occurred as shown. It is difficult to be certain that minor degrees of growth hormone deficiency are not present if there are not adequate previous growth records.

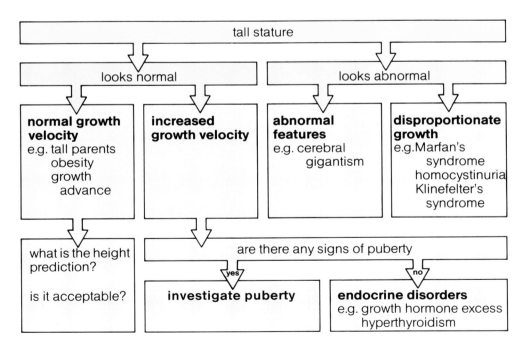

Treatment of Tall Stature

1 measure height and make a height prediction.

2 if height prediction is considered excessive, introduce sex steroids in large doses before the adolescent growth spurt.

Fig. 16.30 Flow diagram to evaluate tall stature.

Fig. 16.31 Table of the major ways of managing tall stature.

TALL STATURE ASSOCIATED WITH NORMAL GROWTH VELOCITY

If a child looks normal, and has a normal growth velocity, constitutional tall stature is usually present (see Fig. 16.32). Obese children are often taller than average for their age, and if maturity is also advanced then puberty may occasionally occur earlier. Tall stature may represent a considerable handicap and, if necessary, limitation of growth should be considered by the administration of sex steroids.

TALL STATURE ASSOCIATED WITH INCREASED GROWTH VELOCITY

With increased growth velocity pubertal status should be assessed. If signs of puberty are present, together with accelerated skeletal maturation, this should be investigated. Precocious sexual development (Fig. 16.33) should be differentiated from pseudo-precocious puberty, where excessive androgen and oestrogen production results from a tumour in the ovary, testis or adrenals, or to congenital adrenal hyperplasia. In precocious puberty the linear growth and bone maturation are advanced, and height often above average, although the final height is likely to be reduced.

Growth Hormone Excess

An excess of growth hormone in childhood or adolescence causes gigantism (Fig. 16.34), but bone age is not advanced. The pituitary fossa may be enlarged, and a growth hormone secreting tumour may be present. Growth hormone (GH) levels are raised, contrasting with levels in constitutional tall stature. Clinically, the disease is characterised by extremely rapid linear growth, overgrowth of soft tissues and metabolic changes similar to those observed in older acromegalic patients. Treatment is aimed at reducing the excessive growth hormone secretion. Radiotherapy, dopamine agonists (such as bromocriptine) or trans-sphenoidal removal of the tumour are the possible treatment modalities to be considered, as for acromegaly (see Chapter 3).

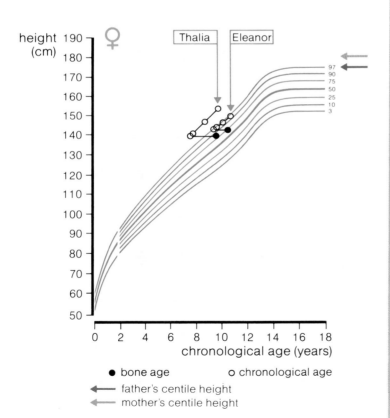

● bone age   ○ chronological age

◄── father's centile height
◄── mother's centile height

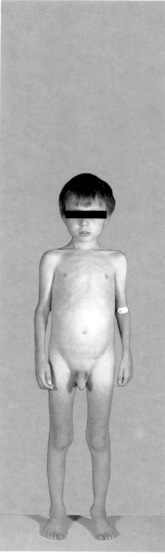

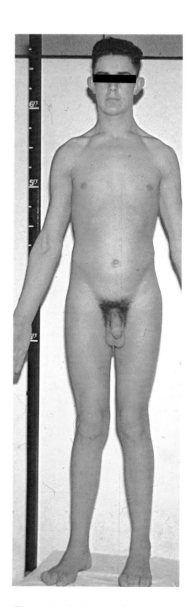

Fig.16.32 Height distance chart of two sisters with constitutional tall stature brought for assessment by their tall mother. Since Eleanor's bone age is less advanced than Thalia's, her eventual height will probably be greater. Provided their growth velocity is normal (thus excluding other diagnoses) whether oestrogen is used to reduce their final height is not so much a medical decision as a social decision.

Fig. 16.33 Photograph of an 8-year-old child with precocious puberty and tall stature, which are associated with a cerebral tumour.

Fig. 16.34 Example of a 16-year-old patient suffering from gigantism. GH is raised and bone age is not advanced indicating that his eventual stature will be abnormally tall.

Hyperthyroidism

An increase in growth rate associated with advanced bone age is seen in hyperthyroid children and also in hypothyroidism overtreated with thyroxine. The diagnosis is made by measuring the T_4, FTI and T_3 levels, and a TRH test should be carried out where doubt still exists. A photograph of a hyperthyroid girl next to her hypothyroid twin sister is shown in Figure 16.35.

TALL STATURE ASSOCIATED WITH AN ABNORMAL APPEARANCE

Sotos Syndrome

Children with Sotos syndrome have a large elongated head, prominent forehead, large ears and jaws, elongated jaw and coarse facial features. Most have subnormal intelligence. These children have normal GH secretion and no evidence of thyroid, adrenal or gonadal dysfunction.

Marfan's Syndrome

Patients with Marfan's syndrome (Fig. 16.36) usually are well above average in height but within the normal range. They have long limbs with narrow hands and long slender fingers. Their arm span is greater than their height and the lower segment is much greater than the upper segment. Hyperextensible joints, kyphoscoliosis, rib cage deformities and dislocation of the lens are also present. Death from a dissecting aneurysm may occur in early adult life.

Homocystinuria

This is caused by an absence of the enzyme cystathionine synthetase. Phenotypically, patients resemble those with Marfan's syndrome but they usually have mental retardation, and there is a tendency for them to die from thrombotic disorders. Lenticular dislocation also occurs, usually in a downward direction.

Klinefelter's Syndrome

Affected patients (see Fig. 16.37) have an XXY karyotype, a tendency to be tall and also display eunuchoid features. Seminiferous tubule dysgenesis, gynaecomastia and small pea-sized testes are present.

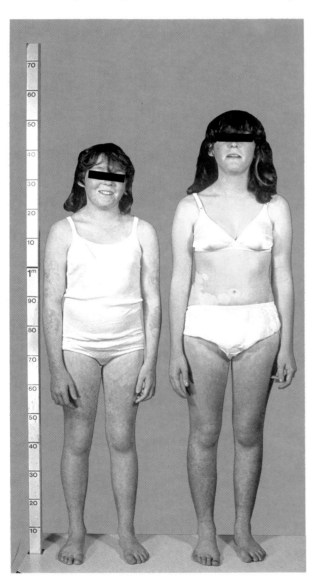

Fig. 16.35 Photograph of a girl (right) whose tall stature is caused by excessive thyroid activity. Her twin sister (left) suffers from hypothyroidism and is consequently short for her age.

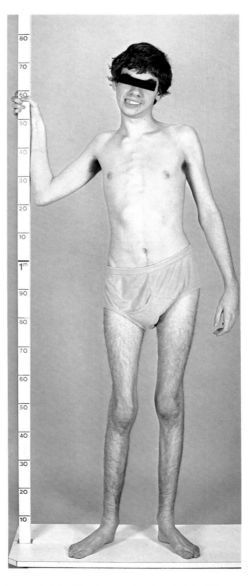

Fig. 16.36 Photograph of a child with Marfan's syndrome. Arm span is greater than height and the limbs are long with slender hands and fingers. The cause of death in these patients is usually a dissecting aneurysm in early adult life.

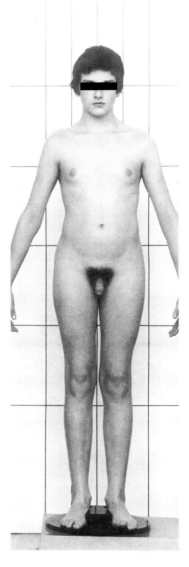

Fig. 16.37 Photograph of a patient with Klinefelter's syndrome. Patients are tall with gynaecomastia and small firm testes.

16.13

Abnormalities of growth represent a frequent cause of referral to the endocrine clinic. The approach to the management of these patients is summarised in Figure 16.38. The importance of accurate anthropometry cannot be overemphasized and, in the early assessment, it is mandatory to establish the parental pattern of growth and also the age at which puberty was entered. The mid-parental height adjusted for the sex of the patient enables the clinician to gain an estimate of the expected final height of the individual and, by using a height distance chart, to determine whether the child is on course to achieve this. The estimation of skeletal maturity, usually by radiography of the child's wrist, is essential in the assessment of growth prognosis of the likely final height.

Follow-up measurements should also be carried out at a minimum of six-monthly intervals, allowing the growth velocity to be calculated. The growth velocity is a most important clue as to the pattern of growth taking place. Abnormality of growth velocity requires systematic investigations directed at the diagnosis of systemic or endocrine pathology.

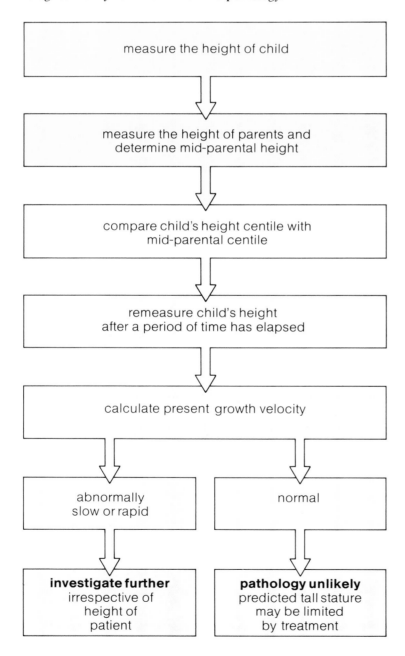

Fig. 16.38 Summary of essential steps in the assessment of growth disorders.

17 Calcium and Common Endocrine Bone Disorders

David A Heath, MB,ChB,FRCP

HORMONAL CONTROL OF CALCIUM METABOLISM

Calcium metabolism is under the control of a variety of hormones. The most important of these are parathyroid hormone (PTH) and vitamin D which act on the intestine, bone and kidney. In this way serum calcium concentration is maintained between very closely defined limits (Fig. 17.1) – normally 2.20-2.65 mmol/l.

Parathyroid hormone is produced first as a larger precursor molecule, pre-pro-PTH, which is initially cleaved to pro-PTH and then to the secreted eighty-four amino acid polypeptide PTH. The major stimulus to secretion is hypocalcaemia. Once secreted, PTH is metabolised into a variety of smaller fragments, many of which are devoid of biological activity (Fig. 17.2). PTH acts predominantly on the kidneys to increase calcium resorption in the tubule, although calcium resorption in bone is also increased by PTH. It also acts on the renal tubule to decrease phosphorous resorption.

Vitamin D is present in two forms, cholecalciferol (vitamin D_3) which is formed predominantly in the skin by the action of ultraviolet light and ergocalciferol (vitamin D_2), a synthetic compound which is used to fortify some foods. In normal situations over ninety per cent of vitamin D originates in the skin, with dietary sources being relatively unimportant. The parent vitamin D has little biological activity and thus has to be metabolised to a biologically active compound. Both cholecalciferol and ergocalciferol are handled identically, firstly by conversion to 25-hydroxy vitamin D in the liver which the kidney subsequently converts to either 1,25-dihydroxy vitamin D or the inactive metabolite 24,25-dihydroxy vitamin D (Fig. 17.3).

The active metabolite is 1,25-dihydroxy vitamin D which acts on the gut to facilitate calcium absorption in the small intestine. It is essential for bone formation – probably by helping to provide the appropriate concentrations of minerals at the site of calcification. When present in excess it stimulates bone resorption and causes hypercalcaemia. The ability of the kidney to switch between the production of active and inactive metabolites plays an important part in the fine control of calcium metabolism.

Calcitonin is a peptide containing thirty-two amino acids and is produced by the parafollicular C-cells of the thyroid gland. It has actions which, in many respects, are the reverse of PTH, since it inhibits bone resorption and lowers serum calcium. In humans, it has not yet been shown to have an important role in calcium homeostasis and only produces hypocalcaemia in situations of increased bone turnover, for example in Paget's disease.

Calcium is present in the blood in three forms – ionised, protein-bound and complexed calcium. Ionised calcium is the physiologically active form and accounts for nearly half of the total calcium. The only other major component is the protein-bound calcium, where calcium is bound predominantly to albumin and, to a lesser and variable degree, to globulins. Ionised calcium is more difficult to measure routinely and most measurements of serum calcium only give an estimate of the total calcium. For this reason, any change in the serum proteins induced by disease, dehydration or venous stasis can alter the total serum calcium (Fig. 17.4). Any measurement of serum calcium should therefore be accompanied by a simultaneous measurement of the serum proteins.

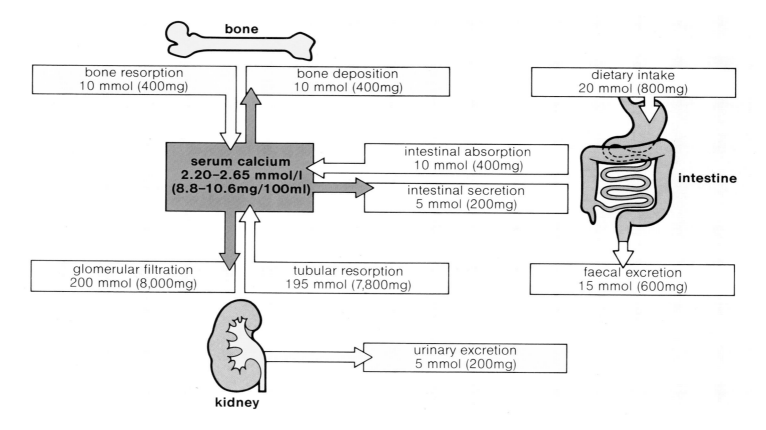

Fig. 17.1 Diagram illustrating the mechanisms of calcium homeostasis. Serum calcium is controlled by the hormonal regulation of calcium flux across the intestine, bone and kidney. The figures shown are daily values.

parathyroid gland

pre-pro-PTH

pro-PTH

NH$_2$ | 1 | 32 PTH | 84 | COOH

serum

NH$_2$ | 1 | 32 | 84 | COOH
intact PTH
active

NH$_2$ | 1 | 32 | amino-terminal fragment
active

32 mid-molecule fragment
inactive

32 | 84 | COOH
inactive

84 | COOH
carboxy-terminal fragment
inactive

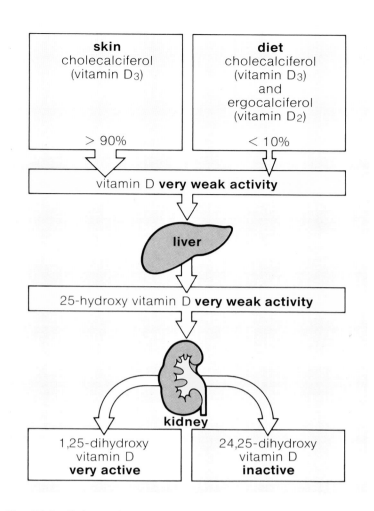

Fig. 17.2 Schematic representation of PTH production and metabolism. The eighty-four amino acid polypeptide PTH is produced from a larger precursor molecule. The intact molecule, the ends of which are designated amino-(NH$_2$) and carboxy-(COOH) terminals, is cleaved to yield a variety of fragments. Only those fragments with the first thirty-two amino acids intact have biological activity; therefore inactive fragments predominate in serum.

Fig. 17.3 Schematic representation of vitamin D metabolism. Skin is the major source of vitamin D. Metabolism by the liver and kidneys leads to the production of the very active metabolite 1,25-dihydroxy vitamin D. The kidney can also produce an inactive metabolite, 24,25-dihydroxy vitamin D.

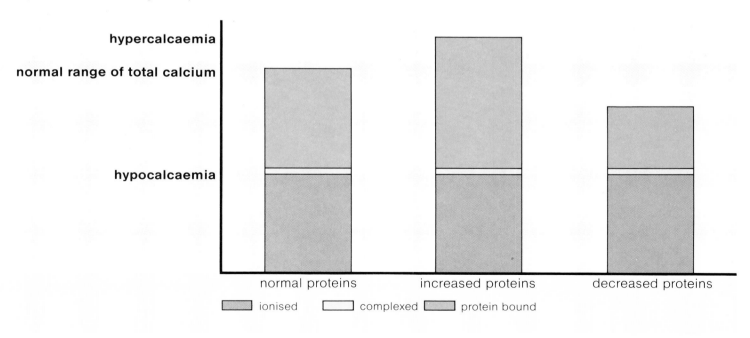

Fig. 17.4 Diagrammatic representation of changes in serum protein concentration on total serum calcium. Marked changes in serum proteins may alter total serum calcium and simulate hyper- or hypocalcaemia. Increased levels of proteins occur in prolonged venous stasis, dehydration and myelomatosis. Common causes of hypoproteinaemia are malignancy and nephrotic syndrome. In each situation above the ionised calcium is normal.

HYPERCALCAEMIA

The causes of hypercalcaemia are shown in Figure 17.5. Surveys have shown that the cause of the hypercalcaemia in the vast majority of cases is either malignancy or hyperparathyroidism, other causes accounting for less than five per cent of the total. Irrespective of the cause of the hypercalcaemia the symptoms are as shown in Figure 17.6.

Hypercalcaemia of Malignancy

Hypercalcaemia is a relatively common complication of malignancy, although it is rare when the disease is not disseminated. The tumours most commonly associated with hypercalcaemia are listed in Figure 17.7. The prevalence of hypercalcaemia in various malignant states is shown in Figure 17.8.

The cause of hypercalcaemia in malignancy is uncertain at present. In many cases it is likely that the tumour produces a humoral agent but that this factor is not PTH. The concentrations of PTH in hyperparathyroidism and malignancy are shown in Figure 17.9. The results obtained vary with different assays and some assays may show up to twenty per cent of malignant cases with an apparently elevated PTH concentration. There is, however, increasing evidence that the substance measured is usually not PTH. Although experimental evidence supports the involvement of prostaglandins and osteoclastic activating factor in some cases of hypercalcaemia, it seems likely that other, as yet uncharacterised, agents are involved in the vast majority of cases.

The presence of the malignant state is usually clear from the history, examination or basic investigation of the patient. There is no specific biochemical abnormality associated with malignant hypercalcaemia, although the disseminated nature of the disease often causes the serum protein and liver function to be deranged (Fig. 17.10).

Wherever possible, specific treatment should be directed at the primary malignant disease; if successful, this will correct the hypercalcaemia. Even when treatment of the malignant process is impossible, treatment of the hypercalcaemia should be considered as this can greatly improve the quality of the patient's life. Adequate hydration is of paramount importance and, when hypercalcaemia is moderate or severe, intravenous fluids are mandatory. At least 6-8 l of fluid may be required daily in the initial management. Potassium supplements are almost always necessary as hypokalaemia frequently develops. Adequate hydration alone is often sufficient to alleviate severe symptoms so that the need for other emergency measures is rare. In less severe hypercalcaemia, or to maintain the effects of initial emergency treatment, an effective oral treatment should be given. At present, the most effective agent is oral phosphate given in doses of 1-2g daily. While effective in perhaps seventy-five per cent of patients, gastrointestinal side-effects are very common and thus significantly limit its clinical role. Oral steroids (e.g. prednisolone 20-40 mg daily) are more readily tolerated but effective in only half the cases. The dose administered should be the lowest effective dose. The successful treatment of a case of severe hypercalcaemia is shown in Figure 17.11.

Causes of Hypercalcaemia

common
malignancy
hyperparathyroidism

uncommon
thyrotoxicosis
vitamin D poisoning
sarcoidosis
familial hypocalciuric hypercalcaemia

rare
Addison's disease
milk-alkali syndrome
acute renal failure
phaeochromocytoma
vasoactive intestinal peptide (VIP)-
  secreting islet cell tumours
tuberculosis
thiazide diuretics
immobilisation
idiopathic hypercalcaemia of infancy

Fig. 17.5   Table showing the causes of hypercalcaemia.
Malignancy and hyperparathyroidism account for ninety-seven per cent of the causes of hypercalcaemia.

Symptoms of Hypercalcaemia

tiredness and lethargy
polyuria, nocturia and polydipsia
nausea, vomiting and constipation
proximal muscle weakness
drowsiness, psychosis and coma

Fig. 17.6   Table of the symptoms found in hypercalcaemia.
All symptoms are non-specific and often mimic disorders of other systems. Only routine measurement of serum calcium will bring most cases to light. Mild hypercalcaemia is often asymptomatic.

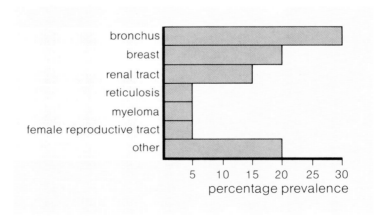

Fig. 17.7   Hypercalcaemia and malignancy. The tumour sites in a series of consecutive cases of malignancy complicated by hypercalcaemia are shown. Over seventy-five per cent of the cases had obvious evidence of metastases. After Fisken et al., Quarterly Journal of Medicine 1980; 49: 405-418, by permission of the publishers, Oxford University Press.

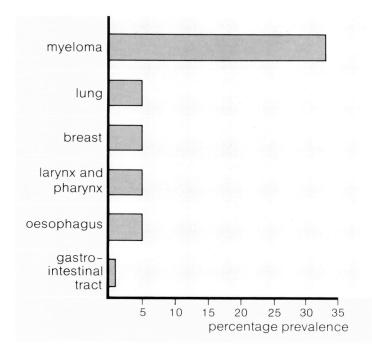

Fig. 17.8 The prevalence of hypercalcaemia in various malignant states. Varying prevalence rates are found depending upon when the studies were performed. The rates shown are those found in hospital in-patients admitted for investigation or treatment. Much higher rates are found in autopsy studies. After Fisken et al., Quarterly Journal of Medicine 1980; 49: 405-418, by permission of the publishers, Oxford University Press.

Malignancy as a Cause of Hypercalcaemia

history

weight loss

haemoptysis or haematuria

examination

lymphadenopathy

palpable mass

basic investigations

anaemia

high erythrocyte sedimentation rate (ESR)

low albumin

high globulin

abnormal liver function tests

abnormal chest radiograph

Fig. 17.10 Clues to the diagnosis of hypercalcaemia of malignancy. Most cases of hypercalcaemia of malignancy have obvious evidence of the malignant state which is apparent on initial evaluation of the patient.

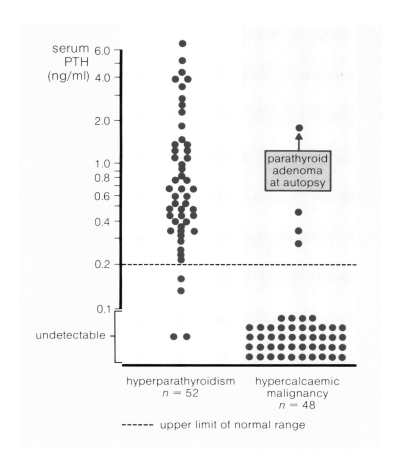

------ upper limit of normal range

Fig. 17.9 Serum PTH concentrations in hyperparathyroidism and malignancy. In this particular assay, normal PTH levels are rarely measurable. Most patients with primary hyperparathyroidism have elevated values, but this is rare in hypercalcaemic malignancy. Other assays may show 'normal' values in both hyperparathyroidism and malignancy. The coincidental occurrence of malignancy and primary hyperparathyroidism is well described.

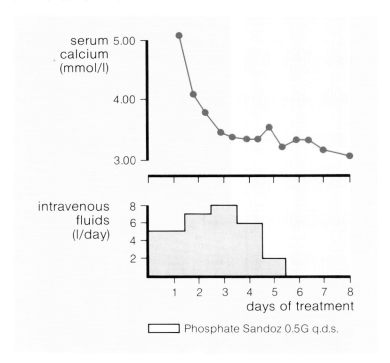

Fig. 17.11 Graph showing the treatment of severe hypercalcaemia with oral phosphates. These values were taken from a patient with carcinoma of the breast who was semiconscious on admission. Marked clinical improvement occurred with rehydration; this allowed subsequent oral phosphate treatment to be given to control the hypercalcaemia.

17.5

Primary Hyperparathyroidism

Primary hyperparathyroidism is the clinical condition produced by the inappropriate over-production of PTH. It occurs in increasing frequency with age and affects women three times more commonly than men. Most patients are aged over fifty years.

In the vast majority of cases there is no obvious explanation for the autonomous PTH over-production. Rarely, there may have been a previous disease present which caused prolonged hypocalcaemia (e.g. malabsorption or renal failure). This acts as a stimulus to the parathyroid glands which attempt to correct the hypocalcaemia and produce secondary hyperparathyroidism. Very occasionally this appears to lead to hypercalcaemia which becomes permanent (termed tertiary hyperparathyroidism).

Multiple Endocrine Neoplasia (MEN) Syndromes

MEN type 1	MEN type 2a	MEN type 2b
hyperparathyroidism	hyperparathyroidism	medullary thyroid carcinoma with marfanoid habitus and mucosal neuromas
pancreatic islet cell tumours	medullary thyroid carcinoma	
pituitary tumours	phaeochromocytoma	

Fig. 17.12 Table of the multiple endocrine neoplasia (MEN) syndromes. These syndromes are inherited as autosomal dominant conditions. Parathyroid hyperplasia is common and phaeochromocytomas are usually bilateral. Clinical features rarely develop within the first two decades except in MEN type 2b where childhood presentation is more common.

The Changing Presentation of Hyperparathyroidism in Britain

	percentage presentation			
	bone disease	renal disease	other	asymptomatic
Dent 1962	31	57	12	0
Pyrah et al. 1966	35	40	25	0
Watson 1974	13	47	32	8
O'Riordan 1978	12	45	26	17
Barnes 1984	5	23	42	30
Mundy et al. 1980	0	7	36	57

Fig. 17.13 The changing presentation of hyperparathyroidism. Major series reported from Britain are listed. Bone and renal presentations, previously common, are now becoming unusual. Cases of asymptomatic patients with tiredness and lethargy are now the rule. The first five series were all surgical. The final series (Mundy et al., 1980) represents cases diagnosed by following up all known cases of hypercalcaemia; many were not referred for surgery.

Diagnosis of Primary Hyperparathyroidism

essential tests	tests of occasional use
elevated serum calcium	hand radiographs
clinical exclusion of malignancy and other known causes of hypercalcaemia	hydrocortisone suppression test
	urinary calcium measurements
an elevated or high normal PTH concentration	family screening

Fig. 17.14 The diagnosis of primary hyperparathyroidism. Non-parathyroid causes of hypercalcaemia are usually clinically obvious and rarely associated with elevated PTH levels. Although radiological changes of hyperparathyroidism are unusual today, they are diagnostic of the disease when present. In this situation the hands are the most commonly affected part of the skeleton.

Hyperparathyroidism is the most common component of the multiple endocrine neoplasia (MEN) syndromes (Fig. 17.12) which are familial disorders with dominant inheritance. MEN type 1 consists of combinations of hyperparathyroidism, islet cell tumours and pituitary tumours. MEN type 2 consists of combinations of hyperparathyroidism, medullary carcinoma of the thyroid and phaeochromocytomas which are usually bilateral. Such forms of hyperparathyroidism are more often associated with hyperplasia of all four parathyroid glands and are rare.

Until recently, hyperparathyroidism was almost exclusively a disease characterised by renal stones or bone disease. With the advent of biochemical screening these two presentations have become less common, being replaced by either asymptomatic patients or by a group with very non-specific symptoms – especially excessive weakness. The change in presentation of patients in several studies during the past fifteen years is shown in Figure 17.13. All were surgical patients except in the last series, which reported hyperparathyroid patients discovered by evaluating all hypercalcaemic subjects detected by the laboratories serving all the hospitals of a major city. From this last survey, the incidence of hyperparathyroidism has been estimated to be approximately five hundred per million of the population per year.

As mentioned earlier, when malignancy is the cause of hypercalcaemia it is usually clinically obvious; this is also true of other rarer causes of hypercalcaemia. Therefore, the patient who has neither clinical, radiological or biochemical evidence of malignancy, nor thyrotoxicosis nor sarcoidosis, will nearly always be suffering from hyperparathyroidism. The finding of an elevated or high-normal PTH concentration will confirm the diagnosis. If in such a situation the PTH concentration is low, then the possibility of an occult malignancy or one of the other rarer causes of hypercalcaemia should be considered (Fig. 17.14).

Other biochemical tests are rarely helpful in differentiating between the causes of hypercalcaemia. When doubt as to the cause persists, a hydrocortisone suppression test may be helpful. Should the serum calcium revert to normal when hydrocortisone (40 mg eight-hourly for ten days) is given, then hyperparathyroidism is a very unlikely cause of the hypercalcaemia (Fig. 17.15). Failure to suppress does not, however, prove the diagnosis of hyperparathyroidism since fifty per cent of cases of hypercalcaemia of malignancy fail to suppress.

Radiological evidence of hyperparathyroidism is relatively uncommon but, when present, is diagnostic of the disease. If present, the hands are nearly always affected, with subperiosteal erosions being seen, especially on the radial side of the phalanges (Fig. 17.16).

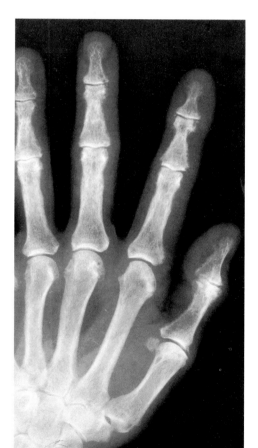

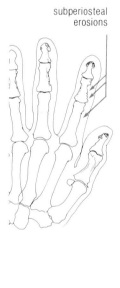

Fig. 17.15 Hydrocortisone suppression test: graph showing serum calcium levels in two patients during hydrocortisone administration. Two patients were given 40 mg of hydrocortisone eight-hourly for ten days and their serum calcium was regularly checked. Patient 'a' failed to respond and had primary hyperparathyroidism. Such a response is not diagnostic of hyperparathyroidism as fifty per cent of hypercalcaemic malignancies also fail to respond. Patient 'b' had sarcoidosis, but similar responses may occur in vitamin D intoxication. His calcium levels rapidly decreased to the normal range; such a response is exceptional in hyperparathyroidism.

Fig. 17.16 Hand radiograph in primary hyperparathyroidism. The classical change is the development of subperiosteal erosions (more marked along the radial border of the phalanges) giving the cortex of the phalanges a very ragged appearance. Bone cysts may also occur, as may chondrocalcinosis.

Definite Indications for Parathyroidectomy

symptomatic disease

i.e. marked tiredness, muscle weakness

complications of the disease

i.e. renal stones, bone disease

young age irrespective of symptoms

Fig. 17.17 Table listing indications for parathyroidectomy. All young patients or those with significant symptoms or complications of the disease should be offered parathyroidectomy. No drug therapy has been shown to control the hyperparathyroid state. The alternative to surgery is observation with no treatment.

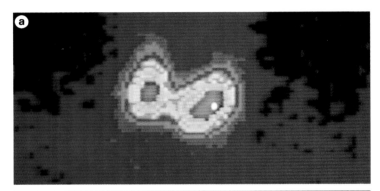

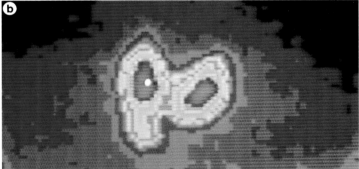

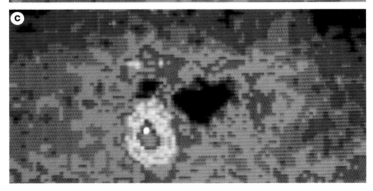

Fig. 17.18 Technetium: thallium subtraction scans used in the localisation of a parathyroid adenoma. An initial technetium scan (a) is performed to delineate the thyroid. This is followed by a thallium scan (b) which localises in both thyroid and parathyroid glands. A computer subtracts the technetium counts from the thallium counts leaving counts localised solely in the parathyroid adenoma (c). This technique is successful in approximately sixty per cent of cases.

In the past, all patients with hyperparathyroidism were treated surgically. The recognition of many elderly patients with few or no symptoms has more recently led to a change in this policy. At present surgery is offered to all patients with significant complications of the disease, for instance renal stones, bone disease, resistant peptic ulceration and to all young patients irrespective of their symptoms (Fig. 17.17). Prior to surgery a number of techniques have been tried in an attempt to localise the parathyroid tumour, but most have been inaccurate. More recently, the combined scanning of the neck with technetium and thallium has led to an accurate pre-operative localisation of parathyroid adenomas in approximately sixty per cent of cases (Fig. 17.18). If operations are performed by an experienced parathyroid surgeon the lesions are virtually always found, making pre-operative localising techniques of dubious value in the previously unoperated case. In nearly ninety per cent of cases a single parathyroid adenoma will be found and removed. In approximately ten per cent all four parathyroid glands are hyperplastic (Fig. 17.19). In such a situation, most surgeons now perform total parathyroidectomy with autotransplantation of one gland into the forearm.

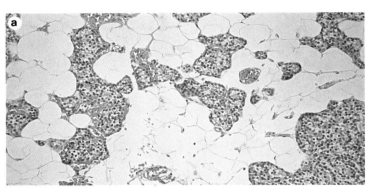

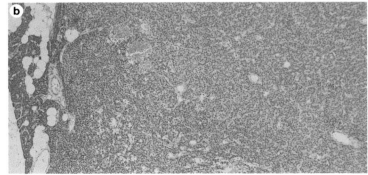

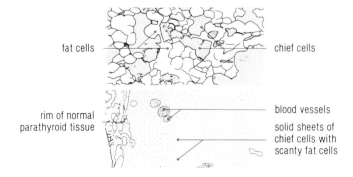

fat cells — chief cells

rim of normal parathyroid tissue — blood vessels

solid sheets of chief cells with scanty fat cells

Fig. 17.19 Histological appearance of the parathyroid glands. Normal parathyroid tissue is shown in view (a) and a parathyroid chief adenoma is shown in view (b). There is a deficiency of fat cells in the adenoma together with a rim of compressed normal parathyroid tissue. Haematoxylin and eosin stain, magnification ×100. By courtesy of Prof. E.L. Jones.

Occasionally two adenomas are found. Parathyroid carcinoma is extremely rare.

Following successful parathyroidectomy, serum calcium levels usually fall to normal within twenty-four hours. Mild, asymptomatic hypocalcaemia frequently develops but is usually self-limiting (Fig. 17.20). Occasionally, more severe hypocalcaemia develops postoperatively, especially when bone disease is present. In this situation, both intravenous calcium and high dose vitamin D therapy are necessary for a period which rarely exceeds two to four weeks. Very occasionally permanent hypoparathyroidism ensues. In experienced surgical hands recurrent laryngeal palsy is a rare complication.

Current opinion is that it is unnecessary to operate on elderly patients with few or no symptoms. Various medical treatments have been tried to control the hypercalcaemia. Although oral phosphate, cellulose phosphate and diphosphonates may control the hypercalcaemia, they do not affect the hyperparathyroid state and there is no evidence that they are beneficial to the patient. Medical treatment therefore involves the monitoring of the patient's biochemistry and well-being.

Familial Hypocalciuric Hypercalcaemia

Familial hypocalciuric hypercalcaemia (FHH) or familial benign hypercalcaemia has only been recognised during the past decade. In many respects it closely mimics mild primary hyperparathyroidism from which it may be difficult to differentiate. There is a tendency towards hypocalciuria and the hypercalcaemia is rarely corrected by parathyroidectomy. The exact abnormality in FHH is unclear. There is evidence to support both an abnormality of renal calcium handling and parathyroid function.

FHH was first recognised in patients thought to have hyperparathyroidism in whom parathyroidectomy did not correct the hypercalcaemia. Subsequent studies showed them to have a relative hypocalciuria and other hypercalcaemic family members. Very few patients complained of any symptoms and the condition was usually found during biochemical screening. When specifically questioned, hypercalciuric family members are more likely to complain of mild, non-specific symptoms such as tiredness, weakness, headache and arthralgia (Fig. 17.21). Affected subjects do not appear to have an increased incidence of renal stones or bone disease. However, there does appear to be an increased incidence

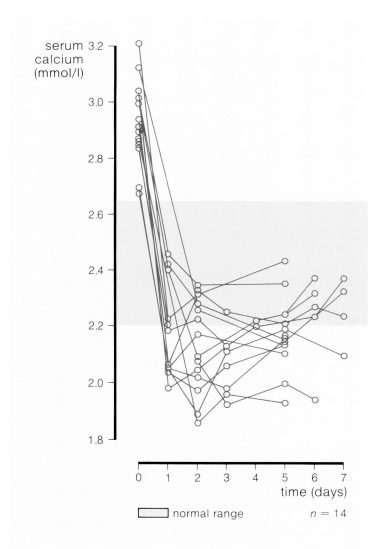

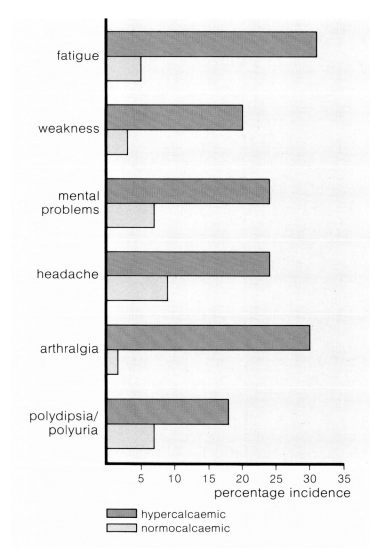

Fig. 17.20   Graph showing the biochemical response to successful parathyroidectomy. A significant fall in serum calcium always occurs the day after surgery and, unless the pre-operative calcium is very high, serum calcium levels should descend to the normal range. Mild hypocalcaemia, usually asymptomatic, occurs subsequently and is usually self-limiting. In the presence of bone disease, postoperative hypocalcaemia may be more severe and prolonged.

Fig. 17.21   Table of symptoms in patients affected with familial hypocalciuric hypercalcaemia. Hypercalcaemic family members are compared with normocalcaemic members. The symptoms listed above were more common in affected members. Redrawn from Marx S J et al., Medicine 1981; 60: 397-412, by permission of the publishers Williams and Wilkins Co., Baltimore.

of recurrent pancreatitis in adult members and severe neonatal hypercalcaemia in new-born infants. FHH is inherited as an autosomal dominant disorder with complete penetrance and affected members are hypercalcaemic from birth (Fig. 17.22).

This distinguishes it from familial hyperparathyroidism where patients very rarely manifest hypercalcaemia during the first two decades.

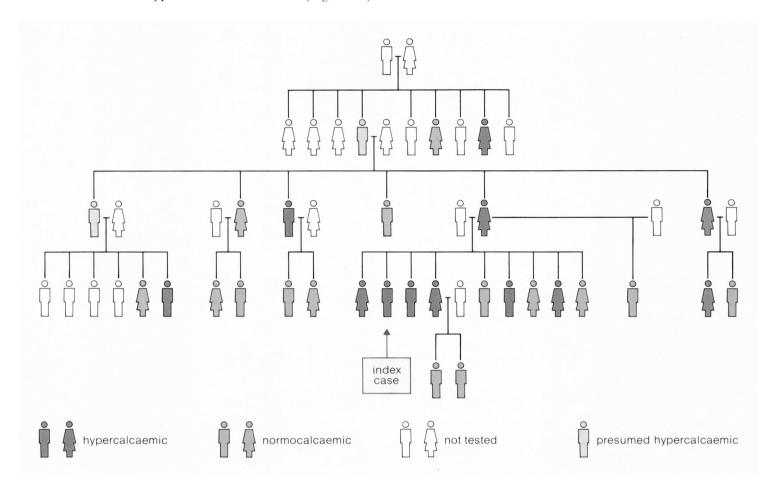

Fig. 17.22 Inheritance of familial hypocalciuric hypercalcaemia. The index case presented with a renal stone, hypercalcaemia and elevated PTH concentrations. He remained hypercalcaemic after two parathyroid explorations. Family studies then revealed hypocalciuria and hypercalcaemia in approximately half the relatives tested, including some children.

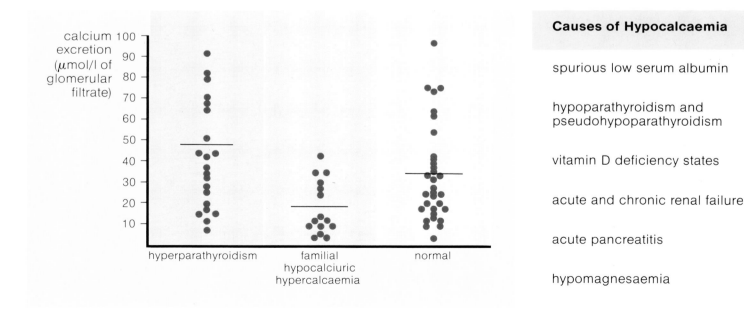

Fig. 17.23 Urinary calcium excretion in familial hypocalciuric hypercalcaemia. Urinary calcium excretion, however measured, tends to be lower in FHH than in hyperparathyroidism. There is, however, a marked overlap in values between the two conditions.

Causes of Hypocalcaemia

spurious low serum albumin

hypoparathyroidism and pseudohypoparathyroidism

vitamin D deficiency states

acute and chronic renal failure

acute pancreatitis

hypomagnesaemia

Fig. 17.24 Table showing the causes of hypocalcaemia.

At present, the best biochemical clue to the pre-operative diagnosis of FHH is the finding of hypocalciuria (Fig. 17.23). Even then there is a significant overlap between the two groups. Serum magnesium tends to be towards the high side of normal, while serum phosphate and chloride levels tend to be intermediate between those seen in hyperparathyroid patients and normal subjects. PTH concentrations are usually within the normal range but have been reported to be mildly elevated in up to twenty-five per cent of affected individuals. The diagnosis of FHH should be suspected in all asymptomatic hypercalcaemic individuals who do not have raised urinary calcium levels. This is particularly important in young individuals who will proceed to parathyroidectomy even if totally asymptomatic. If doubt exists, attempts should be made to screen family members and, wherever possible, both parents should be tested. The finding of hypercalcaemic hypocalciuric children within a family is virtually diagnostic of the condition.

The principal reason for making an early diagnosis of FHH is to avoid parathyroid surgery which virtually never corrects the hypercalcaemia. No specific therapy is yet available and, as patients are usually asymptomatic, the best policy is continued observation.

Rarely, infants of an affected parent may be symptomatically affected at birth. This usually presents as failure to thrive, with severe hypercalcaemia and marked hyperparathyroid bone disease. The condition responds to early total parathyroidectomy although there is now some evidence it may improve spontaneously with time.

Other Causes of Hypercalcaemia

Causes of hypercalcaemia other than hypercalcaemia of malignancy, primary hyperparathyroidism and FHH are uncommon and account for about three per cent of cases of hypercalcaemia seen in clinical practice (see Fig. 17.5). In the vast majority of these, the other causative medical condition is obvious, for example thyrotoxicosis, sarcoidosis or high-dose vitamin D therapy. When these conditions are not obvious, the possibility of such a condition being present should be considered if the serum PTH is not elevated and hypercalciuria is present. Suppression of the hypercalcaemia with high dose steroids may occur; this is very unusual in hyperparathyroidism. In sarcoidosis the serum 1,25-dihydroxycholecalciferol may be inappropriately elevated while the patient is hypercalcaemic.

HYPOCALCAEMIA

The causes of hypocalcaemia are shown in Figure 17.24. Excluding spurious hypocalcaemia due to low serum proteins, hypocalcaemia is a rarer biochemical abnormality than hypercalcaemia.

Hypoparathyroidism

The commonest forms of hypoparathyroidism result from surgical procedures to the neck. Transient hypocalcaemia is commonly seen after parathyroidectomy and less so after thyroidectomy. Permanent hypoparathyroidism is rare unless three or more parathyroid glands are damaged or removed. It commonly occurs after total laryngectomy. Very occasionally, the condition presents many years after the operation.

Rarely, the condition is idiopathic when evidence of an auto-immune disorder may be present. In such cases there is a higher incidence of hypothyroidism, hypoadrenalism, diabetes mellitus and cutaneous monilial infections.

Hypoparathyroidism following neck operations is usually present two to five days postoperatively. Symptoms include paraesthesiae, especially circumoral and in the extremities, followed by muscle cramps and, if severe, by fits. Increased muscle and nerve irritability produce the clinical signs attributed to Chvostek and Trousseau (Fig. 17.25). When hypoparathyroidism occurs many years after surgery, or in the idiopathic form, the onset is far more insidious. Tiredness, malaise, muscle cramps and epileptic fits are common. Cataracts may also develop.

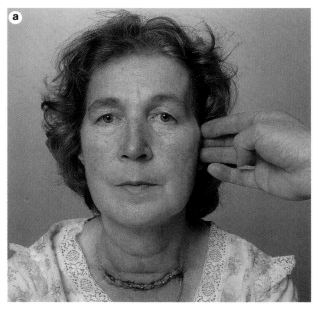
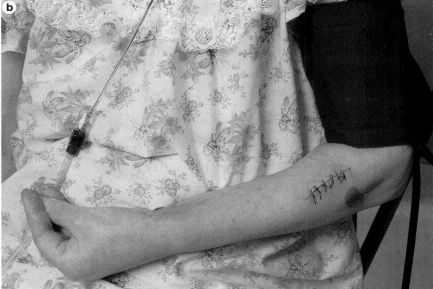

Fig. 17.25 The clinical signs of hypocalcaemia. Chvostek's sign (a) is elicited by tapping over the facial nerve and producing a contraction of the upper lip muscles. Trousseau's sign (b) is produced when a sphygmomanometer cuff is inflated to above systolic pressure for up to three minutes. This lady had four-gland hyperplasia and developed transient postoperative hypocalcaemia. All four glands were removed and pieces from one auto-transplanted into the forearm. The site of the transplantation can be clearly seen.

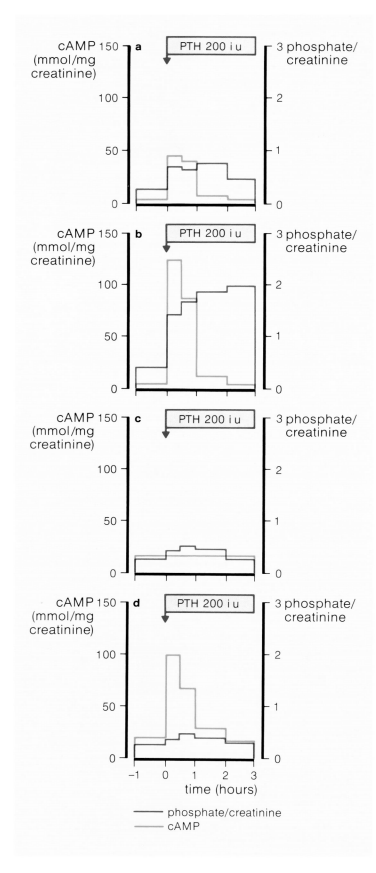

Fig. 17.26   Urinary cAMP and phosphate excretion in hypoparathyroidism and pseudohypoparathyroidism. PTH is injected intravenously at time t = 0. Urine is collected for the hour prior to the injection and for the next three hours. Urinary cAMP, phosphate and creatinine are measured. The responses shown are as follows: (a) normal response, (b) idiopathic hypoparathyroidism, (c) pseudohypoparathyroidism type 1 (no cAMP or phosphate response) and (d) pseudohypoparathyroidism type 2 (good cAMP response but no phosphaturia).

The finding of hypocalcaemia and hyperphosphataemia in the absence of renal failure is virtually diagnostic of hypoparathyroidism. PTH levels are low or undetectable but, following an injection of PTH, patients are able to respond normally by increasing their plasma and urinary cAMP and urinary phosphate (Fig. 17.26).

Following neck surgery, mild asymptomatic hypocalcaemia is self-limiting and requires no treatment. When symptomatic, it can usually be controlled with intravenous calcium injections. When severe or permanent, treatment with vitamin D is necessary which can be given either as calciferol in a dose of around 100,000 iu daily or as one of the potent vitamin D metabolites such as 1α-cholecalciferol (Alfacalcidol) 1-2μg daily or 1,25-dihydroxy vitamin D (Calcitriol) 0.5-2μg daily. Additional calcium supplements are not usually necessary but regular checks of the serum calcium are required for the duration of the therapy.

Pseudohypoparathyroidism

This is a rare, inherited condition often associated with a characteristic appearance – obesity, a round face, short fourth and fifth fingers, cerebral calcification and mental subnormality (Fig. 17.27). The biochemical changes are identical to those seen in hypoparathyroidism but patients show a resistance to injected PTH. This demonstrates a defect in the PTH receptor or postreceptor mechanisms. Two variants of the disease have been described – type 1 where PTH fails to produce an increase in urinary cAMP and phosphate, and type 2 where cAMP, but not phosphate, excretion increases (Fig. 17.26). Pseudo-pseudohypoparathyroidism shows the characteristic appearance of pseudohypoparathyroidism but with normal biochemistry.

Rickets and Osteomalacia

The effects of vitamin D deficiency on the growing skeleton produce rickets, a disease predominantly of the metaphyseal and epiphyseal area of bones. In the adult, osteomalacia ensues.

Although vitamin D is present in our diet, most vitamin D present in the body is synthesised in the skin as a result of exposure to ultraviolet light. In the past, vitamin D deficiency in Britain was confined to the overcrowded slum areas of major cities affected by serious industrial air pollution. With slum clearance and increasing control of air pollution, rickets and osteomalacia had virtually disappeared from this country. They have re-emerged in the Asian community in Britain, chiefly affecting those with increased vitamin D requirements – neonates, growing children and adolescents, also pregnant women (Fig. 17.28). Studies on apparently healthy Asians often show them to have low vitamin D concentrations in the blood. The exact explanation for the high prevalence of vitamin D deficiency in Asians is unclear. Simple dietary deficiency or inability to produce vitamin D in the skin are not the sole explanation, since it is particularly associated with those with a vegetarian diet and high chapatti intake.

Vitamin D deficiency remains rare in non-Asians in Britain. It may, however, complicate malabsorptive states associated with upper intestinal disorders, for example Crohn's disease and small bowel resection, pancreatic disease (e.g. chronic pancreatitis), cystic fibrosis, and liver disease (e.g. primary biliary cirrhosis). More recently, vitamin D deficiency has been recognised in the elderly population of all ethnic groups in Britain. This is particularly common in those old people who are confined to home and presumably arises from inadequate exposure to sunlight. The size of the clinical problem remains to be ascertained and much controversy surrounds the possible role of vitamin D deficiency in the aetiology of hip and wrist fractures in the elderly.

The presentation of vitamin D deficiency depends upon the age of the affected individual (Fig. 17.29). Intra-uterine deficiency of vitamin D leads to babies who are small for their weight with a greater tendency to hypocalcaemia and neonatal fits. Such babies fail to thrive and have a higher perinatal mortality. When the deficiency is particularly severe, gross radiological changes may be present with multiple fractures and craniotabes.

In growing children the cardinal feature is bone pain and deformity. Pain is particularly common in the knees. Although present at rest, it is usually worse on exercise which may consequently be avoided. Knock-knees or, less commonly, bow-legs may develop (Fig. 17.30). The wrists are often swollen and tender. Short stature is common.

In adults, women are usually affected, especially during or after pregnancy. Diffuse bone pain, especially arising from the ribs, back and pelvis, is the commonest symptom. Pseudofractures are common and affect particularly the pelvis and femoral necks where they cause the pain, and hence the difficulty in walking. Muscle weakness affecting almost exclusively the proximal muscles adds to the walking difficulty and combines to produce a classical waddling gait.

In addition to these presentations, severe hypocalcaemia can occur in all age groups, and the first presentation of the disorder may be epileptic fits. For this reason it is wise to measure the serum calcium in all Asian patients presenting with epilepsy.

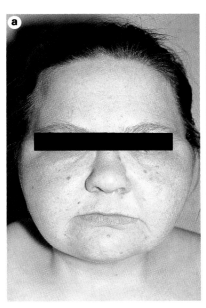
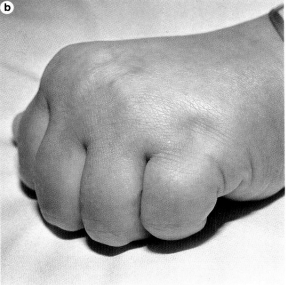

Fig. 17.27 Clinical photographs of a patient with pseudo-hypoparathyroidism. Typical round facies characteristic of pseudohypoparathyroidism can be seen in photograph (a). View (b) shows a dimpled knuckle as a result of a shortened fifth metacarpal. By courtesy of Dr D. Hosking.

Patients at Risk of Vitamin D Deficiency in Britain

Asians:
especially neonates, growing children, adolescents and pregnant women

elderly:
especially the housebound

those with:
small bowel, pancreatic, and liver disease

Fig. 17.28 Groups at risk of vitamin D deficiency in Britain. The above groups are more likely to develop vitamin D deficient states than the normal population.

Presentation of Vitamin D Deficiency

neonates
failure to thrive;
hypocalcaemic fits

growing children
bone pain and deformity,
especially lower limbs; fits

adults
bone pain especially ribs,
back and pelvis;
waddling gait; fits

Fig. 17.29 Table showing the cause of presentation of vitamin D deficiency in neonates, children and adults.

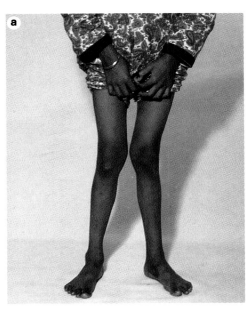
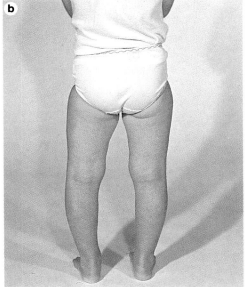

Fig. 17.30 Photographs showing knock-knees and bow-legs in rickets. The Asian boy with knock-knees (a) has simple vitamin D deficiency. In view (b) the girl, being white, was unlikely to have vitamin D deficiency and was subsequently found to have hypophosphataemic rickets.

Awareness of those groups most at risk is of primary importance. Clinical examination is often normal unless skeletal deformities are present. Biochemically, the most typical changes are a serum calcium level at the lower limit of normal, a slightly reduced serum phosphate concentration and an elevated serum alkaline phosphatase. Occasionally marked hypocalcaemia can occur. Frequently, calcium and phosphate levels may be within normal limits with only an abnormal alkaline phosphatase. Such changes are difficult to interpret in children, where an elevated alkaline phosphatase is the rule during rapid growth, and also in the elderly, where an elevated alkaline phosphatase is frequently seen in asymptomatic and often unrecognised Paget's disease. Radiological changes, when present, are diagnostic. In children, the most prominent changes take place at the metaphyseal end of growing bones, particularly at the wrist and knee. The epiphysis becomes widened and the metaphysis is expanded and irregular (Fig. 17.31). In adults, the classical change is the development of pseudofractures or Looser's zones (Fig. 17.32). These are translucent zones passing through the cortex of the bone. They usually occur in the rami of the pelvis, femoral necks, ribs and borders of the scapulae. In addition to these changes, those of secondary hyperparathyroidism may develop, especially sub-periosteal erosions. Bone biopsy is a relatively non-invasive technique when a core of bone can be taken either from the iliac crest or wing of the pelvis. Histologically, the amount of osteoid is increased and is usually associated with increased osteoclastic activity due to secondary hyperparathyroidism (Fig. 17.33).

Prevention of vitamin D deficiency should be the prime aim. Vitamin D supplements should be considered for all pregnant Asian women, babies and adolescents. Patients with intestinal, pancreatic and liver disease may also require extra supplements. Prevention and treatment of established disease can almost always be accomplished with small oral doses of the vitamin. Infants should be given vitamin drops (usually as part of a multivitamin preparation) to provide 400 iu/day. Older children and adults should be treated with calcium and vitamin D tablets (BNF). Each tablet contains 500iu of vitamin D. One tablet daily is adequate for prophylaxis, while two or three tablets daily are appropriate for treatment. Such treatment regimes are completely safe and do not require biochemical monitoring. Treatment should last for six to nine months or until the period of increased vitamin requirements has passed. Simple vitamin D deficiency should never be treated with the very potent vitamin D metabolites.

Rarer Forms of Rickets and Osteomalacia
Vitamin Dependent Rickets
This is a recessively inherited disease producing an identical biochemical, radiological and histological picture to that seen in vitamin D deficiency rickets. The disease fails to heal on small doses of vitamin D but complete resolution occurs when larger doses of around 50,000 iu per day are given. The condition is thought to result from impaired 1α-hydroxylation in the kidney.

Vitamin D Resistant Rickets
Under this classification there occurs a variety of diseases characterised by marked hypophosphataemia, phosphaturia, normocalcaemia and a resistance even to massive doses of vitamin D. Various forms of inheritance have been described, the commonest being either an autosomal dominant or a sex-linked inheritance. One form of the disorder, Fanconi's syndrome, is associated with multiple proximal tubular abnormalities including glycosuria, phosphaturia, amino-aciduria and renal tubular acidosis. It is likely that the primary defect in all these conditions is a defect of phosphate transport and the basis of treatment is frequent phosphate supplementation in order to maintain a normal serum phosphate. Such treatment induces hypocalcaemia and secondary hyperparathyroidism. This is counteracted by moderate vitamin D supplements.

An identical clinical syndrome can be seen with certain rare tumours, usually of the skin or muscle, and is called tumoral or oncogenic rickets. Hypophosphataemia is again marked and complete removal of the tumour allows resolution of the disease.

Renal Failure
Hypocalcaemia may occur in both acute and chronic renal failure. In acute renal failure, hypocalcaemia results primarily from phosphate retention causing the complexing of calcium into insoluble compounds. Added to this, in chronic renal failure the the kidney is unable to produce 1,25-dihydroxy vitamin D. This leads to the development of rickets or osteomalacia. Hypocalcaemia induces a secondary hyperparathyroidism response, so that the clinical disease seen in long-standing chronic renal failure is a variable mixture of osteomalacia and parathyroid bone disease. More recently it has been realised that aluminium retention may play a part in the bone disease of chronic renal failure, the aluminium being derived from two sources – tap water used in dialysis, or from the use of oral aluminium salts used as phosphate binders in an attempt to lower the elevated serum phosphate. The aluminium localises in the calcification front of the bone and causes a failure of bone formation and severe osteomalacia.

Renal osteodystrophy causes generalised bone pain and profound proximal muscle weakness. Radiological changes of either osteomalacia or hyperparathyroidism, or both, are usually present. A particularly common feature is the occurrence of areas of both sclerosis and diminished bone density. This produces the so-called 'rugger jersey spine' in the vertebrae (Fig. 17.34).

Trials are under way to see if the prophylactic use of active vitamin D metabolites will prevent or minimise the development of the disease. Established disease can be treated with either 1α-cholecalciferol or 1,25-dihydroxycholecalciferol. Careful monitoring is required as hypercalcaemia can be readily produced. Paradoxically, the cases which appear to respond best are those with more obvious parathyroid bone disease and minimal osteomalacia. The occurence of severe osteomalacia resistant to treatment with vitamin D metabolites should raise the possibility of aluminium toxicity. Bone biopsy may help, as specific stains for aluminium are now available. To avoid this disorder many centres now use de-ionised water for dialysis and alternative phosphate binders to aluminium hydroxide are being sought.

Finally, parathyroidectomy may be required to control the severe bone disease that is resistant to other treatments – especially when hypercalcaemia (tertiary hyperparathyroidism) develops.

Acute Pancreatitis
Hypocalcaemia may occur during the early stages of acute pancreatitis. When severe it is associated with a poor prognosis. The precise aetiology of the disorder is unclear. Pancreatitis is an unusual but well-recognised presentation of hyperparathyroidism. In such cases the serum calcium may be normal during the acute attack and only elevated after the pancreatitis has resolved.

Hypomagnesaemia
Hypomagnesaemia can lead to the secondary development of hypocalcaemia. The hypocalcaemia is extremely resistant to

treatment but can be completely corrected by magnesium supplements. The reason for the hypocalcaemia is twofold: firstly, there is a failure to secrete PTH in the hypomagnesaemic state and this is coupled with a peripheral resistance to the action of PTH.

Severe hypomagnesaemia is uncommon but may be seen in severe diarrhoeal states, especially small bowel resections, and chronic alcoholism. On rare occasions a primary magnesium absorptive defect occurs. Recently, hypomagnesaemia has been reported during prolonged aminoglycoside therapy and with cisplatinum therapy.

Serum magnesium should be measured in any situation where magnesium deficiency may occur or where hypocalcaemia is resistant to conventional therapy. Magnesium supplements, initially intravenous, lead to a rapid correction of the hypocalcaemia.

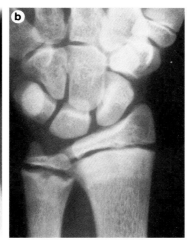

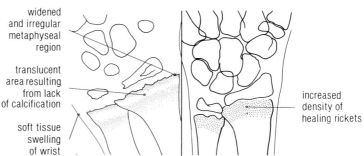

Fig. 17.31 Radiological appearance of rickets before and after treatment. In (a) the metaphysis is widened and the ends of the bone are very irregular. Behind this is a translucent zone due to a lack of calcification. During healing (b) the translucent zone, seen in (a), calcifies heavily to produce a band of increased density. By courtesy of Dr K. Shah.

widened and irregular metaphyseal region

translucent area resulting from lack of calcification

soft tissue swelling of wrist

increased density of healing rickets

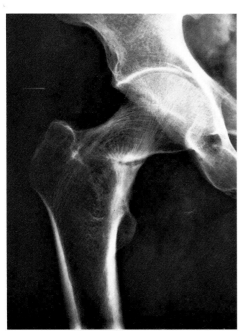

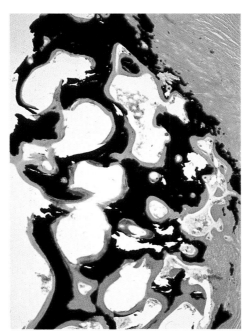

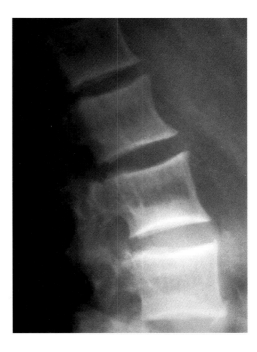

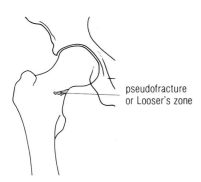

pseudofracture or Looser's zone

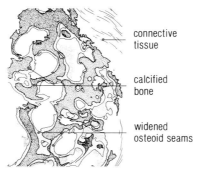

connective tissue

calcified bone

widened osteoid seams

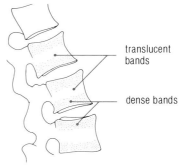

translucent bands

dense bands

Fig. 17.32 Radiological appearance in osteomalacia. In adults, the classical change is the development of pseudofractures or Looser's zones.

Fig. 17.33 Histology of bone in osteomalacia. The calcified bone is shown black with thickened osteoid seams lining the bone red. Van Kossa's stain, magnification ×16. By courtesy of Prof. E.L. Jones.

Fig. 17.34 Radiological appearance in renal osteodystrophy. Central translucent bands bounded by denser bone give a 'rugger jersey' appearance.

17.15

OTHER COMMON BONE DISEASES

Osteoporosis

Osteoporosis is a decrease in the bone mass appropriate for the patient's age and sex. This definition implies that there are normally changes in bone mass with age and between the sexes.

One of the problems of osteoporosis is the accurate measurement of bone mass. In routine radiography an approximate twenty-five per cent decrease in bone mass is required before changes can be readily detected; with very careful standardisation and attention to detail this figure can be reduced to ten per cent. Using bone densitometry (in which the ability of gamma rays to penetrate bone is measured) one can detect changes in bone mass of between five and ten per cent, but this technique can only readily be applied to changes in bone mass at the distal forearm. More accurate techniques for measuring total body calcium remain research procedures. Whichever technique is used, it can be shown that bone mass is roughly constant until the fifth decade when bone mass begins to fall progressively, especially in females where the rate of fall is four to five times more marked than in males (Fig. 17.35).

The major cause of bone loss in females is thought to be the post-menopausal decline in circulating oestrogen levels (Fig. 17.36). For this reason, osteoporosis is more likely to occur in women with a premature menopause (e.g. bilateral oöphorectomy) or where oestrogen levels are naturally low (e.g. in Turner's syndrome).

Generalised osteoporosis may also be seen in a variety of other conditions including steroid excess states (Cushing's disease and steroid therapy) and thyrotoxicosis. Localised osteoporosis may be seen in any situation where a bone is immobilised (e.g. in a fracture) or where local inflammation is present (e.g. in rheumatoid arthritis).

In the absence of complications osteoporosis is basically asymptomatic, being detected only as a chance finding. Symptoms are primarily related to fractures. These particularly relate to the wrist, femoral neck and vertebrae. Fractures of the wrist and femoral neck are usually related to obvious trauma and the frequency with which they occur increases rapidly with age. Vertebral fractures are often unrelated to recognisable trauma and are associated with the sudden onset of severe localised back pain which may take four to six weeks to settle. With each fracture there is often an obvious reduction in standing height and the development of kyphosis.

Standard radiographs remain the mainstay in detecting established disease, and show decreased bone density and an increased trabecular pattern. Affected vertebrae show varying degrees of wedging (Fig. 17.37). Routine blood tests are normal apart from an occasional elevated alkaline phosphatase at times of fractures.

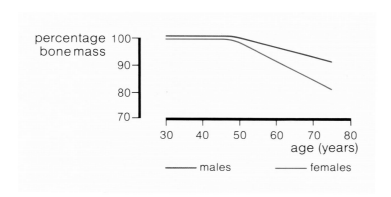

Fig. 17.35 **Graph showing the reduction in bone mass in males and females with age.**

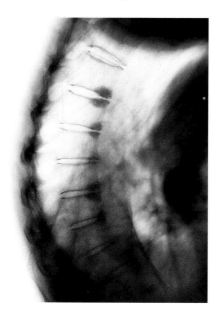

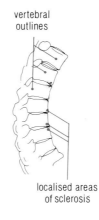

vertebral outlines

localised areas of sclerosis

Fig. 17.37 **Radiological appearance in osteoporosis.** The vertebrae are very translucent with only the outline of the bone being clearly seen. Most of the vertebrae are wedge-shaped and localised areas of sclerosis, occasionally seen in this area, are present.

Causes of Osteoporosis	
generalised osteoporosis	**localised osteoporosis**
postmenopausal women	
hypo-oestrogenic states e.g. Turner's syndrome	immobilisation e.g. fracture
corticosteroid excess states	
thyrotoxicosis	inflammatory disease e.g. rheumatoid arthritis
hypogonadism	

Fig. 17.36 **Table showing the causes of both general and local osteoporosis.**

Bones Affected in Paget's Disease	
common pelvis, sacrum, femur, skull, tibia, vertebrae	**uncommon** ribs
	rare fibula, mandible
less common scapula, humerus, clavicle, patella, radius, ulna, os calcis	**very rare** metatarsals, metacarpals, phalanges

Fig. 17.38 **Bones liable to be affected in Paget's disease.**

Disease prevention would obviously be ideal. The evidence is very strong that cyclical oestrogen therapy instituted at or around the menopause reduces the loss of bone mass. However, there are no techniques available to detect those women who are at risk of developing symptomatic osteoporosis twenty to thirty years later. At present, relatively few healthy menopausal women are being offered long-term oestrogen therapy.

The management of established disease is controversial. Obviously, any aetiologically important condition or therapy should be dealt with wherever possible. A variety of treatments have been suggested as therapies for established disease. They include oestrogens, vitamin D, calcium supplements, anabolic steroids, PTH and calcitonin. The evidence for most, if not all these claims is lacking. In the elderly, evidence of osteomalacia should be sought and treated appropriately.

Paget's Disease

Paget's disease is associated with the production of abnormal bone-containing areas of both increased osteoclastic and osteoblastic activity. In Britain, it is a common disorder in elderly people. Over the age of fifty years approximately five per cent of the population have radiological evidence of the disorder – the figure rising with increasing age. Also, within Britain there is a geographical variation with the highest incidence in the north-west of England. Paget's disease is uncommon in Asian, Oriental and African races living in Britain. The aetiology of the condition is unknown, although virus-like particles have been found within the osteoclast of Pagetic bone. However, the vast majority of people with Paget's disease are completely asymptomatic.

In the majority of patients the diagnosis of Paget's disease is made as a chance radiological finding during the investigation of other conditions. The commonest symptom is a dull, persistent pain arising from the affected bone. The bones liable to be affected are listed in Figure 17.38. Deformity of bones is not uncommon together with enlargement and abnormal curvature of bones (Fig. 17.39). Affected bones are more likely to fracture with the fracture frequently passing cleanly across the bone, the so-called 'chalk-stick' fracture. Nerve compression may occur and this particularly affects the eighth cranial nerve which, together with Pagetic involvement of the bones of the inner ear causes deafness. Very rarely an osteogenic sarcoma may develop in affected bone (Fig. 17.40). This is usually associated with a sudden increase in local pain and swelling.

Osteoarthritis is almost invariably associated with Paget's disease and involves bones close to a joint. In such situations, it

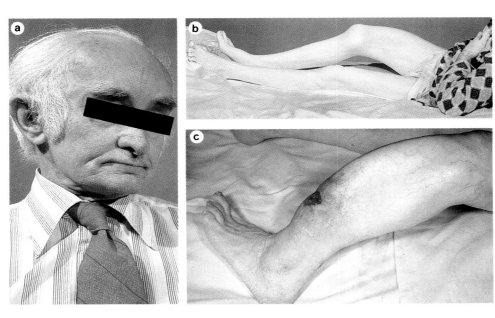

Fig. 17.39 Bone deformity in Paget's disease. Photograph (a) shows marked enlargement of the cranium with normalised facial bones – a hearing aid can be seen. View (b) shows the anterior bowing of the femur and view (c) marked bowing of the tibia with overlying ulceration.

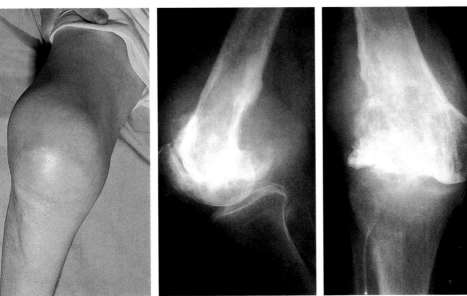

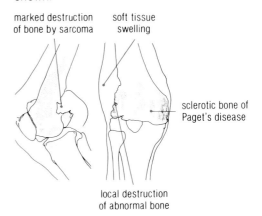

Fig. 17.40 Development of osteogenic sarcoma in Paget's disease. Painful swelling developed in the knee two years after the diagnosis of Paget's disease. Marked bone destruction and soft tissue swelling can be seen on the radiographs shown.

marked destruction of bone by sarcoma

soft tissue swelling

sclerotic bone of Paget's disease

local destruction of abnormal bone

17.17

may be impossible to decide which disorder is responsible for the patient's symptoms.

The diagnosis is based mainly upon the radiological findings. Films show expanded bone of an abnormal texture, often with adjacent areas of sclerosis and resorption (Fig. 17.41). The expansion of bone helps to distinguish the changes from those of sclerotic secondaries. The serum alkaline phosphatase is usually increased, as may be the acid phosphatase. Urinary hydroxyproline is increased, thus indicating the increased bone turnover. Isotope scans show increased uptake of the isotope in affected bone. These changes can easily be mistaken for secondary deposits.

Asymptomatic patients require no treatment. Pain should initially be treated with simple analgesics. When symptoms are not controlled by simple measures two specific treatments of Paget's disease are available. The first effective treatment available was calcitonin. Salmon calcitonin is most frequently used. Subcutaneous injections are often associated with a sensation of warmth and nausea. Symptoms do not begin to improve for four to six weeks, and one third of patients relapse despite good initial control. The other available treatment is the use of disphosphonate drugs; the only one currently generally available is sodium etidronate (Didronel). The drug is given in a daily dose of 5 mg/kg/day, 400 mg being a commonly used dose. The drug has to be given separately from food or milk which inhibit its absorption. Symptoms improve after four to six weeks and an initial course of nine months' treatment is given. Treatment is then stopped to minimise the risk of osteomalacia which may be produced by long-term therapy. After termination of the therapy a proportion of patients remain in long-term remission. Neither treatment cures Paget's disease and there is no evidence that either prevent the development of complications.

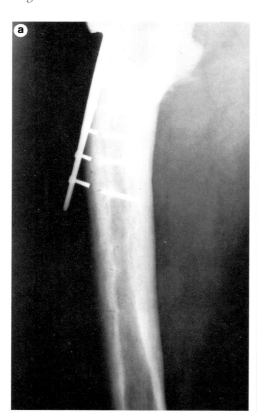

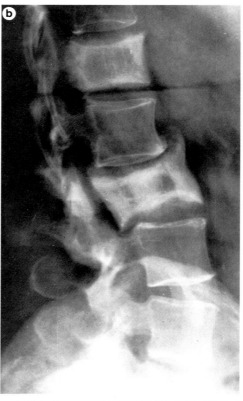

Fig. 17.41 Radiological appearance of the femur, vertebrae and skull in Paget's disease. Radiograph (a) shows the involvement of a femur which has fractured in the past. Deformity has fractured the pins of the plate. The cortex is thickened and there are multiple 'fissure fractures' involving the convex surface of the bone. In radiograph (b) several vertebrae are involved. The affected bones are both sclerotic and enlarged. This differentiates it from sclerotic secondaries where the bones are not enlarged. Changes in the skull (c) include thickening of the cortex and the presence of round areas of sclerotic bone in the vault. Basilar invagination is also present with the odontoid peg, which should be below McGregor's line, being considerably above it.

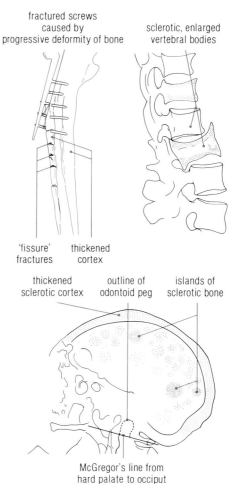

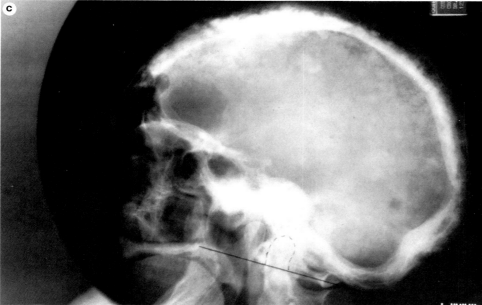

17.18

18 Hypoglycaemia and Insulinomas

Vincent Marks, MA, DM, FRCP, FRCPath

Hypoglycaemia is a biochemical description (Fig. 18.1). Although it has many causes, all are the result of an imbalance between the rate of glucose entry into the glucose pool and its rate of removal.

THE GLUCOSE POOL IN HEALTH

The size of the glucose pool is normally tightly controlled by a number of quasi-independent homeostatic mechanisms co-ordinated by a hypothetical master centre, possibly located in the hypothalamus (Fig. 18.2).

Although the exact size of the glucose pool is determined by both the volume of extracellular fluid and its glucose concentration, in practice it is only the latter that varies. The glucose pool rarely exceeds 27g (0.15 M) even after ingestion of a meal containing up to 360g (2.00 M) of glucose in the form of starch or sucrose. It does not normally decrease below 13g (0.075 M) even after prolonged fasting. The only route by which glucose normally enters the glucose pool is through the hepatic vein, which receives glucose either from hepatocytes during fasting or from the gut (via the portal vein) in the absorptive phase of a meal. During fasting, when the peripheral plasma insulin concentration falls below the level required to stimulate or permit free entry of glucose into insulin-dependent cells (e.g. muscle, fat and connective tissues), outflow from the glucose pool is restricted to non insulin-dependent tissues (mainly the brain and erythron). After feeding, and during the absorptive period, insulin is secreted by the B-cells of the pancreas (Fig. 18.3) in response to: (i) nervous impulses arising in the gut wall, (ii) hormones liberated by endocrine cells in the intestinal mucosa and (iii) a rise in arterial glucose concentration. This has the effect of: (a) decreasing glucose output by the liver and increasing its uptake and conversion into glycogen, (b) increasing outflow from the glucose pool into glucose-dependent tissues and (c) producing a large positive arterio-venous (a-v) glucose difference across the forearm and other peripheral tissues.

Depending upon the integrity and speed of response of the homeostatic mechanism, only a small rise in arterial blood glucose concentration may be observed after ingestion of a meal. This is not always seen in venous blood which may, under certain circumstances, show a postprandial fall in blood glucose concentration to below fasting levels. In situations where the glucose homeostatic mechanism becomes overwhelmed by excessively rapid absorption of glucose, the glucose pool can expand sufficiently to result in glucosuria. This may occur following precipitate entry into the duodenum (e.g. secondary to pyloric incompetence) or by reduced insulin secretory capacity. In the post-absorptive state the glucose needs of the body are confined almost

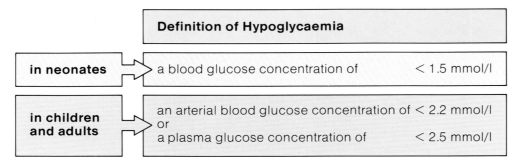

Fig. 18.1 Definition of hypoglycaemia. Hypoglycaemia is a biochemical description which may or may not be accompanied by associated symptoms.

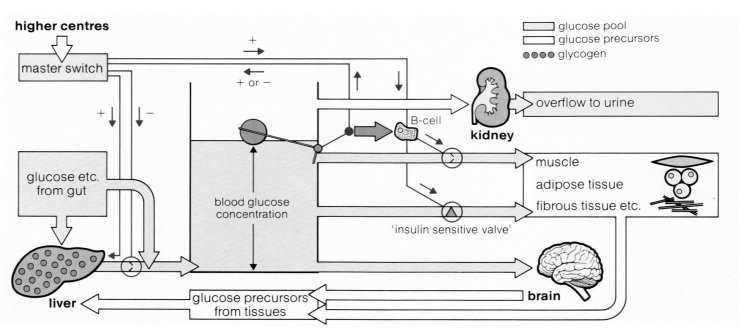

Fig. 18.2 Schematic representation of the autoregulatory control of the size of the blood glucose pool. Glucose homeostasis is presented as a self-regulating plumbing system. Blood glucose concentration rises as glucose enters the blood from the intestine. This, in turn, activates insulin secretion by direct action on the pancreas and also through higher centres. Consequently glucose inflow from the liver (from glycogen) is reduced and outflow into the tissues is increased. During fasting: (i) glucose inflow from the gut ceases, (ii) blood glucose concentration reaches basal levels, (iii) insulin secretion and outflow of glucose into the tissues almost ceases and (iv) glucose release from the liver (glycogen) is activated so that inflow exactly balances outflow into the brain and erythron. The 'insulin sensitive valve' can be activated by both endogenous and exogenous insulin.

exclusively to those of the erythron and the brain. These needs are met by hepatic release of glucose into the circulation either by the breakdown of preformed glycogen (glycogenolysis) or by synthesis (gluconeogenesis) from glucose precursors. Gluconeogenesis occurs predominantly from lactate, pyruvate, alanine and glycerate which have been released into the circulation by somatic tissues (e.g. the brain and erythron) during fasting.

HYPOGLYCAEMIA

Hypoglycaemia results when glucose outflow from the glucose pool is not balanced by glucose inflow from the liver. It most commonly arises from impaired hepatic glucose release under the influence of modest amounts of insulin. Under these circumstances the basal glucose outflow into the tissue is normal or slightly raised and there is no glucose inflow from the gut. In rare cases, hypoglycaemia results from the taking of pharmacologically large doses of exogenous insulin, or from drug-induced endogenous insulin release. The outflow from the glucose pool is therefore accelerated (by opening of a hypothetical 'insulin sensitive valve' – see Fig. 18.2) such that it cannot be counterbalanced by hepatic glucose release, thus hypoglycaemia ensues.

NEUROGLYCOPENIA

Regardless of the immediate cause of hypoglycaemia (i.e. reduced glucose output by the liver or increased glucose uptake by the tissues or a combination of both) most of the ensuing symptom complexes (neuroglycopenia) are caused by alterations in cerebral metabolism. The nature and severity of the neuroglycopenia depend largely upon the speed at which blood glucose levels fall and whether habituation to hypoglycaemia has taken place. The symptoms of acute neuroglycopenia (Fig. 18.4) vary from slight to markedly unpleasant and are commonly experienced by patients with insulin overdose. The symptoms of subacute neuroglycopenia are relatively unobtrusive and may be more apparent to others than to the patient himself. Subacute neuroglycopenia is the type most commonly produced by overdosage with sulphonylureas, or by disease causing 'spontaneous' hypoglycaemia. Chronic neuroglycopenia and hyperinsulin neuropathy, both very uncommon syndromes, almost invariably result from persistent hypoglycaemia secondary to insulinoma or, in rare cases, from overenthusiastic treatment of diabetes by insulin. Normoglycaemic neuroglycopenia can be produced experimentally by 2-deoxyglucose and other substances that impair intraneuronal glucose metabolism. It can also be produced spontaneously in children, and possibly adults, by certain viral infections of the central nervous system which interfere with glucose transport to the brain.

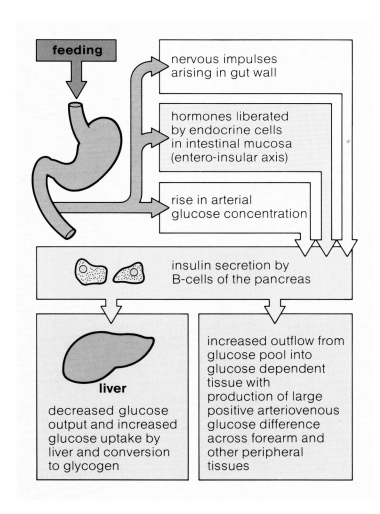

Neuroglycopenic Syndromes

acute neuroglycopenia
Sweating, malaise, anxiety, tachycardia, circumoral and/or carpal paraesthesia, unsteadiness, sleepiness progressing to stupor and coma; abnormal EEG present throughout: rapidly reversed by intravenous glucose but not by saline.

subacute neuroglycopenia
Lack of concentration, sleepiness, lassitude, inactivity progressing to stupor and coma; abnormal EEG throughout: rapidly reversed by intravenous glucose but not saline.

chronic neuroglycopenia (very rare)
Progressive mental deterioration simulating schizophrenia, depression or, most often, dementia; EEG may be normal. No immediate effect produced by glucose; partially reversible by permanent restoration of normoglycaemia.

normoglycaemic neuroglycopenia (very rare)
Caused by impaired intraneuronal glucose metabolism. Symptoms are a combination of those of acute and subacute neuroglycopenia and are partially or wholly relieved by sustained hyperglycaemia.

hyperinsulin neuropathy (extremely rare)
Paraesthesia in hands and feet, muscular weakness and wasting, fasciculation, reduced ankle jerks and high CSF protein concentration. Episodic, acute or subacute neuroglycopenia is common and chronic hypoglycaemia is invariably present.

Fig. 18.3 Hypoglycaemic effect of insulin. Insulin secretion by the B-cells is stimulated during feeding and absorption of food by (i) the nervous impulses arising from the gut, (ii) hormones secreted by endocrine cells in the intestinal mucosa and (iii) a rise in arterial blood glucose and amino-acid concentrations, or both.

Fig. 18.4 Features of the various neuroglycopenic syndromes. Acute neuroglycopenia is rare in patients with 'spontaneous' hypoglycaemia.

FUEL CONSUMPTION BY THE HUMAN BRAIN

Under normal circumstances the human brain consumes approximately 120-130g of glucose per day which constitutes its main, if not sole, source of energy. During prolonged fasting or starvation it can metabolise ketones (e.g. aceto-acetate and β-hydroxybutyrate) as its main fuel (Fig. 18.5). In children, the switch from glucose to ketones as the main source of cerebral energy may occur as little as twenty-four hours after withdrawal of food.

The supply of fuel to various parts of the brain is determined not only by its concentration in the plasma but also by blood flow. Simultaneous reduction of both can lead to impairment of cerebral function even when there is no discernable abnormality in either one alone. This probably accounts for the inability of many elderly subjects to withstand lowering of their blood glucose concentrations to levels that are well tolerated by younger people. Similarly, it explains why elderly diabetic patients with unilateral cerebrovascular disease, who have been rendered hypoglycaemic by insulin, occasionally present with hemiplegia that is rapidly reversed by intravenous glucose.

GLUCOSE HOMEOSTASIS

A popular, if simple, way of looking at glucose homeostasis is to consider it as the result of a balance between the action of hormones and metabolic processes that increase blood glucose concentrations and those that decrease it. The most important are shown in Figures 18.6 and 18.7. Many more are known, but their physiological significance is not.

Amongst the hypoglycaemic hormones insulin is by far the most important. In rare cases, however, in patients with an inborn inability to form insulin from proinsulin and in proinsulin-secreting islet-cell tumours, proinsulin is the dominant circulating hypoglycaemic hormone. Of the hypoglycaemic hormones, both insulin and proinsulin act by reducing hepatic glucose output and, when present in higher concentrations, by increasing glucose uptake by insulin-dependent tissues. Gastric inhibitory polypeptide (GIP) is probably the most important gut hormone in the regulation of insulin secretion in response to the ingestion of food; it does not affect glucose homeostasis directly but stimulates insulin secretion. Somatomedin-C (IGF 1) is one of a group of substances displaying non-suppressible insulin-like activity (NSILA).

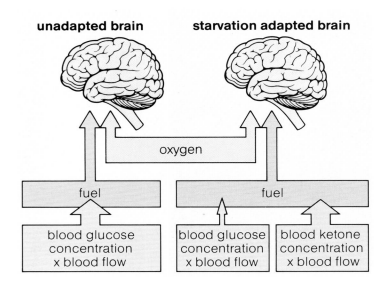

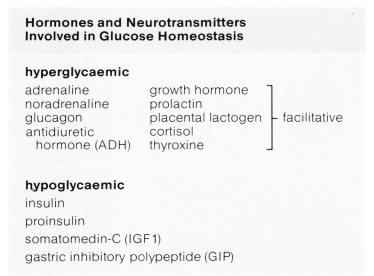

Fig. 18.5 Fuel utilisation by the human brain. Although the brain normally uses glucose as its sole fuel it can adapt. It uses β-hydroxybutyrate and aceto-acetate in infants, and also in adults during starvation.

Fig. 18.6 Possible hormones and neurotransmitters involved in glucose homeostasis.

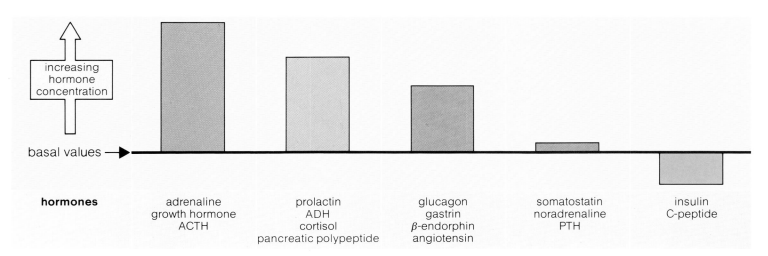

Fig. 18.7 Changes in plasma hormone concentrations produced by acute insulin-induced hypoglycaemia in healthy subjects. Relative magnitude and direction of change in the plasma concentrations of various hormones produced by acute hypoglycaemia are shown. Chronic hypoglycaemia produces smaller or no changes at all except in insulin and C-peptide levels.

These substances were originally identified by their insulin-like actions which included an increase in glucose uptake by isolated tissues *in vitro*. They were subsequently recognised to function as tissue growth factors of which somatomedin-C is thought to be the most important. Whether somatomedin-C and other growth factors present in human plasma exert hypoglycaemic effects *in vivo* is uncertain at the present time.

Pharmacologically, glucagon is the most potent of the hyperglycaemic hormones, but it does not play an essential role in raising blood glucose concentrations even after induced depression by exogenous or endogenous insulin (Fig. 18.8). It works exclu-sively through the liver by liberating glucose from preformed glycogen, by increasing glycogenolysis and, to a lesser extent, by gluconeogenesis from glucose precursors (Fig. 18.9). Antidiuretic hormone (ADH or vasopressin) and adrenaline are also potent glycogenolytic agents. However, it is doubtful whether adrenaline has a glycogenolytic effect at physiological concentrations. Nor-adrenaline, liberated at sympathetic nerve terminals in the liver, promotes glycogenolysis and liberation of glucose by hepatocytes through adrenoceptor activation. Growth hormone, prolactin, placental lactogen, cortisol and thyroxine indirectly impede glucose utilisation and promote its outflow from the liver.

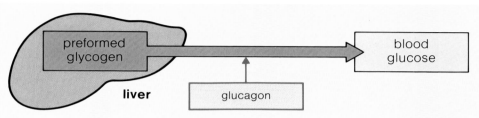

Fig. 18.8 Hyperglycaemic effect of glucagon. Glucagon works only on preformed glycogen to produce a rise in blood glucose. Thus it does not cause hyperglycaemia if the liver is already depleted of glycogen, for example, by prolonged fasting or alcohol intake.

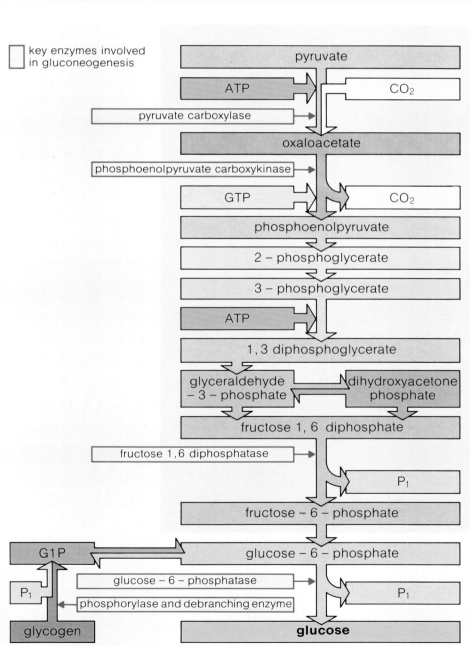

Fig. 18.9 Pathways of gluconeogenesis and glycogenolysis. Only those enzymes unique to the above pathways and not shared by glycolysis and gluconeogenesis are shown.

CLINICAL CLASSIFICATION OF HYPOGLYCAEMIA

Several conditions which may be confused clinically with hypoglycaemia and its associated symptomatology are listed in Figure 18.10. There are many ways of classifying hypoglycaemia clinically; the most useful is into 'fasting' hypoglycaemia and 'stimulative' hypoglycaemia. The former, as its name implies, is provoked by fasting. The latter occurs only in response to a particular stimulus: iatrogenic, drug-induced hypoglycaemia, certain rare inborn errors of metabolism, as well as reactive hypoglycaemias, belong to this category. The main pathological causes of hypoglycaemia and their main clinical manifestations are shown in Figure 18.11. Except in cases of inappropriate insulin secretion, factitious hypoglycaemia and rebound hypoglycaemia, an historical event or physical abnormality can usually be found to account for the hypoglycaemia – although this often emerges only after a long and thorough investigation.

Clinical Conditions which may be Confused with Hypoglycaemia

hysteria	vaso-vagal attacks or faint
anxiety neurosis	brain tumour
depression	angina pectoris
alcoholic and drug intoxications	narcolepsy
epilepsy	syndrome of Klein and Levine

Fig. 18.10 Clinical conditions which may be confused with hypoglycaemia.

Main Causes of Hypoglycaemia

type	example
fasting hypoglycaemia	
inappropriate insulin secretion	insulinoma and nesidioblastosis
factitious hypoglycaemia	surreptitious insulin or sulphonylurea administration
drug and alcohol-induced hypoglycaemia	alcohol, aspirin, β-blockers
non insulin-producing tumours	fibrosarcomas, carcinomas of stomach, adrenal, colon, prostate and breast
liver, heart or kidney failure	
endocrine disease	adrenocortical insufficiency, hypopituitarism
inborn errors of metabolism	glycogen storage disease types 1, 3 and 4; maple syrup urine disease; hereditary fructose intolerance
carbohydrate deprivation (especially in children)	'ketotic hypoglycaemia of children'
symptomatic neonatal hypoglycaemia of diverse aetiology	
stimulative	
rebound 'reactive' hypoglycaemia	post-gastrectomy, alcohol-induced or 'idiopathic'(rare)
iatrogenic	
overtreatment with insulin	
overtreatment with sulphonylureas non-metabolised metabolised	chlorpropamide glibenclamide

Fig. 18.11 Table of the main causes of clinical hypoglycaemia. These may be divided into three types: fasting, stimulative and iatrogenic hypoglycaemia.

FASTING HYPOGLYCAEMIA

Insulinoma

This is a rare but important cause of hypoglycaemia and occurs with an incidence of approximately one case per million of the population per year. Hypoglycaemia and its associated neuro-glycopenia is the presenting, and usually only discernable, ab-normality. Characteristically, there is a history, often of several years standing, of episodic alterations in consciousness lasting from a few minutes to several hours, with increasing frequency and severity. Symptoms frequently occur in the morning before breakfast and commonly include difficulty in waking. Measure-ments of the blood glucose concentration after an overnight fast almost always reveal hypoglycaemia (Fig. 18.12), provided they are performed on at least three occasions. In suspected cases, glucose determinations can be carried out, during attacks at home, using filter paper blood spots and a sensitive, specific and precise hexokinase method. Sometimes episodes of hypoglycaemia occur only as a result of rigorous exercise. An association with fasting or abstinence from food is seldom remarked upon spontaneously, although, paradoxically, because rebound (stimulative) hypo-glycaemia is also common in this disease, a causal relationship to eating and drinking may be mentioned. Weight gain and loss occur with almost equal frequency, although in rare instances patients can present with seemingly simple but intractable obesity as their sole complaint. Diagnosis depends upon the demonstration of symptomatic fasting hypoglycaemia in the presence of in-appropriately high plasma insulin and C-peptide concentrations. This is virtually pathognomonic of either endogenous hyper-insulinism due to insulinoma in adults (and also children over the age of two years), or of functional hyperinsulinism (nesidio-blastosis) in infants and babies under the age of two years.

Peripheral venous plasma insulin concentrations are usually less than 30mu/l after an overnight fast in healthy subjects, but can be higher in obese, but seemingly otherwise fit individuals, and those with a variety of disorders none of which, apart from insulinoma, are associated with hypoglycaemia. Several factors determine the plasma insulin level in the blood, one of the most important being the arterial blood glucose concentration; a reduction in this leads to a fall in plasma insulin concentration. Consequently, hypoglycaemia almost invariably inhibits endo-genous insulin secretion; this in turn leads to a peripheral venous plasma insulin concentration of less than 5mu/l. The average half-life of insulin in the circulation is between five and ten minutes. Patients who suffer from insulinoma demonstrate inappropriate hyperinsulinaemia whilst they are hypoglycaemic on some occasions, though rarely on all (Fig. 18.13). Factitious hypoglycaemia is usually associated with inappropriate hyper-insulinaemia during hypoglycaemic episodes. All other types of spontaneous hypoglycaemia occur in conjunction with appropri-ately low plasma insulin concentrations.

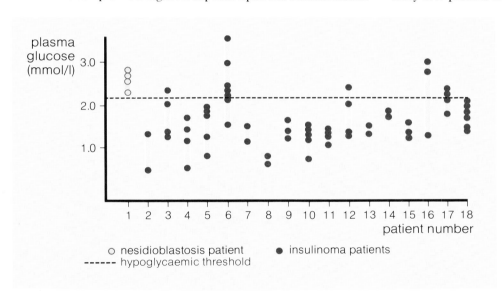

Fig. 18.12 Overnight fasting blood glucose levels in patients with insulinoma compared with those with 'nesidioblastosis'. Seventeen patients with insulinoma and one with 'nesidioblastosis' are shown. Each block represents one patient and each dot the blood glucose concentration measured on one morning. Large differences in blood glucose concentration in the same individual on different occasions can be seen.

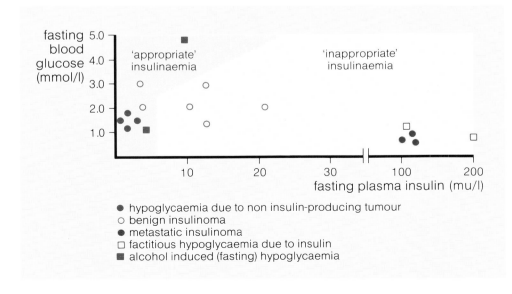

Fig. 18.13 Relationship of fasting plasma insulin to fasting blood glucose in several types of spontaneous hypoglycaemia. Plasma insulin and blood glucose concentrations collected from patients with different types of hypo-glycaemia are shown.

Approximately fifteen per cent of all insulinomas are metastatic and they are usually associated with the highest and most inappropriate insulin levels during hypoglycaemia. Large and spontaneous fluctuations in peripheral venous plasma insulin concentrations often occur in patients with insulinomas (Fig. 18.14). An appropriately low plasma insulin level in the presence of fasting hypoglycaemia does not, in itself, exclude an insulinoma although one inappropriately high concentration is highly suggestive of this diagnosis. Extensive hepatic insulin extraction from portal venous blood can lead to hypoglycaemia by inhibition of glucose release, while peripheral venous plasma insulin concentrations remain appropriately low (Fig. 18.15). Random plasma insulin measurements, except in the presence of chemically established hypoglycaemia, are of no diagnostic value.

Endogenous insulin is derived from its precursor proinsulin (Fig. 18.16). Proinsulin is synthesised on the rough endoplasmic reticulum in the pancreatic B-cells and is then enzymatically cleaved in the β-granules to form two peptides, insulin and C-peptide, which are released simultaneously into the circulation following an insulinotrophic stimulus. Proinsulin has many of the biological properties of insulin itself but only at approximately ten per cent of the molar potency. Intracellular cleavage of proinsulin into the two peptides is usually complete and very little or no proinsulin normally enters the circulation, even in response to intensive B-cell stimulation. However, in the presence of benign or malignant neoplastic B-cell transformation, intact proinsulin or proinsulin-like components (PLC), having similar molecular size and immunoreactivity to proinsulin (but differing in tertiary structure) may be released into the circulation. On rare occasions, proinsulin and PLC account for most, or even all, of the insulin immunoreactivity measurable in peripheral venous plasma. The measurement of proinsulin and PLC as a percentage of total insulin immunoreactivity in peripheral venous plasma may be helpful in the differential diagnosis of obscure cases of fasting hypoglycaemia (Fig. 18.17).

The C-peptide of proinsulin is released from the B-cell with insulin in equimolar amounts. Under basal conditions, that is at low levels of secretory activity, peripheral venous plasma C-peptide concentrations are five to six times higher than those of insulin on a molar basis. This results from the slower rate of removal of C-peptide from the circulation which is cleared mainly by the kidneys. In contrast, insulin is cleared more rapidly by the liver. C-peptide has a half-life in the circulation of approximately thirty minutes, except in renal failure when it may be greatly prolonged.

Plasma C-peptide levels closely follow those of insulin but, because of a larger pool size and slower turnover rate, large fluctuations are less common. Overnight fasting peripheral venous plasma C-peptide levels generally fall within the range 1.5-3μg/l since they are related to the prevailing blood glucose levels. In the presence of hypoglycaemia, venous plasma C-peptide concentrations are invariably less than 1.2μg/l except in the presence of endogenous hyperinsulinism (Fig. 18.18) caused by insulinoma or functional hyperinsulinism of childhood (nesidioblastosis).

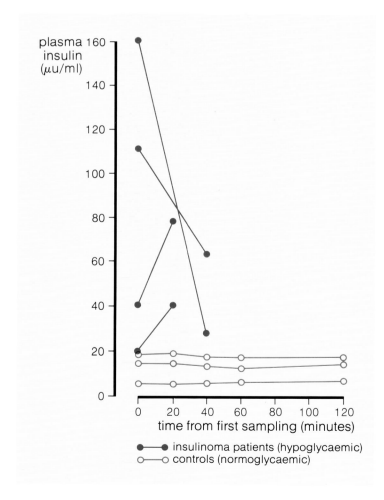

Fig. 18.14 Spontaneous fluctuations of fasting plasma insulin concentrations in four patients with insulinomas compared with three healthy controls.

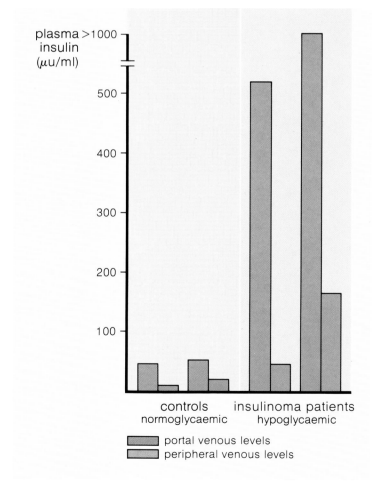

Fig. 18.15 Fasting portal and peripheral venous plasma insulin concentrations during abdominal surgery in two insulinoma patients and two control subjects.

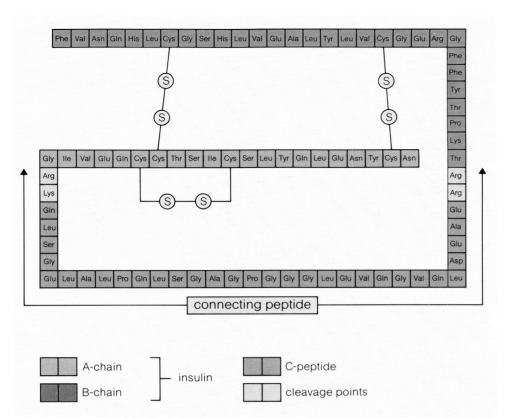

Fig. 18.16 Diagrammatic representation of the structure of human proinsulin. This molecule is enzymatically cleaved to yield two peptides, insulin and C-peptide, following an insulinotrophic stimulus.

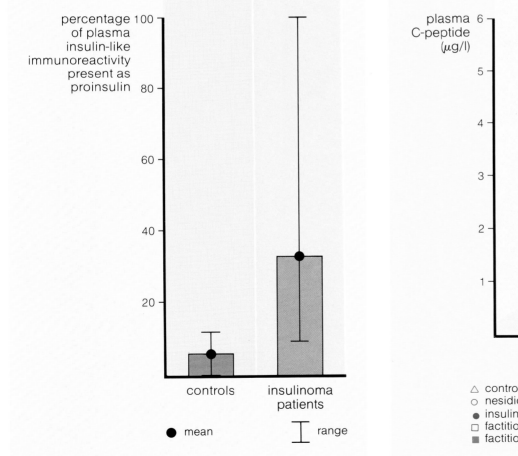

Fig. 18.17 Proportion of immunoreactive insulin present as proinsulin in blood from healthy subjects and patients with insulinomas.

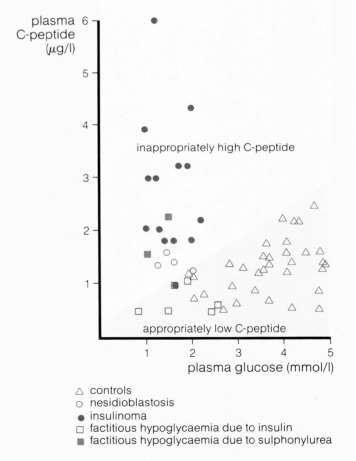

Fig. 18.18 Comparison of fasting plasma glucose and C-peptide concentrations in healthy control subjects and patients with various types of hypoglycaemia. Each symbol represents a single individual.

Patients with hypoglycaemia secondary to diseases other than endogenous hyperinsulinism show appropriate suppression of plasma C-peptide levels by hypoglycaemia. This occurs regardless of whether it is produced 'spontaneously' or by deliberate injection of insulin. C-peptide concentrations are not suppressed, however, in hyperinsulinism resulting from an insulinoma. This is the basis of the insulin hypoglycaemia test (Fig. 18.19) which can be used as a screening test for insulinomas. This test is neither very sensitive (at least twenty-five per cent of patients with proven insulinomas having a false negative response with C-peptide suppression in response to insulin); nor is it very specific since false positive responses can occur in renal failure, and also in situations where insufficient time has elapsed for initially high plasma C-peptide levels to fall below $1.2\mu g/l$ before termination of the test. This situation may arise either in the event of troublesome or distressing neuroglycopenia or where spontaneous recovery has occurred.

The main clinical usefulness of plasma C-peptide assay is in the differentiation of endogenous from exogenous (factitious) hyperinsulinism (Fig. 18.20). It is uninformative, and may be misleading in factitious hypoglycaemia due to surreptitious sulphonylurea self-administration.

In children with functional hyperinsulinism (nesidioblastosis) plasma insulin and C-peptide measurements are less likely to reveal inappropriate insulin secretion than in adults with insulinomas.

Plasma β-hydroxybutyrate concentrations are low in children who are hypoglycaemic secondary to functional (endogenous) hyperinsulinism. This is regardless of whether peripheral plasma insulin concentrations are inappropriately high or not, in contrast to those whose hypoglycaemia results from other causes (Fig. 18.21). In adults the measurement of plasma β-hydroxybutyrate is of less value in distinguishing the various causes of hypoglycaemia.

Functional Hyperinsulinism

Functional hyperinsulinism of childhood (nesidioblastosis) is a condition in which B-cell function is disturbed; this leads to the development of hypoglycaemia and inappropriate hyperinsulinaemia. This condition does not have a well-defined histopathological basis since the diffuse B-cell hyperplasia (which is not necessarily confined to well-demarcated islets of Langerhans and which was once thought to be causally related to the functional disturbance, and thus diagnostic of nesidioblastosis) occurs in many normal babies who never experience spontaneous hypoglycaemia. The syndrome of functional hyperinsulinism of childhood varies in intensity. In its mildest form, there is a transient lowering of blood glucose concentration and minimal inappropriate hyperinsulinaemia with slight, temporary neuroglycopenia during the first few days of life. In its most extreme form, gross intra-uterine hyperinsulinism with associated obesity is present at birth, followed by intractable symptomatic hypoglycaemia leading immediately to severe, permanent brain damage or death unless treatment is instituted at once. Usually the baby has a normal appearance at birth and nothing untoward happens until the child is in its second or third month of life, when failure of mental development or the onset of fits brings it to medical attention. Some cases are familial, especially those in which leucine sensitivity is a feature. Whilst of no discernable pathological significance, leucine sensitivity is pathognomonic of functional hyperinsulinism of childhood.

Nesidioblastosis must be distinguished from other types of neonatal hypoglycaemia – in many of which it is an epiphenomenon of little clinical importance (Fig. 18.22).

Treatment of functional hyperinsulinism varies from the introduction of frequent feeding through to the institution of combined diazoxide-chlorothiazide treatment (Fig. 18.23) or to total pancreatectomy in the most refractory cases. Spontaneous recovery is almost invariable during the first ten to fifteen years of life in children who respond to dietary or diazoxide-chlorothiazide treatment. Thus treatment must be discontinued from time to time, under strict supervision, to see whether spontaneous recovery has occurred.

Fig. 18.19   Patterns of plasma C-peptide behaviour observed during insulin-induced hypoglycaemia in patients with insulinomas or renal failure.

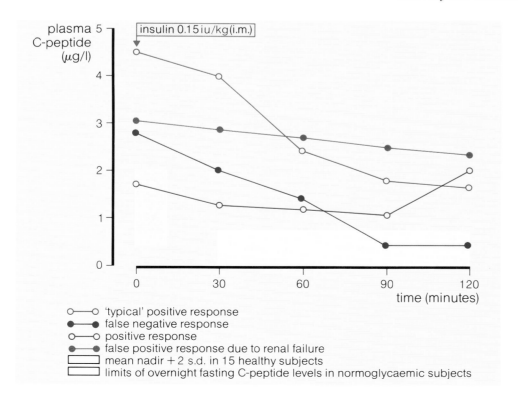

plasma C-peptide (μg/l)

insulin 0.15 iu/kg (i.m.)

time (minutes)

○——○ 'typical' positive response
●——● false negative response
○——○ positive response
●——● false positive response due to renal failure
☐ mean nadir + 2 s.d. in 15 healthy subjects
☐ limits of overnight fasting C-peptide levels in normoglycaemic subjects

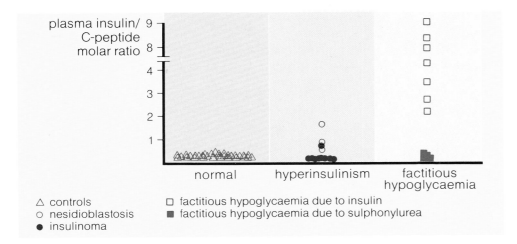

Fig. 18.20 Plasma insulin: C-peptide molar ratios after an overnight fast in control subjects or during hypoglycaemia in patients with endogenous or self-induced hyperinsulinism.

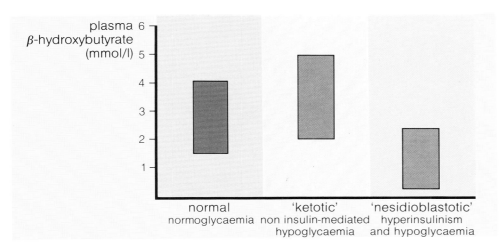

Fig. 18.21 Fasting plasma β-hydroxybutyrate concentrations. Concentrations in healthy children are compared with those in children with either nesidioblastotic (insulin-mediated) or 'ketotic' (non insulin-mediated) hypoglycaemia.

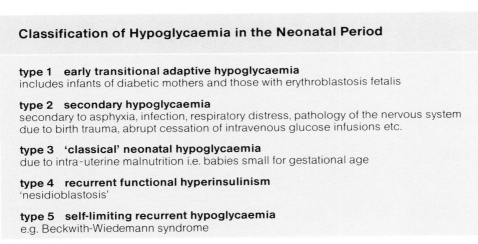

Fig. 18.22 Classification of hypoglycaemia developing in the neonatal period.

Classification of Hypoglycaemia in the Neonatal Period

type 1   early transitional adaptive hypoglycaemia
includes infants of diabetic mothers and those with erythroblastosis fetalis

type 2   secondary hypoglycaemia
secondary to asphyxia, infection, respiratory distress, pathology of the nervous system due to birth trauma, abrupt cessation of intravenous glucose infusions etc.

type 3   'classical' neonatal hypoglycaemia
due to intra-uterine malnutrition i.e. babies small for gestational age

type 4   recurrent functional hyperinsulinism
'nesidioblastosis'

type 5   self-limiting recurrent hypoglycaemia
e.g. Beckwith-Wiedemann syndrome

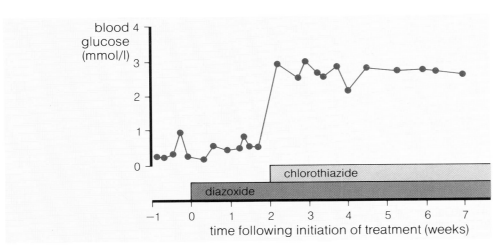

Fig. 18.23 Effect of treatment with diazoxide alone and in combination with chlorothiazide on fasting blood glucose concentration in a hypoglycaemic child. This child's hypoglycaemia was caused by 'nesidioblastosis'.

18.11

Summary of Management of Hyperinsulinism

The sequential steps in the diagnosis of hyperinsulinism are summarised in Figure 18.24. This condition almost invariably results from neoplastic transformation of the B-cells of the islets of Langerhans when the onset is after the age of one year, and functional hyperinsulinism of infancy when it occurs before this age. Extremely rare cases of 'adult nesidioblastosis' have been reported and, in several, a history of hypoglycaemia commencing in childhood has been found. Cases of 'adult nesidioblastosis' are clinically and biochemically identical to those with discrete insulinomas.

Surgical ablation of insulinomas is followed by complete remission except in unusual cases of metastatic growth in which palliative therapy with diazoxide-chlorothiazide may be used to give symptomatic relief for up to ten years. Chemotherapy with streptozotocin, tubercidin or 5-fluorouracil is sometimes successful in staving off death from hypoglycaemia but is rarely curative.

Hypoglycaemia Due to Non-Insulinomas

Several tumour types have been responsible for the production of symptomatic hypoglycaemia, the commonest being fibrosarcomata, and carcinomas of the gut, adrenal, breast and prostate, although all such cases are rare. In a minority, hypoglycaemia is the presenting symptom, the symptomatology being often indistinguishable from that of an insulinoma. The various mechanisms underlying the hypoglycaemia produced by these tumours is poorly understood. Some of the more plausible suggestions are shown in Figure 18.25. Although ectopic insulin production may play a causative role in some cases, the evidence is unconvincing and, in the overwhelming majority, plasma insulin and C-peptide levels are appropriately depressed during spontaneous or induced hypoglycaemia.

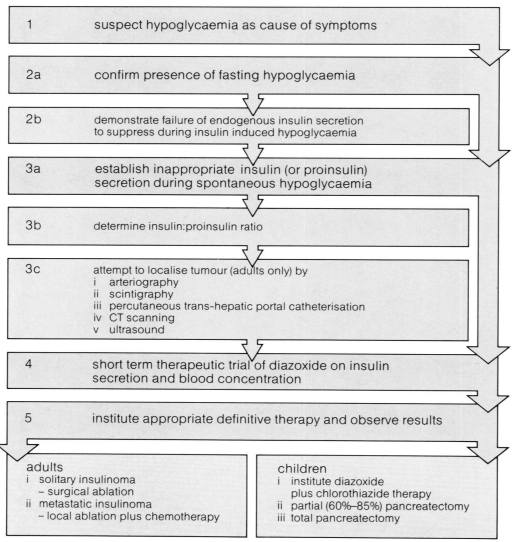

Fig. 18.24 Sequence of events in the diagnosis and treatment of hyperinsulinism.

1   suspect hypoglycaemia as cause of symptoms

2a   confirm presence of fasting hypoglycaemia

2b   demonstrate failure of endogenous insulin secretion to suppress during insulin induced hypoglycaemia

3a   establish inappropriate insulin (or proinsulin) secretion during spontaneous hypoglycaemia

3b   determine insulin:proinsulin ratio

3c   attempt to localise tumour (adults only) by
     i   arteriography
     ii   scintigraphy
     iii   percutaneous trans-hepatic portal catheterisation
     iv   CT scanning
     v   ultrasound

4   short term therapeutic trial of diazoxide on insulin secretion and blood concentration

5   institute appropriate definitive therapy and observe results

adults
i   solitary insulinoma
   – surgical ablation
ii   metastatic insulinoma
   – local ablation plus chemotherapy

children
i   institute diazoxide plus chlorothiazide therapy
ii   partial (60%–85%) pancreatectomy
iii   total pancreatectomy

Fig. 18.25 Mechanisms postulated to explain the production of hypoglycaemia by non insulin-secreting tumours.

Postulated Mechanisms of Hypoglycaemia Production by Non Insulin-Secreting Tumours

excessive and unregulated consumption of glucose by the tumour
secretion of an unidentified insulin-like substance
production of excessive amounts of somatomedin-C (IGF1)
release of a somatostatin-like substance with inhibitory effects on secretion of
   counter-regulatory hormones
inhibition of glycogenolysis
interference with gluconeogenesis

REBOUND (REACTIVE) HYPOGLYCAEMIA

It has been known for more than sixty years that administration of a large glucose load (as a twenty per cent solution) usually results in an early rise in blood glucose concentration in most healthy subjects. This is followed by a late rebound fall, often to hypoglycaemic levels. The rise in blood glucose concentration is more marked in arterial than in venous blood (Fig. 18.26) due to greatly increased glucose uptake by peripheral tissues. This occurs in response to arterial hyperglycaemia and hyperinsulinaemia secondary to alimentary and other insulin stimulatory influences. The increase in glucose difference provoked by oral glucose ingestion persists throughout the absorptive phase. However, arterial glucose levels may only slightly exceed fasting values for much of this period because of accelerated glucose removal from the glucose pool which, in some circumstances, may be faster than glucose entry from the gut. Under these conditions, genuine arterial hypoglycaemia may occur and produce acute neuroglycopenic symptoms. Most commonly, venous blood glucose concentrations fall to well below fasting levels and are of no physiological importance. However, they have been extensively misconstrued in the past as indicative of 'rebound' hypoglycaemia and, as such, responsible for the vague non-specific symptomatic disturbances experienced by many people undergoing prolonged laboratory investigations, regardless of their nature.

The exact time at which the nadir in venous blood glucose concentration occurs following ingestion of an oral liquid glucose load depends upon several factors, the most important being gastric emptying (Fig. 18.27). In situations of excessively rapid gastric emptying such as pyloric incompetence, or in the presence of a hyperactive entero-insular axis, the nadir in venous blood glucose concentration may occur as early as two hours after ingestion of the liquid glucose load. In most healthy subjects, however, the nadir occurs after 210-240 minutes at a time when individuals with an early nadir are already undergoing a hyperglycaemic rebound. A serious misunderstanding of the value of oral glucose loading as a diagnostic tool has arisen because of: (i) the use of population means rather than necessary reference values to compare sick and healthy subjects and (ii) the use of venous rather than arterial blood glucose concentrations as the main indicator of postprandial glucose homeostasis.

Ingestion of solid meals consisting mainly or wholly of digestible carbohydrate is not usually associated with such large fluctuations in arterial or venous blood glucose concentrations. However, large a-v glucose differences may occur, giving an appearance of 'reactive' hypoglycaemia if venous blood alone is sampled. For this reason, arterial or, more practically, capillary blood should be sampled when 'reactive' hypoglycaemia is suspected as the cause. The most favourable time to take a blood sample is during a spontaneous symptomatic episode. This can be readily achieved by instructing patients to absorb capillary blood from a finger prick onto filter paper impregnated with boric acid and to dry it rapidly by heat or blowing air onto it. The filter paper can then be sent by post or any other convenient method to a laboratory equipped to make accurate and precise blood glucose measurements on 10μl of blood or less. Only if blood collected and assayed under these circumstances reveals a low blood glucose concentration can a diagnosis of reactive hypoglycaemia be seriously entertained.

Many patients with fasting hypoglycaemia present with symptoms which may be attributed (with or without associated exercise) to reactive hypoglycaemia. The true cause may only emerge after detailed examination during fasting.

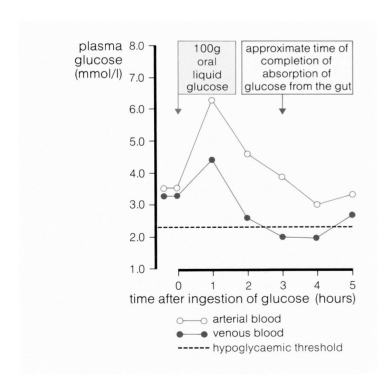

Fig. 18.26 Mechanism of apparent production of spontaneous reactive hypoglycaemia by oral glucose when venous blood is used for sampling. Plasma glucose values are taken from one patient. The disparity between arterial and venous plasma glucose levels can be seen.

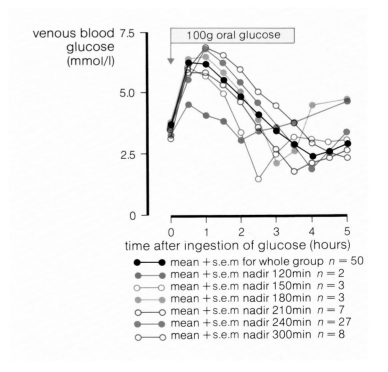

Fig. 18.27 Venous blood glucose levels in fifty healthy subjects. Each was given a 100g oral glucose load and grouped according to the time at which the nadir occurred. In two subjects the lowest venous blood glucose level was observed at 120 minutes following glucose loading; however, in twenty-seven it was at 240 minutes and in eight it was 300 minutes.

Contrary to former belief, reactive hypoglycaemia is not premonitory of non insulin-dependent diabetes. In practice, the commonest cause of reactive hypoglycaemia, for which no other cause can be found, is rapid gastric emptying – usually as a result of gastro-duodenal surgery. Very occasionally no patho-anatomical cause can be found. Excessive secretion of insulin in response to hyperactivity of the entero-insular axis, though an attractive idea, has not been established as a cause of reactive hypoglycaemia. However, the ingestion of a low carbohydrate diet for as little as one week markedly increases the propensity to develop symptomatic reactive hypoglycaemia in response to a large, rapidly absorbed liquid glucose load. This may also occur when an oral glucose tolerance test is performed on an inadequately prepared patient, who has either made a self-diagnosis of hypoglycaemia on the basis of misinformation, or who has interrupted his self-imposed carbohydrate restriction by drinking a large volume of a carbonated soft drink containing up to ten per cent by weight of sucrose or invert sugar. A special example of this occurs when the sugar drink is consumed with alcohol, for instance, when gin and tonic or whisky and ginger ale is consumed on an empty stomach which is not followed by ingestion of a meal. An example of this occurring in a healthy subject who drank three different types of drink at lunch time, after eating a standard breakfast some four

hours earlier, is shown in Figure 18.28. The addition of alcohol to the sucrose-containing drink produced an exaggerated insulinaemic response and severe, though transient, symptomatic reactive hypoglycaemia. This response did not occur, however, when fructose or saccharine was substituted for sucrose as the sweetening agent. Reduction of the amount of sucrose ingested is accompanied by a reduction in the incidence of symptomatic reactive hypoglycaemia, which occurs in up to twenty per cent of subjects when 60g sucrose is ingested with alcohol, but not when ingested alone. Hypoglycaemia is rarely observed at doses lower than 40g. Ingestion of small amounts of predominantly starchy food with alcoholic drink does not abolish (and may even enhance) the propensity to symptomatic reactive hypoglycaemia. This is illustrated in Figure 18.29 where the occurrence of symptomatic hypoglycaemia in an otherwise healthy thirty-year-old woman is demonstrated. On two separate occasions she took a snack providing 40g of alcohol as lager, 40g of carbohydrate and 20g of protein. Hypoglycaemia produced by alcohol in this way results solely from its ability to enhance the insulinotropic effect of glucose. It must therefore be distinguished from the hypoglycaemia produced by alcohol in fasting or under-nourished subjects in whom it produces its effect by inhibition of gluconeogenesis.

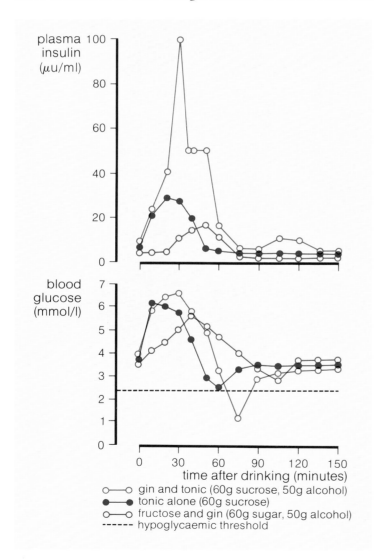

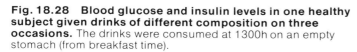

Fig. 18.28 Blood glucose and insulin levels in one healthy subject given drinks of different composition on three occasions. The drinks were consumed at 1300h on an empty stomach (from breakfast time).

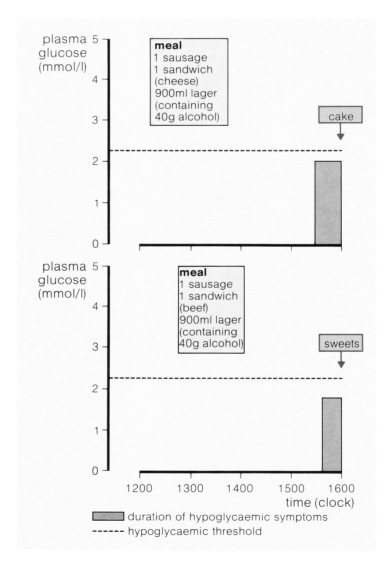

Fig. 18.29 Symptomatic spontaneous alcohol-induced reactive hypoglycaemia. A healthy 30-year-old female was hypoglycaemic in the early afternoon on two separate occasions. This hypoglycaemia was overcome by eating cake or sweets.

19 Ectopic Humoral Syndromes

Louis M Sherwood, MD

CLINICAL MANIFESTATIONS OF MALIGNANCY

Patients with neoplastic disease may present with a variety of clinical problems (Fig. 19.1). A manifestation of the primary lesion such as gastro-intestinal bleeding, a lump or haemoptysis is usually the cause of presentation. However, some patients present only when they have metastatic disease, such as a seizure associated with cerebral metastases from breast or lung cancer, or hepatomegaly due to metastatic carcinoma of the colon. In some cases, the primary lesion may not be detectable even on clinical examination.

In addition to manifestations of primary or secondary lesions, there are many associated manifestations of malignant disease, otherwise known as the 'paraneoplastic syndromes'. This chapter will focus on the subgroup 'endocrine metabolic syndromes' (ectopic humoral syndromes),but there are many other clinical manifestations which may result from the production of a specific protein by the malignant tumour. In the endocrine syndromes, it has been relatively easy to identify specific polypeptides because the known polypeptide hormones have been purified and specific radioimmunoassays developed. However, in patients with other clinical manifestations (e.g. fever, weight loss, neurological syndromes and vascular abnormalities), specific peptides have not yet been identified. It is likely that additional factors are released from tumour tissue and give rise to some of these syndromes; for example, the presence of surface tumour antigens or of antigen-antibody complexes may cause immunological abnormalities such as nephrotic syndrome and joint pains. Nevertheless, as research proceeds, additional factors may be identified which will help to explain some of the common, as well as the uncommon, manifestations of malignancy.

FEATURES OF THE ECTOPIC HUMORAL SYNDROMES

The ectopic humoral syndromes are not isolated curiosities;

indeed, production of peptide hormones by tumours may be the rule rather than the exception (Fig. 19.2). Extensive radioimmunoassay of the serum of patients with malignant disease and of tumour extracts has revealed the widespread presence of some polypeptide hormones. The most predominant of these are adrenocorticotrophic hormone (ACTH) and its precursors, human chorionic gonadotrophin (HCG) and its subunits, calcitonin and antidiuretic hormone (ADH or vasopressin). In some cases, ectopic hormones have even been found in normal tissues (e.g. HCG in the normal testis, liver and colon). Therefore, a knowledge of the pathogenesis of the ectopic humoral syndromes is helpful in understanding not only abnormal cell differentiation (e.g. neoplasia) but also normal cellular growth and differentiation.

Clinical manifestations of ectopic humoral syndromes vary considerably; some patients present with serious metabolic problems, whilst most are asymptomatic. Cushing's syndrome, hypoglycaemia, hypokalaemia, hypercalcaemia and hyponatraemia are clear examples of potentially serious metabolic problems. It is essential to exclude coexisting disorders since, in a patient with a non-endocrine neoplasm in addition to an endocrine disorder, the endocrine abnormality may not result from the tumour itself but from an occult endocrine disorder. For example, hypercalcaemia is not only a common manifestation of certain malignant tumours, it is also a manifestation of the very common endocrine disorder, primary hyperparathyroidism. Venous catheterisation is sometimes useful in establishing the origin of the peptide hormone. Radioimmunoassay of plasma for polypeptide hormones or tumour antigens has so far not been useful in the early diagnosis of malignant disease. In some cases, these measurements are more useful for following the progress of the disease or its recurrence.

CLASSIFICATION OF THE ECTOPIC HUMORAL SYNDROMES

There are several ways of identifying the specific hormone

Clinical Disorders of Malignancy

fever	dermatological
weight loss	renal
immunological and connective tissue related	endocrine-metabolic (ectopic humoral syndromes)
neurological	biochemical
vascular	

Fig. 19.1 Table of the clinical disorders associated with malignancy. These may result from primary or secondary (metastatic) lesions, or from paraneoplastic syndromes.

Ectopic Humoral Syndromes

not isolated curiosities—may be rule rather than exception

give clue to normal and abnormal cell differentiation

patients may be asymptomatic or there may be a serious metabolic problem

coexistence of tumour and endocrine disorder a possibility

so far not useful in the early diagnosis of malignancy

ectopic hormone concentrations may give clue to management

Fig. 19.2 Table listing the features of the ectopic humoral syndromes.

syndrome, some indirect and others direct (Fig. 19.3). Historically, these associations were first defined in patients who had well-recognised endocrine or biochemical disorders and who had concommitant non-endocrine neoplasms. The coexistence of a true endocrine disorder and a non-endocrine neoplasm must first be excluded. In those patients with non-endocrine tumours who have remission of the endocrine or metabolic disorder with treatment (e.g. after surgery, chemotherapy or radiotherapy) but a return of the disorder with recurrence of tumour, it is probable that the diagnosis is an ectopic humoral syndrome. Abnormal hormone levels of a metabolite in the blood or urine, detected by radioimmunoassay, are used to establish the diagnosis. In those organs where it is possible to sample both the arterial and venous sides of the tumour (e.g. the kidney and lung), it may be possible to show an arteriovenous rise in hormone concentration.

The ectopic hormone may be identified by *in vitro* studies of tumour extracts, by bioassay or radioimmunoassay. Using modern techniques, it is also possible to identify from total cytoplasmic RNA the messenger RNA for the hormone, either by cell-free translation of the messenger RNA or by using a cDNA probe for hybridisation studies. It is also possible to show net synthesis and release of the hormone *in vitro* using tumour cells in culture, or by transplanting the tumour into a nude mouse.

PROPOSED MECHANISMS OF ECTOPIC HORMONE PRODUCTION

The pathogenesis of ectopic hormone production is not well understood, and several hypotheses have been proposed to explain the mechanisms involved (Fig. 19.4). One popular hypothesis is that the capacity of non-endocrine tumours to produce hormones is based on the presence of cells derived from neuroectoderm. This is known as the 'APUD' (amine precursor uptake and decarboxylation) hypothesis, and refers to cells with distinct structural and cytochemical characteristics. During embryo-

genesis, cells from the neuroectoderm are thought to migrate to tissues in the endoderm, giving such tissues the capacity to make hormones. The APUD hypothesis usefully explains the hormone production by certain tumours, but not all. Tumours most commonly believed to be APUD in type include oat cell carcinoma of the lung, islet cell tumours, medullary carcinoma of the thyroid, thymoma and certain carcinoids. These tumours produce insulin, calcitonin, ACTH (and its precursors), ADH, gastrin and glucagon. Furthermore, it is believed that tissues may acquire APUD characteristics without necessarily being ectodermal in origin.

A second hypothesis suggests that the capacity of these tumours to make hormones involves a process of de-repression of tumour DNA. Whilst this hypothesis has certain attractive features, it has been impossible to prove or disprove. More recently, Baylin and Mendelsohn (1980) have suggested a forward moving model in which primitive cells have the capacity to undergo cell division, fetal differentiation, then further cell division followed by adult differentiation. When the cells have fetal characteristics, they may have the capacity to produce hormones such as HCG, placental lactogen, carcinoembryonic antigen and alphafetoprotein. If a cell becomes 'locked into' an earlier state of differentiation and proliferates as part of the tumour, it is possible for this cell line to predominate. Mature epithelium, such as in the bronchus or gastrointestinal tract, contains a variety of epithelial cell types. Usually one or two types predominate, but there are also small numbers of cells with endocrine capabilities.

A hypothesis to adequately explain the pathogenesis of the ectopic humoral syndromes must take into account the association between histological type and the hormone produced. It is also true that the hormones produced are not new proteins, but the same polypeptides produced by normal endocrine tissues or their biosynthetic precursors. The hypothesis must also explain the widespread appearance of hormones in tumours and even in normal cells.

Diagnostic Criteria for Ectopic Humoral Syndromes

endocrine or biochemical disorder in a patient with a non-endocrine neoplasm

remission with therapy

return with recurrence

abnormal levels of hormone or metabolite in blood or urine

arteriovenous difference in hormone concentration

test tumour extracts using bioassay or radioimmunoassay

identify tumour mRNA for ectopic hormone in tumour tissue

in vitro synthesis of ectopic hormone from tumour cells

humoral syndrome reproduced in nude athymic mouse by transplanting human tumour

Fig. 19.3 Table showing the diagnostic criteria for the ectopic humoral syndromes.

Proposed Hypotheses of Ectopic Hormone Production

neuroectodermal origin

de-differentiation or de-repression of tumour cell (backward model)

dysdifferentiation of tumour cell (forward model)

Fig. 19.4 Table of three possible mechanisms of ectopic hormone production. All proposed models must explain (i) the correlation between ectopic hormone and histological cell type, (ii) the chemical nature of the hormone produced and (iii) the widespread occurrence of the hormones.

RELATIONSHIP OF TUMOUR TYPE TO HORMONE PRODUCTION

There are distinct associations between certain tumour types and the hormones they produce (Fig. 19.5); a factor which must be explained in a rational pathogenetic theory. For example, oat cell carcinoma of the lung generally produces ACTH and ADH, epidermoid carcinoma of the lung is associated with humoral hypercalcaemia and adenocarcinoma is linked with HCG production. ACTH is, however, produced by all types of lung tumours, but only in oat cell and carcinoid tumours is it associated with functional Cushing's syndrome. It appears that oat cell and carcinoid tumours are capable of releasing active ACTH, whereas other types of tumour of the lung may release ACTH precursors which are biologically inactive. ACTH, insulin, calcitonin and ADH tend to be produced by tumours which have APUD-like characteristics. Conversely, somatomedin, which may be associated with hypoglycaemia, is produced in mesodermal as well as adrenal tumours.

PATHOGENESIS OF CUSHING'S SYNDROME IN VARIOUS DISORDERS

The normal hypothalamo-pituitary-adrenal axis and the site of abnormality in Cushing's syndrome due to primary central nervous system disease, adrenal disorders and the ectopic ACTH syndrome are shown in Figure 19.6. Corticotrophin-releasing hormone (CRH) is produced by the hypothalamus and stimulates ACTH release from the pituitary gland. ACTH then stimulates the adrenal cortex to secrete cortisol, which subsequently feeds back at both the hypothalamic and pituitary level to regulate the secretion of ACTH. A normal circadian variation exists, with ACTH peaking early in the morning and having its nadir late in the evening. This circadian variation is disrupted in disorders associated with Cushing's syndrome. Classical Cushing's disease, as a cause of Cushing's syndrome, results from the over-production of ACTH from the pituitary and, while many patients have ACTH-producing pituitary microadenomas, some evidence suggests that it is initially a hypothalamic disease. There is absence of normal circadian variation in the secretion of ACTH, and elevated levels of cortisol are necessary to suppress pituitary ACTH production. This ultimately leads to hyperplasia of the adrenal glands and Cushing's syndrome. The reverse situation occurs, however, when an adrenal adenoma develops. There is autonomous production of cortisol which suppresses CRH production and pituitary ACTH production. In the ectopic humoral syndrome, there is autonomous production of ACTH by non-endocrine tumours. This has two effects, namely production of bilateral adrenal hyperplasia and Cushing's syndrome, but also suppression of the pituitary and hypothalamus. The latter is complicated by the fact that CRH may also be produced by such tumours, thus making the results of dexamethasone suppression and metyrapone stimulation tests confusing.

ECTOPIC CUSHING'S SYNDROME

The first ectopic syndrome recognised (and one of the most common clinically) is that resulting from ectopic production of ACTH. This occurs most often in patients with tumours of the lungs (oat cell carcinoma), thymus and pancreatic islets. Of these, ectopic ACTH production resulting from carcinoma of the lung is the most common cause of Cushing's syndrome in man, but the clinical manifestations are often different from those of the typical patient (Fig. 19.7). The clinical presentation tends to be dominated by weight loss, muscle weakness, hyperpigmentation, hypertension, peripheral oedema and hirsutism; however, weight gain, centripetal obesity and the usual Cushingoid striae are uncommon. These manifestations appear to be dominated by mineralocorticoid effects. The differences between typical Cushing's disease and ectopic humoral Cushing's syndrome could result from other factors produced by the tumour, debilitation due to malignant disease or the rapidity of the course.

Patients with the ectopic ACTH syndrome tend to be older, with the majority being above the age of fifty years. They have

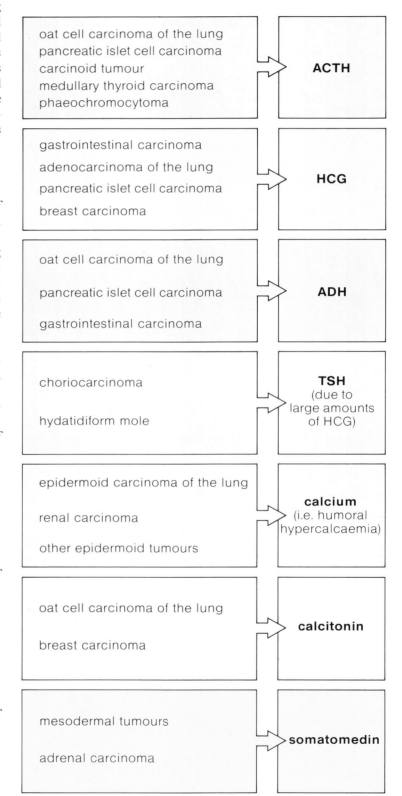

Fig. 19.5 Table indicating the ectopic hormone produced by each tumour type. ACTH is the most common ectopic hormone produced.

extremely high levels of ACTH and correspondingly increased levels of plasma and urinary steroids. Marked hypokalaemic alkalosis and glucose intolerance are often present. These tumours may also produce CRH in addition to ACTH; selective venous catheterisation may often be helpful in differentiating those with ACTH-producing tumours from those patients with hypothalamo-pituitary disease. The hyperpigmentation in patients with ectopic ACTH syndrome results from the melanocyte stimulating activity of ACTH, but also lipotrophin release (this peptide contains the melanocyte-stimulating sequence). If possible, therapy should be directed at the primary tumour. Correction of hypokalaemic alkalosis and hyperglycaemia is important. Blockade of the adrenals with metyrapone (an 11β-hydroxylase inhibitor) and aminoglutethimide (which blocks the conversion of cholesterol to pregnenolone) together with mitotane (op'DDD – an adrenal cytolytic agent) may be useful.

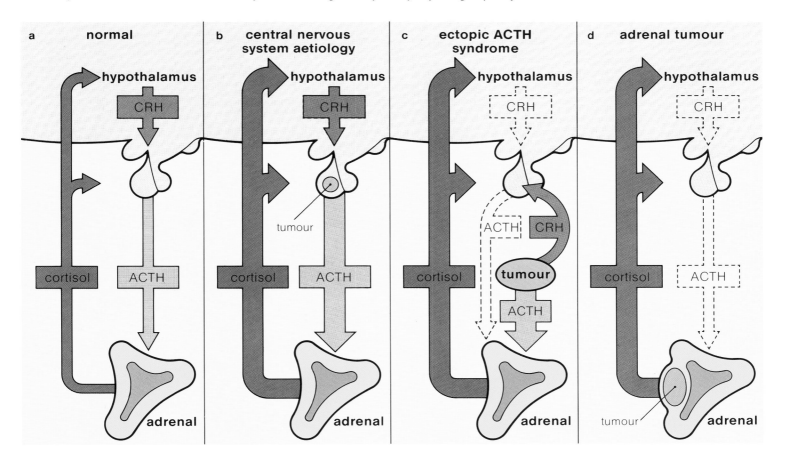

Fig. 19.6   Diagrams illustrating the aetiopathology of Cushing's syndrome. In view (a) the normal feedback mechanism is shown. In pituitary-dependent Cushing's disease (b), caused by a basophil adenoma or hypothalamic abnormality, or both, there is excessive production of ACTH. In view (c), ectopic ACTH production from a tumour leads to raised cortisol production. In view (d) the raised cortisol levels are produced by an adrenal tumour.

Comparison of Clinical Features of Pituitary and Ectopic ACTH Over-Production

characteristics	ectopic	pituitary
age	usually over 50 years	usually under 50 years
sex	predominantly men	predominantly women
anorexia	always	rare
weight loss	usual	rare, often there is weight gain
Cushingoid features	unusual	usual
hypertension	usual	occasional
hyperpigmentation	common	unusual, except post-adrenalectomy
serum potassium	usually low (<3.0mmol/l)	normal or low (usually 3–4 mmol/l)

Fig. 19.7   Table comparing the clinical features of pituitary-dependent Cushing's disease with those of ectopic ACTH-producing tumours.

STRUCTURE AND METABOLISM OF THE ACTH PRECURSOR

The structure of the ACTH precursor is shown in Figure 19.8. There is convincing evidence that ACTH is synthesised from a higher molecular weight precursor known as pro-opiomelanocortin (POMC), which is glycosylated and contains the sequences of ACTH and the β- and γ-lipotrophins. The sequence of β-lipotrophin (89 residues) includes the structure of γ-lipotrophin (1–56), β-endorphin (59–89) and the enkephalins. The data supporting the structure of ACTH and the lipotrophin gene come from two sources. Firstly, radioactive amino acid incorporation into animal and human pituitary cells reveals the presence of higher molecular weight forms of ACTH; the translation product of RNA in cell-free systems yields the precursor. Secondly, the complete structure of the DNA gene has been determined and supports the production of POMC. In addition to data supporting a common precursor, there is also evidence that the metabolism of the precursor may vary in different tissues. For example, it appears that the normal pituitary can process POMC to make ACTH, β-lipotrophin and β-endorphin. This is supported by the fact that serum ACTH as well as lipotrophin and endorphin may be elevated in patients with Addison's disease and Nelson's syndrome. In the *pars intermedia* of animal pituitaries, cleavage occurs at a different position; this yields melanocyte-stimulating hormone (α-MSH) and corticotrophin-like intermediate peptide (CLIP). Differential metabolism is possible depending upon the tissue in which the precursor is present, and presumably also the presence of different enzymes and the position of the secretory granules where the precursor is metabolised. Although ACTH production by neoplasms is widespread, the precursor form of ACTH is usually released into the circulation, and only in tumours which are definitely associated with Cushing's syndrome (e.g. oat cell carcinoma of the lung) is mature ACTH produced.

APUD-TYPE TUMOURS

The neurosecretory-type granules observed in cells of the APUD tumour type are electron-dense granules 10–250nm in diameter (Figs. 19.9 and 19.10). Certain tumours of the lung (oat cell carcinoma and carcinoids), thymic, pancreatic islet, adrenal medulla and argentaffin cells (carcinoid), and also medullary carcinomas, seem to fit this category. These cells have special staining characteristics which include: (i) masked metachromasia and argyrophilia, (ii) the presence of α-glycerol phosphate dehydrogenase and other enzymes, (iii) formaldehyde-induced fluorescence and (iv) the ability to carry out amine precursor uptake and decarboxylation. Immunocytochemical techniques are also successful in localising hormones in these tumours. Suspected 'APUDomas' should be tested for a variety of hormones, even when no clinical symptoms are present, since it is quite common to have multiple hormone production from these tumours. The hormones which tend to be produced are ACTH, lipotrophin, insulin, calcitonin, ADH, gastrin, glucagon, secretin, catecholamines, various biogenic amines (including serotonin and histamine), vasoactive intestinal peptide (VIP), pancreatic polypeptide, prostaglandins and growth hormone releasing hormone (GHRH).

DEVELOPMENT OF ACROMEGALY FROM NON-PITUITARY TUMOURS

In recent years, there has been increasing evidence for the association of acromegaly with non-pituitary tumours that produce GHRH and stimulate the normal pituitary gland to release growth hormone (GH), thereby causing acromegaly (Fig. 19.11). These associations have been found primarily with bronchial carcinoid and pancreatic islet cell tumours associated with clinical acromegaly, pituitary enlargement and elevated GH. In many cases, the tumours have been relatively silent in the face of clinical acromegaly. There are no distinguishing features between acromegaly, which is primarily of pituitary or hypothalamic origin, and the condition in which a non-pituitary tumour stimulates the pituitary through the production of GHRH. Isolation of this factor from such tumours and its structural determination was made by Thorner, Vale and Guillemin (1983) and has led to identification of normal GHRH, a hypothalamic hormone. This growth hormone stimulator, which is forty-four amino acids long, may prove to be a pharmacologically useful agent. Assays for its measurement in plasma have been developed. In every patient with acromegaly, the possibility of an extrapituitary tumour should be considered; therefore, examination of the lung by radiography, together with examination of the pancreas by ultrasound or computerised tomography (CT), is a reasonable clinical approach.

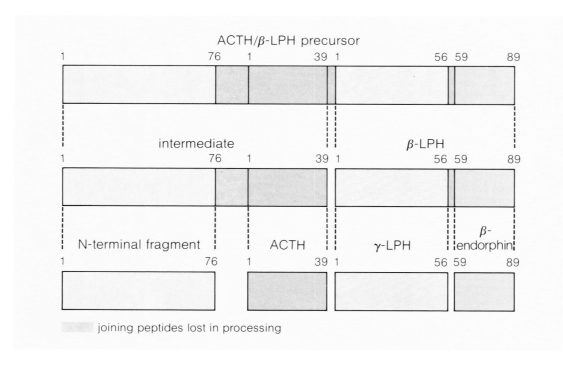

Fig. 19.8 Diagram illustrating the structure and metabolism of the ACTH precursor, pro-opiomelanocortin (POMC). This is cleaved to yield several fragments including pro-γ-MSH, ACTH, γ-LPH and β-endorphin.

ACTH/β-LPH precursor

intermediate β-LPH

N-terminal fragment   ACTH γ-LPH β-endorphin

joining peptides lost in processing

THE PATHOGENESIS OF HYPERCALCAEMIA IN MALIGNANT DISEASE

Hypercalcaemia is very commonly associated with malignant disease. The pathogenesis of hypercalcaemia in these patients is usually based on one of two mechanisms (Fig. 19.12). Firstly, there is metastatic bone disease (and presumably the physical presence of tumour cells) which accounts for excess mobilisation of calcium from the skeleton. Tumours commonly associated with bony metastases and hypercalcaemia include those of the lung, breast and kidney. Prostate carcinoma often metastasises to bone, but it causes osteoblastic rather than osteolytic metastases. In those patients who have metastatic disease to bone without a circulating humoral factor, it is also conceivable that tumour cells may produce local mediators which resorb bone. Candidates for such mediators include prostaglandins of the PGE_2 type as well as osteoclast activating factor (OAF) and others.

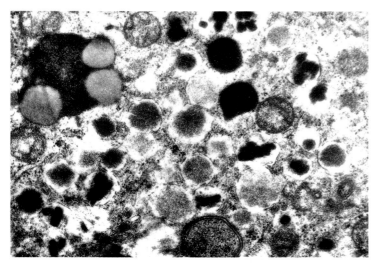

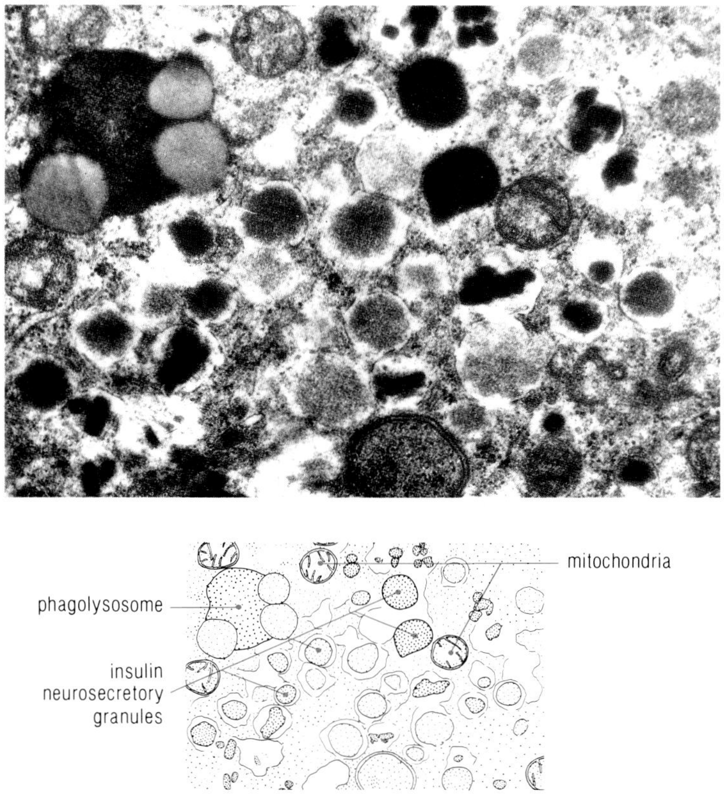

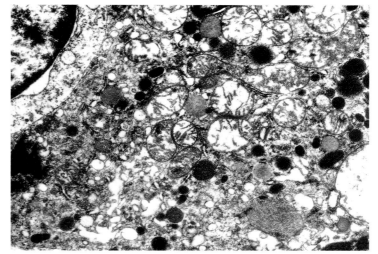

Fig. 19.9 Electron micrograph showing the ultrastructure of an islet cell tumour of the pancreas. This tumour is associated with excessive insulin secretion. The numerous neurosecretory granules are characteristic of a neuroendocrine tumour.

Fig. 19.10 Electron micrograph showing the ultrastructure of an oat cell carcinoma of the lung associated with Cushing's syndrome. The secretory granules containing ACTH are less frequent than in the islet cell tumour; nevertheless they are also characteristic of neuroendocrine cells.

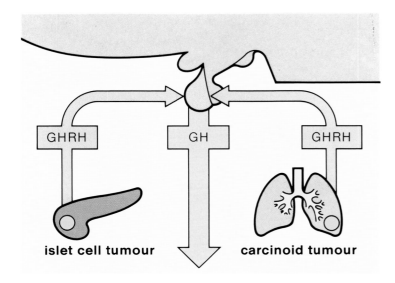

Fig. 19.11 Diagram indicating the neoplasms associated with ectopic growth hormone releasing hormone (GHRH) production. Both carcinoid tumours of the lung and islet cell tumours of the pancreas may produce GHRH; this subsequently leads to overproduction of growth hormone and clinical acromegaly.

Aetiopathology of the Hypercalcaemia of Malignancy

metastatic disease to bone
(with or without local mediators)

humoral factor production

non-PTH cyclic AMP-stimulating factor that binds to the PTH receptor

parathyroid hormone (PTH)

prostaglandin (PGE_2 series)

osteoclast activating factor (OAF)

Fig. 19.12 Table of the pathological mechanisms involved in the hypercalcaemia of malignancy. Hypercalcaemia of malignancy may be secondary to metastatic bone involvement (directly or via local mediators) or secondary to the production of humoral factors (non-metastatic).

Secondly, a different mechanism exists in those patients who have non-endocrine tumours, who may not have metastatic disease but whose hypercalcaemia is associated with the presence of the tumour because of humoral factor production. In these patients, removal of the tumour often results in correction of the hypercalcaemia. For many years there has been active investigation of the pathogenesis of this disorder, and parathyroid hormone (PTH) has been invoked as the most obvious cause. At present, there are a few reports indicating that PTH itself, or something behaving immunologically like it, is present in some non-endocrine tumours (particularly squamous cell carcinoma of the lung and renal cell carcinoma). Those tumours that produce PTH itself probably account for a very small number in the total spectrum of patients with humoral hypercalcaemia of malignancy. In another group of patients, it appears that production of prostaglandins may be a possible pathogenetic factor. Animal sarcoma studies suggest that PGE_2 may be the active prostaglandin involved. In a few instances, hypercalcaemia has been correctable with indomethacin and, in some patients, large amounts of PGE_2 metabolites have been identified in the urine. Even in those patients in whom prostaglandin levels have been elevated, it is not clear whether there is some additional circulating factor responsible. A precise cause and effect relationship for PGE_2 in humoral hypercalcaemia has not been completely established. A third factor which has been identified in some patients as a pathogenetic factor in lymphoma and myeloma is OAF, a peptide found in the supernatant of lymphocyte or plasma cell cultures which can recruit osteoclasts and cause bone resorption. Recently, primary emphasis has been on a non-parathyroid peptide which appears to behave like PTH. This peptide, which is higher in molecular weight than PTH, stimulates renal adenylate cyclase and causes an increase in cyclic AMP. Immunologically, it does not resemble PTH and appears to be a peptide which has hitherto been unrecognised; however, it does bind to the PTH receptor in bone and kidney. A vigorous search is currently underway in several laboratories to identify this peptide.

ECTOPIC HUMORAL SYNDROMES ASSOCIATED WITH GONADOTROPHIN PRODUCTION

Ectopic production of HCG by tumours, particularly from the gastrointestinal tract, is extremely common. Conversely, clinical syndromes related to gonadotrophin production are uncommon. In males with choriocarcinoma and, less frequently, other testicular and lung tumours, there may be gynaecomastia with raised oestrogen production. The increased levels of oestrogen found in these patients may be the result of HCG-mediated secretion of oestradiol by the testis, although oestrogen can also be formed by aromatisation of circulating androgens by the tumour. In young boys, hepatoblastoma has been shown to be associated with precocious puberty due to HCG production. There are usually no symptoms in women whose tumours produce gonadotrophins.

The pituitary glycoprotein hormones, which include follicle stimulating hormone (FSH), luteinizing hormone (LH) and thyroid stimulating hormone (TSH or thyrotrophin), as well as the placental hormone HCG, consist of two non-covalently linked subunits (Fig. 19.13). The alpha subunits of the pituitary hormones are similar, whilst the beta subunits confer specific biological activity. Sensitive radioimmunoassays and radioreceptor assays have been developed for both the combined subunits as well as specific beta subunits. It has been found that isolated production of subunits, especially beta subunits, may be useful as tumour markers; for example, in patients with islet cell carcinoma of the pancreas, beta subunits in the circulation are suggestive of malignancy. In some males with choriocarcinoma or trophoblastic tumours of the testis, and in women with choriocarcinoma or hydatidiform mole, clinical hyperthyroidism has been found. Careful studies of tumour extracts and plasma have indicated that the hormone responsible is probably not TSH but HCG, which is present in extremely large amounts. The small amount of thyrotrophic activity present in the beta subunit of HCG, when it is present in such high concentrations, accounts for the hyperthyroid state.

PANCREATIC TUMOURS

There is a variety of clinical disorders associated with non-beta islet cell tumours, and, also occasionally with other tumours that are known as 'pancreatic cholera' (Fig. 19.14). This syndrome classically includes vigorous watery diarrhoea, hypokalaemia and hypochlorhydria. It may be produced by a variety of substances which include VIP, prostaglandins, secretin, glucagon, gastrin, calcitonin, gastric inhibitory polypeptide (GIP) and pancreatic polypeptide. In addition to stimulating motility of the gut and producing diarrhoea, these substances inhibit gastric acid secretion, thus producing hypochlorhydria. The diagnosis of pancreatic tumours has been facilitated by the development of new techniques such as ultrasound and CT scanning. More recently, a disorder has been identified in which there is excessive production of somatostatin which may inhibit gastric acid production, duodenal

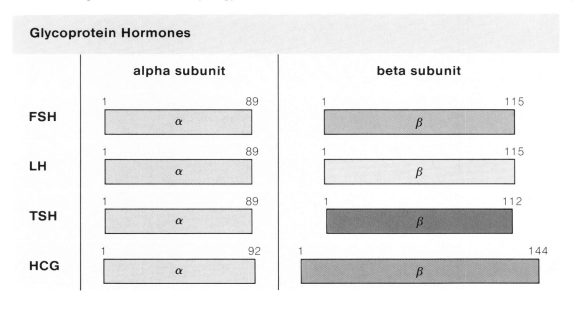

Glycoprotein Hormones

	alpha subunit	beta subunit
FSH	α (1–89)	β (1–115)
LH	α (1–89)	β (1–115)
TSH	α (1–89)	β (1–112)
HCG	α (1–92)	β (1–144)

Fig. 19.13 Diagrammatic representation of the structure of the glycoprotein hormones. These hormones all share a common α-chain (although HCG has an extra three amino acids), and hormone specificity is achieved as a result of differing β-subunit structures. The β-subunit of HCG is similar to that of TSH in that it has a small amount of TSH-like activity.

motility and gall bladder contraction. This leads to gall-stones, inhibition of endocrine pancreatic secretion and the release of gastrin, secretin, insulin and glucagon. The clinical manifestations of a 'somatostatinoma' include abdominal pain, diarrhoea, weight loss, hyperglycaemia and gall bladder disease. A rare disorder in which there is a glucagon-producing tumour is associated with hyperglycaemia as well as a reversible bullous skin eruption called migratory epidermal necrolysis. The aetiology of the eruption is uncertain.

ECTOPIC PRODUCTION OF ANTIDIURETIC HORMONE

There are several hyponatraemic syndromes associated with malignancy; in some instances, ADH has either been extracted from the tumours or the tumours have been shown to produce it *in vitro*. Production of ADH by tumours (Fig. 19.15) may be associated with the clinical disorder SIADH ('syndrome of inappropriate ADH secretion') and causes hyponatraemia. In addition, cerebral metastases, mediastinal tumours or pulmonary infection, renal tubular defects, central nervous system infection, hypothyroidism, cerebrovascular disease, smoking, pain, trauma, emotional stress and the use of drugs (e.g. chlorpropamide and vincristine) may also be associated with SIADH. Tumours associated with ADH production are primarily the oat cell tumour of the lung as well as tumours of the pancreas and upper gastrointestinal tract. Clinical manifestations, which appear in the presence of excess water intake, may include nausea and vomiting, headaches, diplopia, anorexia, confusion and coma. Modern therapy of the syndrome includes the restriction of fluid and, in some cases, the administration of demeclocycline or lithium carbonate. In patients with life-threatening hyponatraemia, intravenous saline may be necessary.

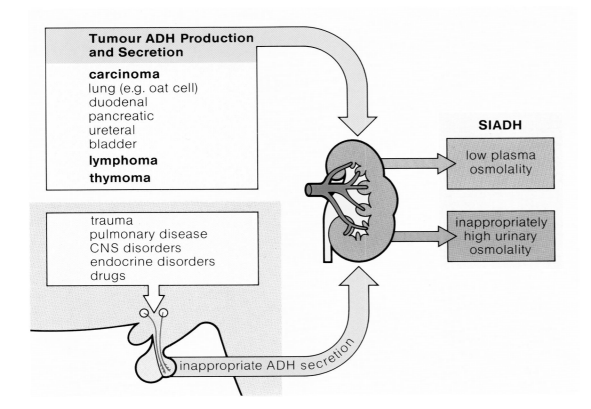

vasoactive intestinal peptide production (VIPoma or Werner-Morrison syndrome)
such 'pancreatic cholera' may also be associated with production of pancreatic polypeptide (in 70% of cases),prostaglandins and calcitonin

glucagon production (glucagonoma)
rash, diarrhoea, anaemia, glucose-intolerance

islet cell tumour

insulin production (insulinoma)
hypoglycaemia

somatostatin production (somatostatinoma)
abdominal pain, diarrhoea, weight loss, hyperglycaemia and gall bladder disease

gastrin production (gastrinoma or Zollinger-Ellison syndrome)
hyperacidity and ulcers, diarrhoea

Fig. 19.14 The clinical effects of islet cell tumours. These tumours can secrete glucagon, insulin, gastrin, somatostatin and vasoactive intestinal peptide. The resultant clinical effects are dependent upon which ectopic hormone is produced.

Tumour ADH Production and Secretion

carcinoma
lung (e.g. oat cell)
duodenal
pancreatic
ureteral
bladder
lymphoma
thymoma

trauma
pulmonary disease
CNS disorders
endocrine disorders
drugs

inappropriate ADH secretion

SIADH

low plasma osmolality

inappropriately high urinary osmolality

Fig. 19.15 Diagram of the factors leading to the syndrome of inappropriate ADH secretion (SIADH). SIADH may be caused by ectopic ADH secretion by a tumour, particularly oat cell carcinoma of the lung. However, brain disorders (e.g. metastases, aneurysms), pulmonary diseases and drugs are also common causes.

POLYPEPTIDE HORMONE SYNTHESIS AND SECRETION

A full understanding of the nature of polypeptide hormone synthesis and release by ectopic tumours requires a detailed understanding of the normal processes of hormone biosynthesis, packaging and secretion from normal endocrine tissues and also the abnormalities that may occur in the patients with malignant disease. The process of transcription and translation in hormone synthesis is shown in Figure 19.16. The initial RNA transcript made from DNA includes areas which are present in the final messenger RNA molecule (exons) as well as areas that are not (introns). Those intervening RNA sequences, or introns, that are removed, often interrupt the sequence of bases coding for the polypeptide being synthesised. The processing of precursor mRNA to mRNA requires the removal of one or more introns and the addition of a polyadenylate tail (normally 50–100 adenosine residues long).

The initial translation product synthesised on the ribosomes includes the peptide coding for the hormone, as well as a 'leader' or 'signal' sequence of between fifteen and twenty-five (or possibly more) amino acids preceding the hormone sequence. This region of the peptide (which is usually hydrophobic) permits the newly synthesised peptide to be transported through the membranes of the endoplasmic reticulum into the subcellular transport system. The 'leader' sequence is cleaved and removed at its junction with the hormone or prohormone as the transport occurs, and the pre-hormone either never appears in the Golgi region or is released from the cell. In several hormones (e.g. insulin, ACTH and PTH), there is an intermediate precursor peptide (e.g. proinsulin, POMC or proPTH). This intermediate peptide is found in the endoplasmic reticulum and may appear in the Golgi region for packaging. The final processing of prohormone to product often takes place in the secretory granule and involves the presence of trypsin-like enzymes which cleave these precursors – usually at lysine or arginine residues.

In addition, those hormones which have carbohydrate are generally glycosylated as the hormone or prohormone is transported from the site of synthesis. In some cases, the precursor (e.g. proinsulin) may be released into the circulation, whilst in others (e.g. proPTH) it is not.

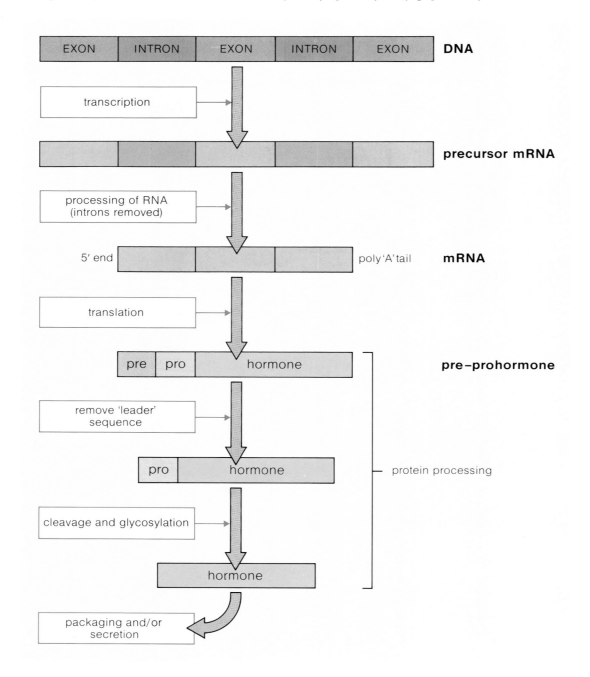

Fig. 19.16 Diagram illustrating the sequence of events in polypeptide hormone synthesis and secretion.

20 Radiology of Endocrine Disease

Janet E Dacie, FRCP, DMRD, FRCR
F Elizabeth White, MRCP, DMRD, FRCR

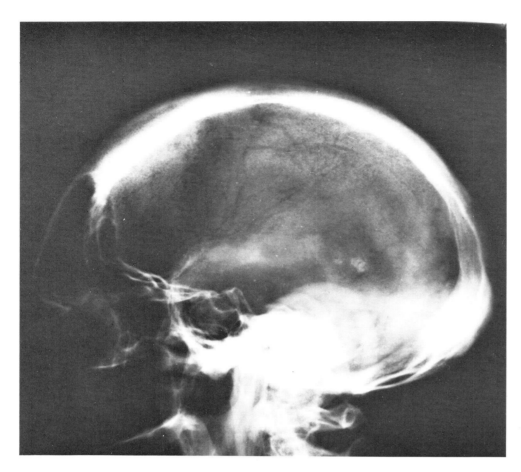

Fig. 20.1 Acromegaly: lateral skull film showing vault changes and a 'ballooned' pituitary fossa. The main role of radiology in the assessment of acromegaly is to confirm the presence of a pituitary tumour and to provide information necessary for treatment and follow-up (see Chapter 21 for a discussion of the radiological assessment of pituitary tumours). Certain characteristic systemic changes do, however, occur in acromegaly and this lateral skull film demonstrates typical diffuse hyperostosis of the calvarium and abnormally large frontal sinuses. A double floor to the pituitary fossa can be seen: one side is of normal contour and the other is grossly expanded ('ballooned'): see Fig. 20.3 for details.

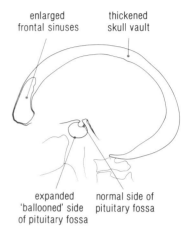

enlarged frontal sinuses   thickened skull vault

expanded 'ballooned' side of pituitary fossa   normal side of pituitary fossa

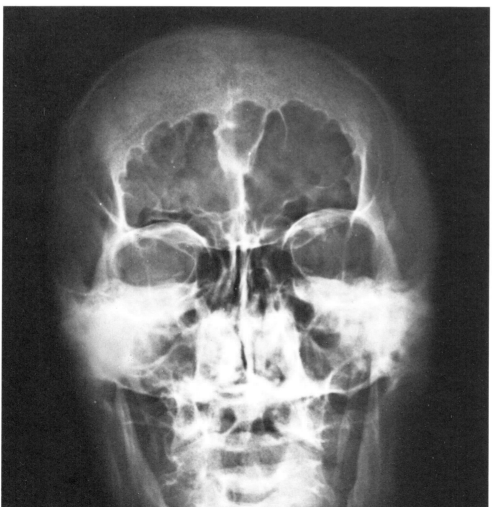

Fig. 20.2 Acromegaly: postero-anterior (PA) skull film showing enlarged frontal sinuses. This PA skull film of the same patient as in Fig. 20.1 demonstrates the marked enlargement of the frontal sinuses. The floor of the pituitary fossa is seen to be grossly enlarged on the right side by a large but asymmetric pituitary tumour.

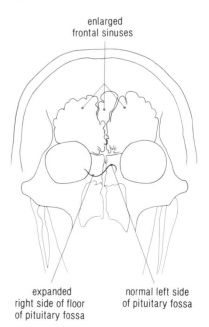

enlarged frontal sinuses

expanded right side of floor of pituitary fossa   normal left side of pituitary fossa

20.2

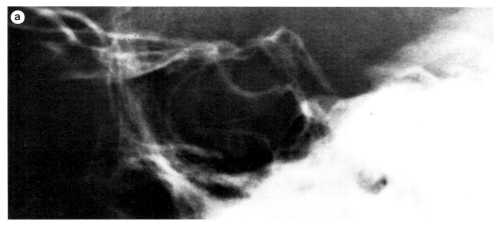

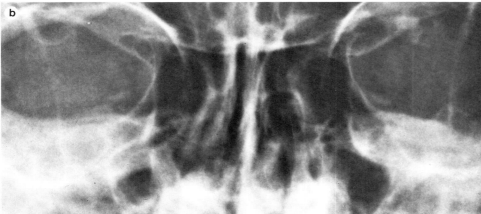

Fig. 20.3 Acromegaly: coned views of 'ballooned' pituitary fossa.
These coned views of the pituitary fossa are of the same patient as in Figs. 20.1 and 20.2 and demonstrate more clearly the gross asymmetric expansion of the right side of the floor of the pituitary fossa.

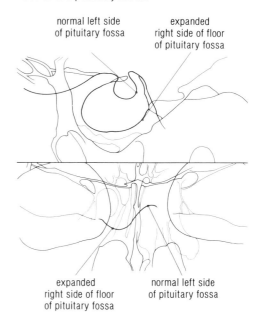

normal left side of pituitary fossa

expanded right side of floor of pituitary fossa

expanded right side of floor of pituitary fossa

normal left side of pituitary fossa

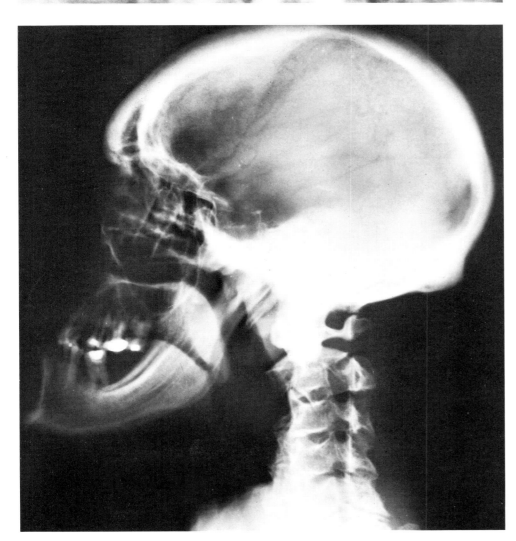

Fig. 20.4 Acromegaly: prognathic jaw.
The lateral skull film of another patient shows characteristic prognathism with increase in the normal angle of the mandible. The pituitary fossa is grossly enlarged and the skull vault is markedly thickened, particularly anteriorly, although in this patient the frontal sinuses are not enlarged.

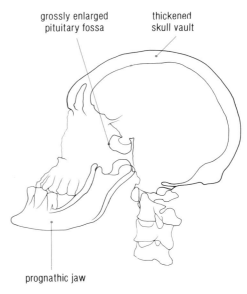

grossly enlarged pituitary fossa

thickened skull vault

prognathic jaw

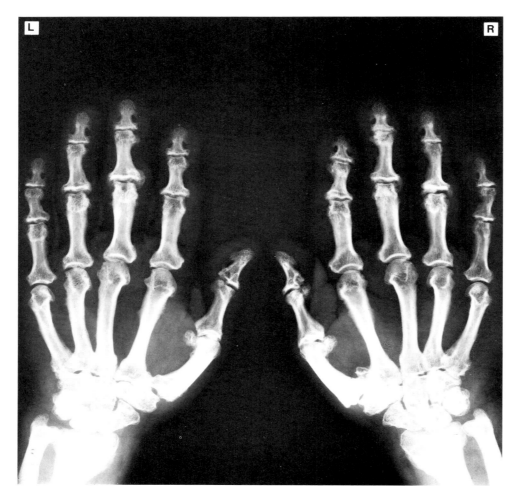

Fig. 20.5 Acromegaly: hands. In acromegaly the hands are large and the classical radiological features include generalised soft tissue thickening, widening of the joint spaces due to hypertrophy of the articular cartilages, prominent muscle insertions particularly along the metacarpal shafts, tufting of the tips of the terminal phalanges and prominent osteophyte formation. In addition, in this patient, degenerative cysts are present in some of the carpal bones, particularly in the right carpus.

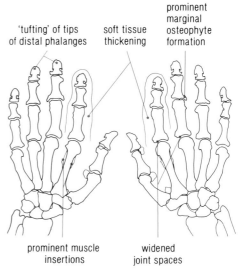

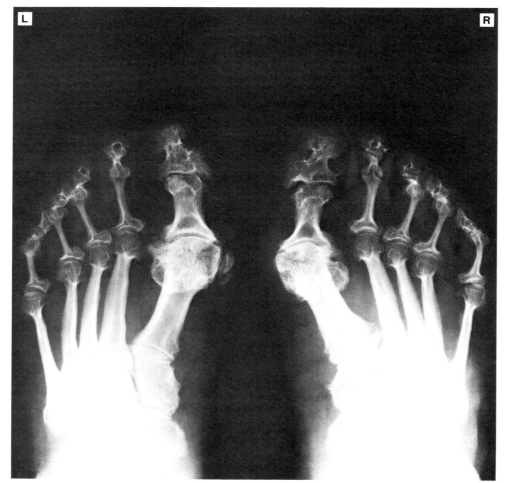

Fig. 20.6 Acromegaly: feet. The radiological changes in the hands in acromegaly are also seen in the feet but, in addition to new bone formation, bone resorption occurs giving rise to typically thinned metatarsals. Thinning of the shafts of the phalanges may also occur, as in this patient.

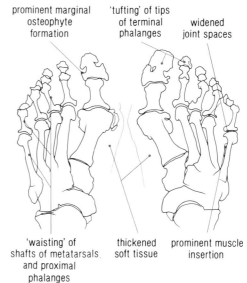

20.4

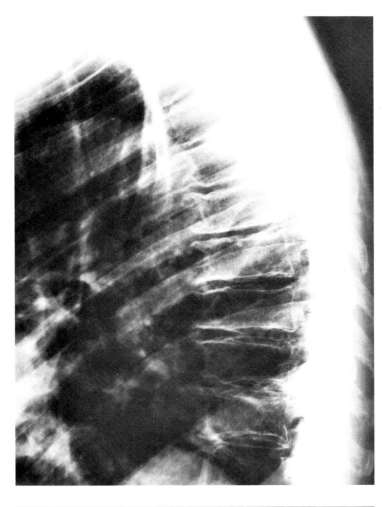

Fig. 20.7 Acromegaly: lateral dorsal spine. In acromegaly new bone formation may occur around the vertebral bodies. This lateral view of the dorsal spine shows such changes at the anterior margins of the vertebrae. The anterior edge of the intervertebral discs can be clearly identified and the vertebral bodies are increased in their anteroposterior diameter. The new bone formation is usually more marked in the dorsal than in the lumbar spine.

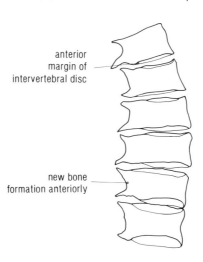

anterior margin of intervertebral disc

new bone formation anteriorly

Fig. 20.8 Acromegaly: lateral lumbar spine. In addition to new bone formation anteriorly this lateral view of the lumbar spine shows prominent marginal osteophyte formation and characteristic scalloping of the posterior margins of the vertebral bodies. Although such scalloping may be seen in the dorsal spine, the lumbar spine is most commonly affected.

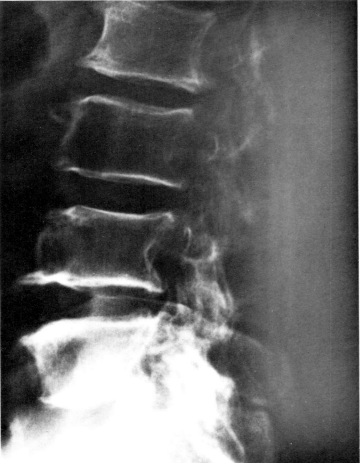

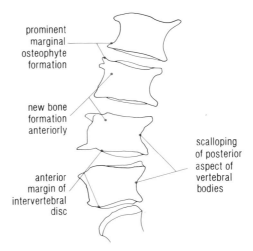

prominent marginal osteophyte formation

new bone formation anteriorly

anterior margin of intervertebral disc

scalloping of posterior aspect of vertebral bodies

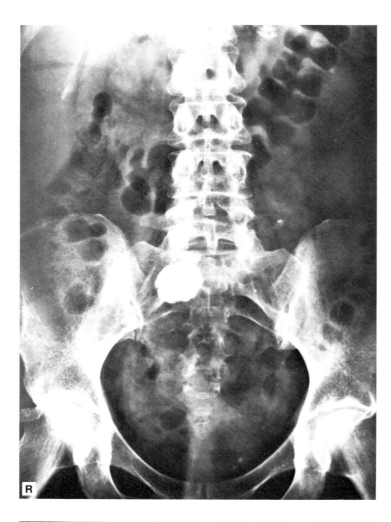

Fig. 20.9 Addison's disease: calcified adrenal glands. This anteroposterior (AP) plain abdominal film demonstrates calcified adrenal glands, seen in some patients with Addison's disease. An identical appearance, however, may be found incidentally in patients without evidence of adrenal disease (the so–called 'idiopathic' calcification of the adrenals).

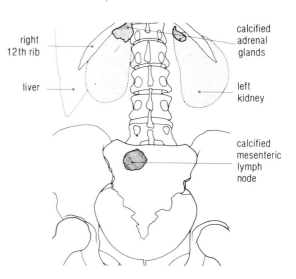

Fig. 20.10 Addison's disease: position of the kidneys demonstrated by intravenous urography. The relationship of the calcified adrenal glands to the upper pole of the kidneys can be better appreciated on intravenous urography. This full length abdominal film was obtained twenty minutes after the injection of intravenous contrast medium (same patient as in Fig. 20.9).

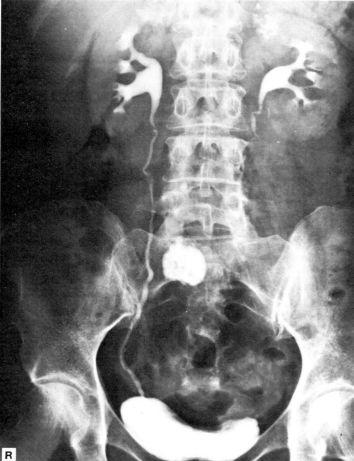

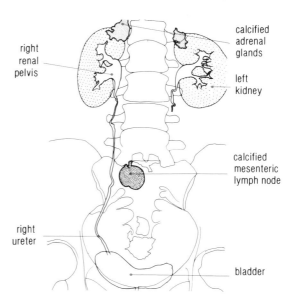

Fig. 20.11 Conn's syndrome: right adrenal adenoma demonstrated by computed tomography (CT) and a normal right adrenal for comparison. Conn's syndrome is caused by either adrenal hyperplasia or an adrenal tumour, the majority of which are small adenomas. The film on the left shows a 1.5 cm tumour in the right adrenal lying between the inferior vena cava (IVC) and the upper pole of the right kidney. Intravenous contrast has been given to enhance the kidney and IVC and to delineate the tumour more clearly. The scan on the right shows a normal right adrenal for comparison. The short adrenal body is situated immediately posterior to the IVC. It divides into two parallel limbs which lie between the liver and right crus of the diaphragm. Venous sampling to measure aldosterone levels may be required to confirm the CT findings and may detect tumours too small to be visualised with CT. Depending upon the machine used for CT scanning, lesions larger than 0.3 – 0.6 cm can usually be detected. Significantly elevated aldosterone levels from both adrenals usually indicate bilateral hyperplasia.

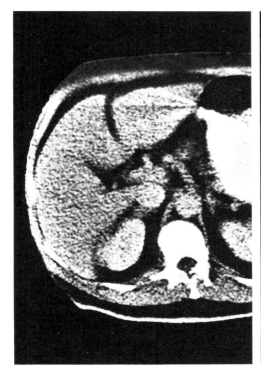
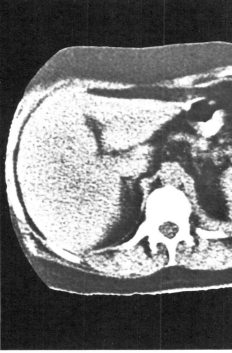
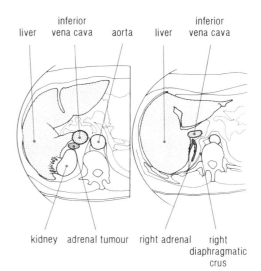

Fig. 20.12 Conn's adenoma in the left adrenal gland: demonstration by venography (with normal venogram for comparison). The film on the left shows the typical venographic appearance of a Conn's adenoma. The catheter tip is in the left adrenal vein and contrast medium has filled veins stretched around a 1 cm tumour in the superior pole of the adrenal gland. This appearance should be compared with the normal venogram shown on the right. Blood for aldosterone estimation should be taken from the adrenal vein prior to venography because of the risk of extravasation of contrast medium during that procedure. Even careful venography carries a small risk of adrenal infarction which could result in adrenal insufficiency if both adrenal glands are compromised.

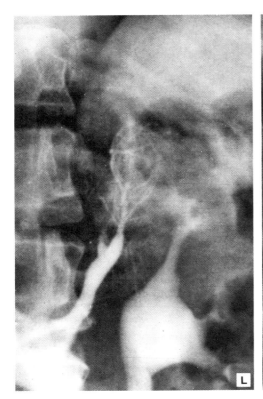
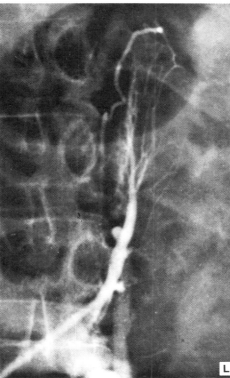
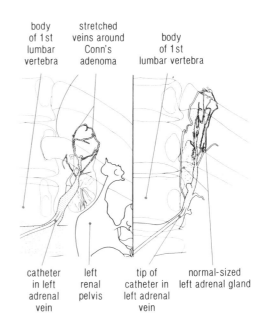

20.7

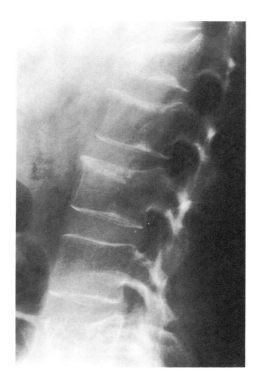 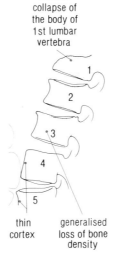

marked
collapse of
the body of
1st lumbar
vertebra

thin
cortex

generalised
loss of bone
density

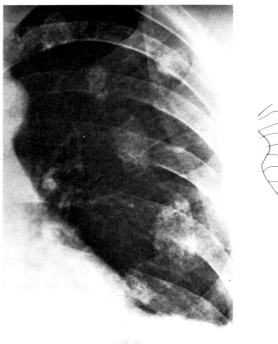

rib fractures

excessive
callus formation

Fig. 20.13 Cushing's syndrome: osteoporosis and vertebral fractures. Cushing's syndrome, when severe, results in generalised osteoporosis and this lateral film of the lumbar spine shows the typical appearance. The bone density is reduced and the cortical margins of the bones are thin. There is marked collapse of the body of the first lumbar vertebra, with marginal condensation of the superior borders of the bodies of the second and third. In the dorsal spine multiple vertebral fractures may lead to a pronounced kyphosis. It should be noted that the radiological appearances of osteoporosis affecting the spine are similar whatever the cause.

Fig. 20.14 Cushing's syndrome: rib fractures. Spontaneous asymptomatic rib fractures are characteristic of Cushing's syndrome and this coned view shows the typical appearance. Multiple rib fractures are surrounded by excessive callus formation. In some patients, in addition to obvious rib fractures, characteristic widening of the anterior ends of the ribs resulting from numerous stress infractions may be seen.

Fig. 20.15 Cushing's syndrome: increased fat deposition demonstrated by chest radiography. Increased fat deposition is characteristic of Cushing's syndrome. This PA chest film shows generalised increase in the soft tissues and poor definition of a slightly enlarged cardiac silhouette. There is also generalised loss of bone density.

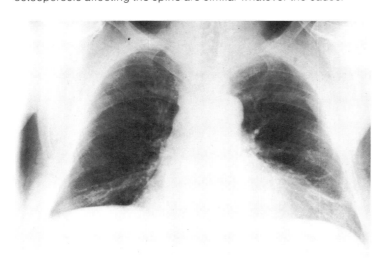

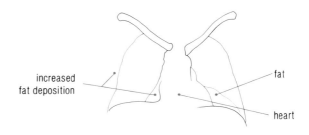

increased
fat deposition

fat

heart

Fig. 20.16 Cushing's syndrome: increased fat deposition demonstrated by CT. The CT scan of the same patient as in Fig. 20.15 shows that the apparent cardiomegaly is due to fat deposition around the heart. There is also fat deposited behind the diaphragmatic crurae.

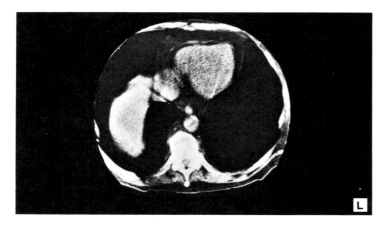

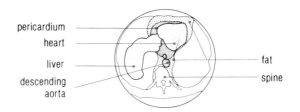

pericardium

heart

liver

descending
aorta

fat

spine

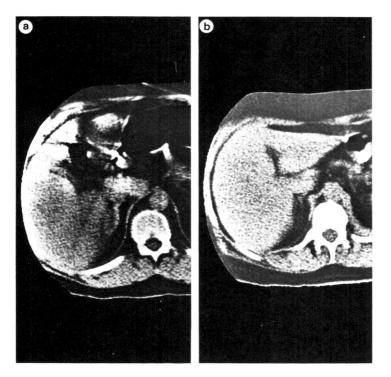

Fig. 20.17 Cushing's syndrome: hypertrophy of the right adrenal demonstrated by CT (with a normal for comparison). Most cases of Cushing's syndrome are caused by increased ACTH production by the pituitary gland; the remainder are due either to an ectopic ACTH-producing tumour or to a primary adrenal tumour (adrenoma or carcinoma). Increased ACTH levels result in adrenal hyperplasia with accompanying hypertrophy. Small changes in size cannot be detected by CT and the adrenals may therefore appear normal. More marked hypertrophy can be shown as in the left picture which shows a hypertrophied right adrenal, the gland being thickened with convex margins, although the normal configuration is retained. A normal right adrenal is shown in the right picture for comparison.

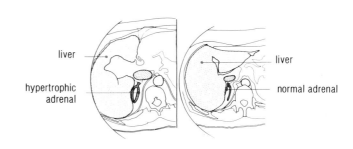

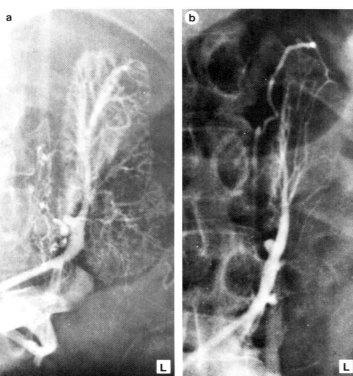

Fig. 20.18 Cushing's syndrome: hypertrophied left adrenal gland demonstrated by venography (with normal venogram for comparison). The left picture shows the venographic appearances of a hypertrophied adrenal gland. The tip of the catheter is in the left adrenal vein and contrast medium has filled small veins within the enlarged gland. A segment of the left renal vein has been partially outlined. The appearances should be compared with those of a normal-sized left adrenal (right picture).

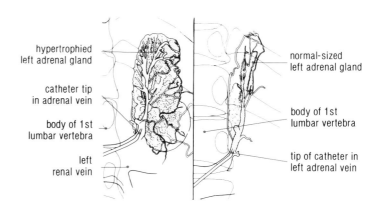

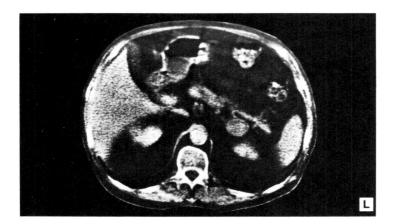

Fig. 20.19 Cushing's syndrome: left adrenal adenoma demonstrated by CT. Adrenal adenomas causing Cushing's syndrome are usually 2-5 cm in size. They are readily detected by CT because of the contrast provided by the abundant retroperitoneal fat which is present in most patients. This scan shows a 3.5 cm rounded mass in the left adrenal clearly outlined by the surrounding fat. It lies between the splenic vein and the upper pole of the left kidney. By courtesy of the British Medical Journal.

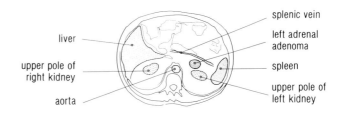

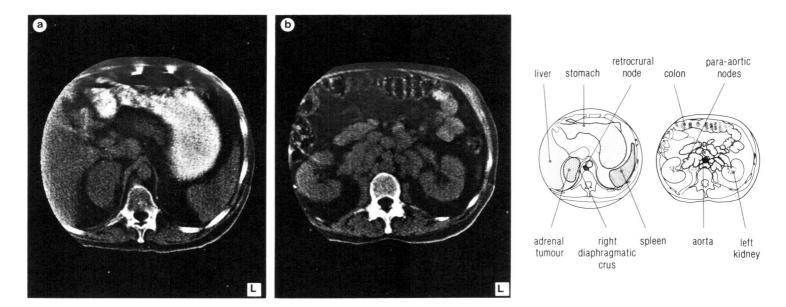

Fig. 20.20 Cushing's syndrome: right adrenal carcinoma with lymph node involvement demonstrated by CT. Adrenal carcinomas are usually 5 cm or more in size, irregular in shape and may contain areas of calcification. The first picture (a) shows a large, irregular right adrenal mass infiltrating the crus of the diaphragm. The second picture (b) is a scan at the level of the renal hilum, showing marked enlargement of the para-aortic nodes consistent with spread from a malignant tumour.

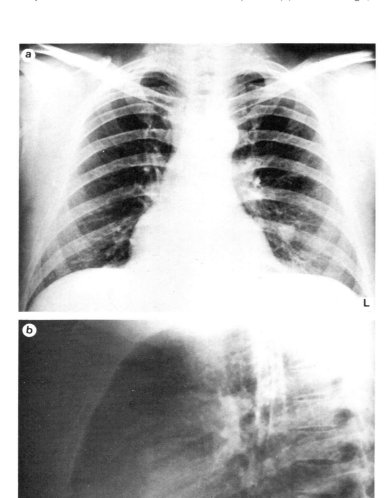

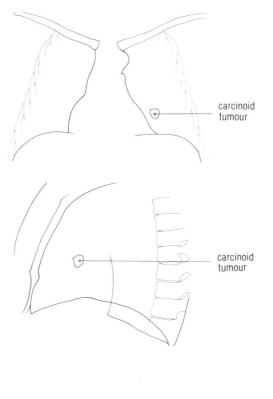

Fig. 20.21 Cushing's syndrome: ectopic ACTH production by a carcinoid tumour of the lung. Cushing's syndrome sometimes results from ectopic ACTH production by tumours, particularly of the lung, thymus or pancreas. Such tumours may be very difficult to locate. Although a few may be detected by conventional radiographic techniques, others require CT scanning or venous sampling for their identification, and some are never found. The PA chest film (a) shows a small mass in the left lower zone. There is some generalised loss of bone density and the patient appears fat. On the lateral view (b) the mass is shown to lie in the lingular segment of the left upper lobe. The patient had Cushing's syndrome secondary to ectopic ACTH production by a benign bronchial carcinoid tumour of the lung.

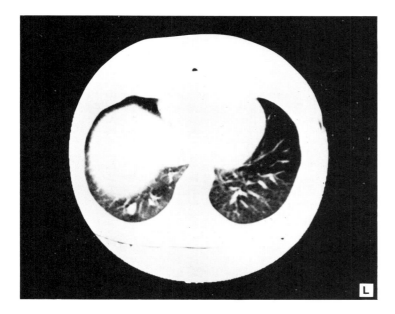

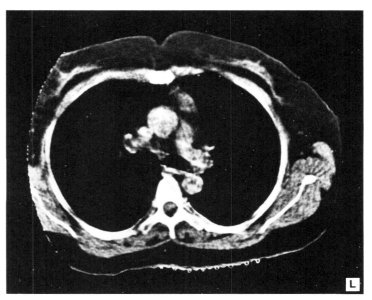

Fig. 20.22 Cushing's syndrome: ACTH-secreting carcinoid tumour of the lung demonstrated by CT. The 7 mm nodule in the right costophrenic recess represents a small malignant carcinoid tumour secreting ACTH. It could not be seen on either chest radiography or conventional tomography. Removal of the tumour cured the patient. By courtesy of the British Medical Journal.

Fig. 20.23 Cushing's syndrome: thymic ACTH-secreting carcinoid tumour demonstrated by CT. Ectopic ACTH can be produced by carcinoid tumours of the thymus. This scan shows a 3 cm ACTH-producing tumour lying just in front of the pulmonary trunk. CT is more sensitive than chest radiography or conventional tomography in detecting abnormalities of the anterior mediastinum. These tumours often enhance after intravenous contrast medium.

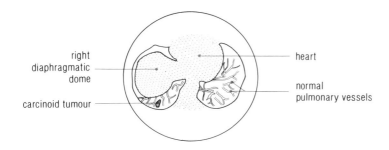

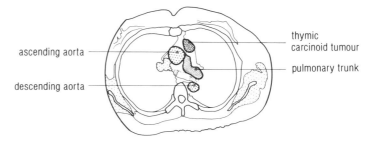

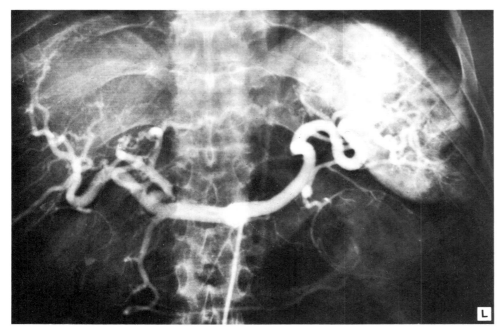

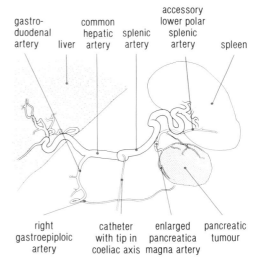

Fig. 20.24 Cushing's syndrome: ectopic ACTH production by an islet cell tumour of the pancreas demonstrated by angiography. This picture shows the arterial phase of a coeliac axis arteriogram. The procedure was carried out to define the blood supply of a pancreatic tumour which had been previously demonstrated by CT. The pancreatica magna artery is enlarged and its branches are stretched over the surface of a large pancreatic tumour. The splenic vein was shown to be patent on later films. At operation a large tumour of the pancreas was removed. Histological examination showed an islet cell tumour which was thought to be malignant. The tumour contained ACTH and the patient was cured of his Cushing's syndrome upon its removal.

20.11

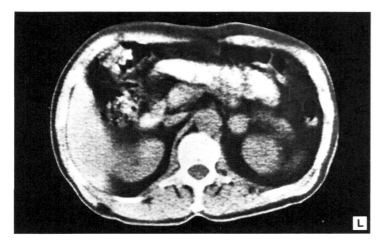

Fig. 20.25 Adrenal phaeochromocytoma: left adrenal tumour demonstrated by CT. Most adrenal phaeochromocytomas can be detected by CT as they are usually 3 cm or more in size. This picture shows a 3 cm homogeneous mass in the left adrenal lying anterior to the upper pole of the left kidney. Larger tumours may contain areas of low density due to central necrosis.

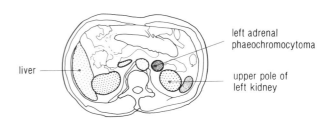

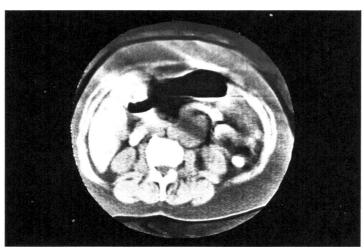

Fig. 20.26 Para-aortic paraganglioma: left para-aortic tumour demonstrated by CT. If an adrenal tumour is not shown on CT in a patient with strong clinical evidence of a phaeochromocytoma, it is likely that the tumour lies at an ectopic site along the sympathetic chain. The majority of such paragangliomata occur in the para-aortic region or around the renal hilum and may be visible on CT. This picture shows a 4 cm tumour lying to the left of the aorta just below the kidneys. A benign paraganglioma was removed at surgery. To detect tumours at other ectopic sites or those too small to be seen on CT, venous sampling for catecholamine levels is required.

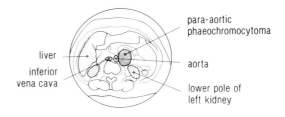

Fig. 20.27 Carotid body tumour: demonstration by angiography. This patient with persistent hypertension after the removal of a left adrenal phaeochromocytoma had elevated levels of catecholamines in the right side of the neck on venous sampling. Subsequent carotid angiography demonstrated a typical carotid body tumour. On this lateral film the carotid bifurcation is seen to be splayed by the tumour which lies between the origins of the internal and external carotid arteries. The blood supply of the tumour arises from the proximal external carotid artery and a tumour blush is present.

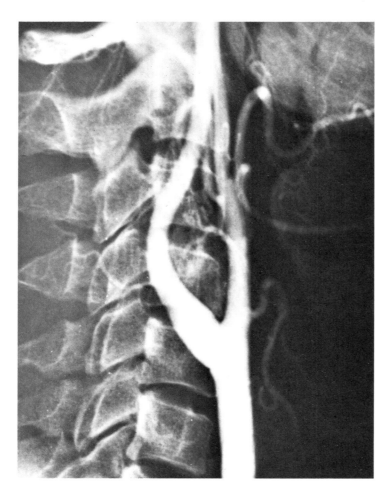

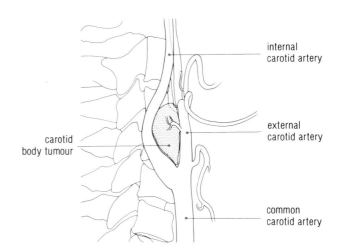

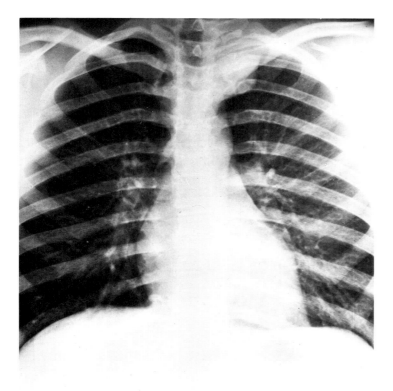

Fig. 20.28 Malignant paraganglioma in the left upper chest.
This PA chest film shows a mass with a well-defined margin lying in the left upper paravertebral region. The patient complained of occasional headaches and sweating but was normotensive. At operation, however, the blood pressure rose steeply while the tumour was being handled. Histological examination showed a paraganglioma which was originally thought to be benign. Seven years later, however, the tumour recurred in the chest and metastatic paraganglioma was found on biopsy of a skull lesion.

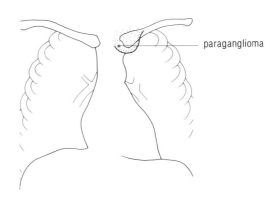

paraganglioma

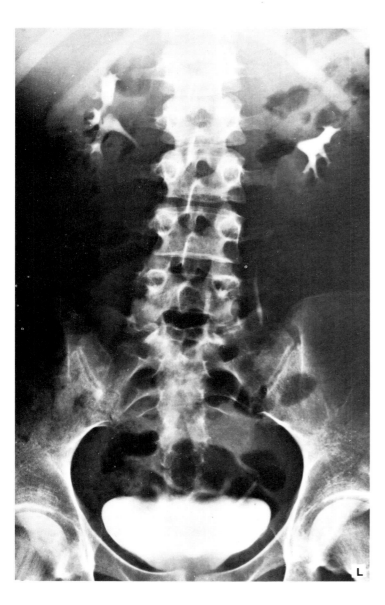

Fig. 20.29 Adrenal phaeochromocytoma: displacement of the kidney demonstrated by intravenous urography.
This patient had a left adrenal phaeochromocytoma which was so large that it caused displacement of the kidney. This full length abdominal film was obtained 20 minutes after the intravenous injection of contrast medium and shows downwards displacement of the left kidney with lateral tilting of the normal oblique orientation of the pelvicalyceal system. The abnormal position of the left kidney should be compared with that of the normal right kidney. In general, intravenous urography is a very unreliable method for investigating suspected adrenal tumours, because only a few can be identified as a tumour blush in the early nephrogram phase and only large tumours will displace the kidney. Further studies in this patient are shown in Fig. 20.31.

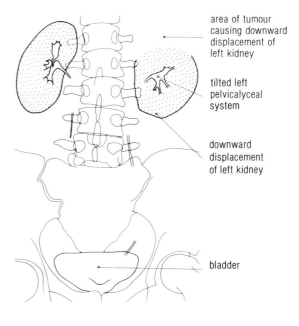

area of tumour causing downward displacement of left kidney

tilted left pelvicalyceal system

downward displacement of left kidney

bladder

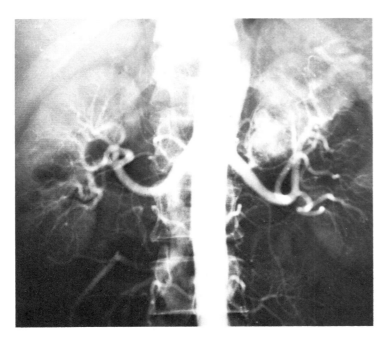

Fig. 20.30 Adrenal phaeochromocytoma: small vascular tumour demonstrated by arteriography. This film from a flush aortogram series shows a vascular phaeochromocytoma of the left adrenal gland. The tumour is supplied from a large inferior adrenal artery which arises from the left renal artery. Because phaeochromocytomas may be relatively avascular, they may be missed at angiography and this investigation has now been largely superseded by CT and venous sampling. Arteriography is hazardous unless adequate medical blockade has been given and the procedure should be undertaken only if really essential. Angiography still has a place in identifying an ectopic phaeochromocytoma located by venous sampling if CT examination is negative.

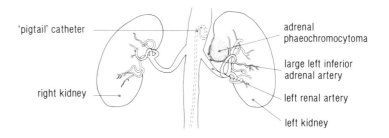

Since invasive investigations (eg aortography) and manipulation of the tumour during surgery may precipitate dangerous and unpredictable pressor crises, it is customary to carefully prepare patients with a phaeochromocytoma before undertaking such procedures. A commonly used regimen consists of administering intravenous phenoxybenzamine by infusion (0.5 mg/kg in 250 ml of 5% dextrose over 2 hours) each day for at least 3 days before the procedure. After the first phenoxybenzamine infusion, propranolol (40 mg 8 hourly orally) is started. This regimen allows the increased vascular tone to relax and prevents the occurrence of severe hypertensive episodes, or hypotension after tumour removal (Ross E.J. et al,1967).

Fig. 20.31 Adrenal phaeochromocytoma: large relatively hypovascular tumour demonstrated by arteriography. These subtraction films of the arterial (a) and early capillary (b) phases of a flush abdominal aortogram were obtained in the same patient as in Fig. 20.29. They show a hypertrophied middle adrenal artery which arises from the aorta and which gives rise to pathological vessels stretched around an 8 cm adrenal mass above the left kidney. The kidney is displaced downwards and flattening of its upper pole can be seen. The double image of the 'pigtail' catheter is due to recoil during the injection of the contrast medium.

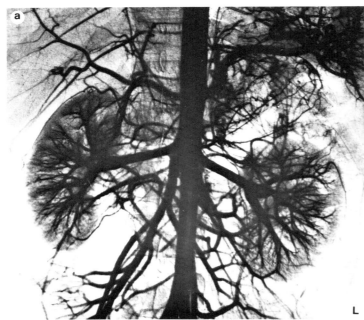

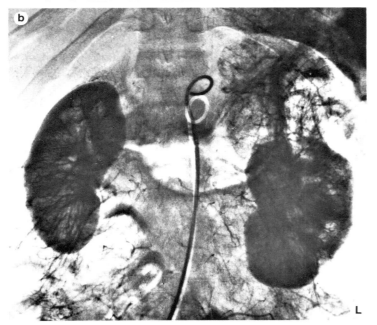

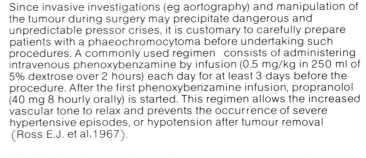

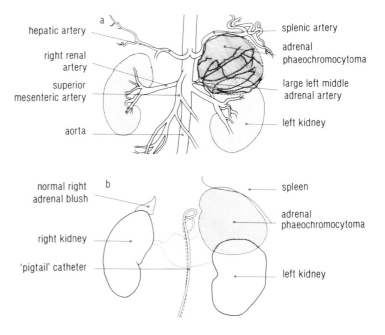

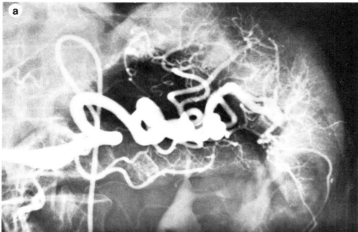

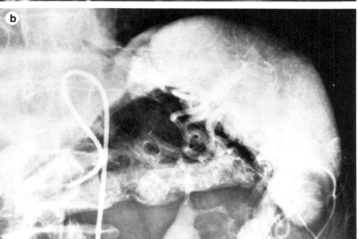

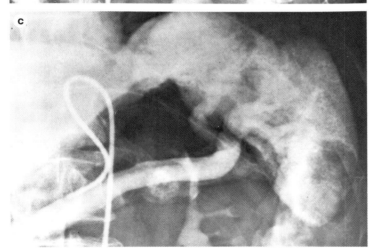

Fig. 20.32 Islet cell tumour of the pancreas: characteristic angiographic appearance. These films from a selective splenic arteriogram demonstrate the typical angiographic appearance of an islet cell tumour of the pancreas. The arterial phase (a) shows a very tortuous splenic artery, reflux of contrast medium retrogradely into the hepatic artery, and a fine mesh of abnormal vessels arising from the transverse pancreatic artery. In the capillary phase (b) a tumour blush is seen distinct from the normal pancreatic blush and this persists into the venous phase (c). Although large pancreatic tumours can be identified by CT, high quality angiography is usually necessary to detect insulinomas as they are often small and may be multiple. Selective or superselective arterial catheterisation is required together with gas distension and paralysis of the stomach to prevent overlap of the stomach wall and the pancreas. Transhepatic venous sampling may be helpful in locating an islet cell tumour if angiography is negative.

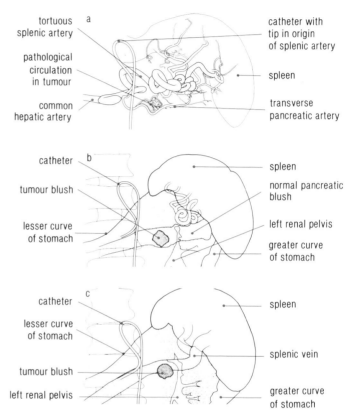

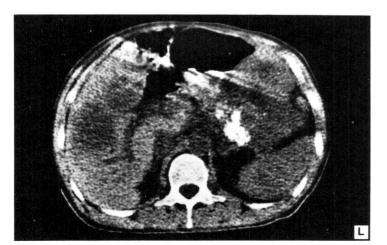

Fig. 20.33 Malignant insulinoma: pancreatic tumour and liver metastases demonstrated by CT. This CT scan shows a large irregular mass arising from the 'tail' of the pancreas which contains areas of amorphous calcification. The air lies in the gastric fundus which is displaced medially by the mass. In addition, there are two low density areas in the liver which represent hepatic metastases. (Islet cell tumour of the pancreas: ectopic ACTH production. See under Cushing's syndrome Fig. 20.24.)

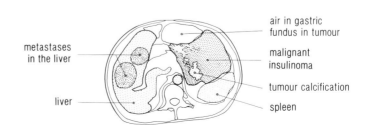

20.15

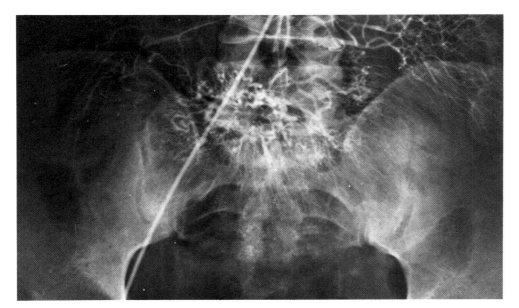

This film from the arterial phase of a superior mesenteric arteriogram demonstrates the typical angiographic appearance of a carcinoid tumour which has invaded the mesentery. Invasion results in thickening and foreshortening of the mesentery and the vessels become very tortuous and are drawn into a characteristic stellate pattern. Arterial narrowing distal to the tumour frequently occurs.

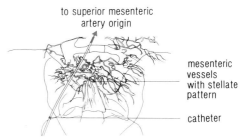

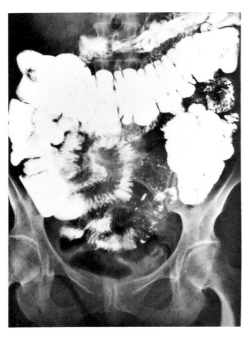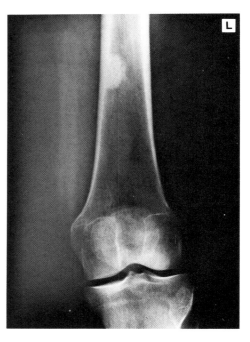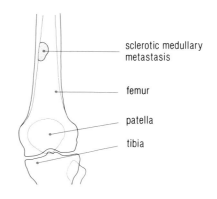

Fig. 20.35 Carcinoid tumour: distal ileal involvement. This 80 minute follow-through film shows an abnormal distal ileum with mesenteric thickening, nodular masses invading the bowel wall, and angulation and tethering of mucosal folds. These appearances are characteristic of carcinoid tumour and reflect invasion by the tumour with an extensive fibroblastic response. Metastatic carcinoma to the mesentery can cause a similar appearance.

Fig. 20.36 Carcinoid tumour: hypervascular hepatic metastases. Hepatic metastases from a carcinoid tumour are characteristically hypervascular and this film of the arterial phase of a coeliac axis arteriogram shows multiple tumour blushes throughout the liver. A similar appearance is produced by other hypervascular hepatic metastases such as those from a renal cell carcinoma.

Fig. 20.37 Carcinoid tumour: sclerotic bony metastasis. Bony metastases from malignant carcinoid tumours are characteristically densely sclerotic. This AP film of the distal femur and knee shows the typical appearance of such an intramedullary lesion. The primary tumour was in the rectum. (Carcinoid tumour: ectopic ACTH production. See under Cushing's syndrome Figs. 20.21 – 20.23.)

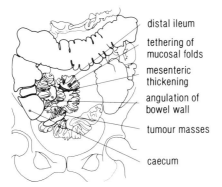

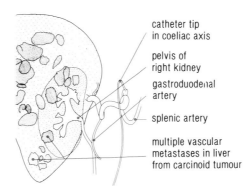

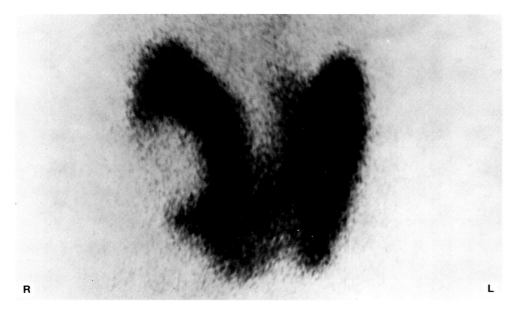

R   L

Fig. 20.38 Thyroid nodule: area of decreased uptake (cold) on isotope scan.
Radionuclide scans (using ^{99m}Tc, ^{131}I, ^{123}I or ^{132}I) can be helpful in the investigation of suspected hyper- and hypothyroidism. In addition, they are useful in determining the activity of a thyroid nodule. This isotope scan shows a cold area in the right lobe of the thyroid. This appearance is most commonly due to a cyst, as was subsequently shown in this patient. Malignant thyroid tumours also show diminished uptake and an ultrasound scan is therefore needed in order to differentiate a cyst from a solid lesion.

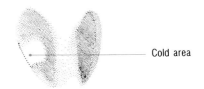

Cold area

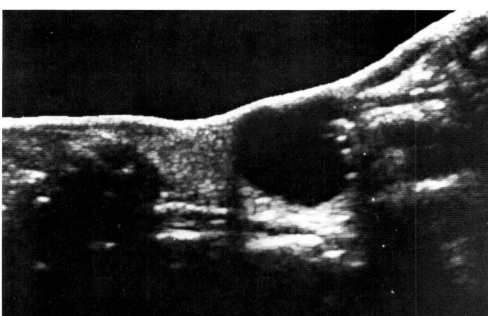

Fig. 20.39 Thyroid cyst: ultrasound scan. This longitudinal ultrasound scan of the right lobe of the thyroid shows a 2.5 cm anechoic area in the lower pole with increased through-transmission of sound behind it. These are the characteristic features of a simple thyroid cyst.

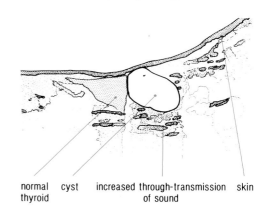

normal   cyst   increased through-transmission   skin
thyroid   of sound

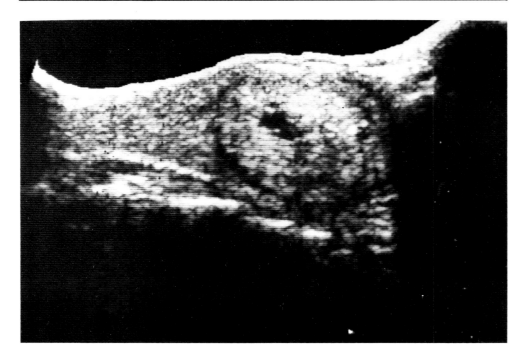

Fig. 20.40 Thyroid tumour: ultrasound scan. This longitudinal scan of the left lobe of the thyroid shows a 3 cm solid but non-homogeneous mass in the lower pole. There is a halo of reduced echogenicity separating the mass from the remainder of the normal thyroid tissue, suggesting that it is encapsulated. This tumour proved to be an adenoma but ultrasound cannot distinguish a benign from a malignant tumour.

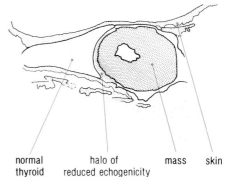

normal   halo of   mass   skin
thyroid   reduced echogenicity

20.17

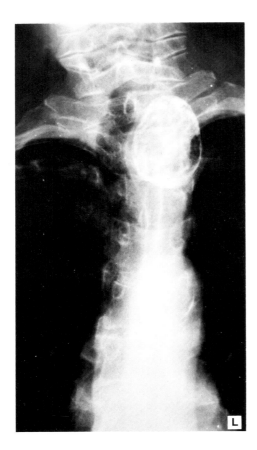
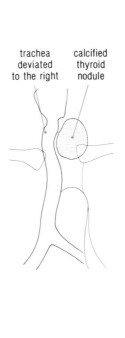

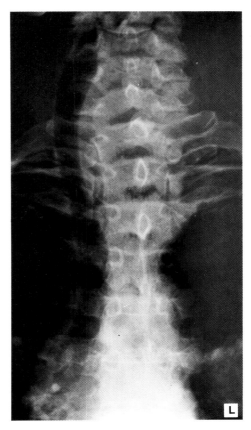
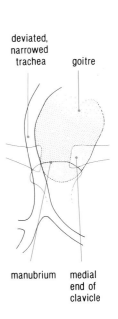

Fig. 20.41 Goitre: calcified thyroid nodule. This AP film of the thoracic inlet shows the typical appearance of a large calcified thyroid nodule which is slightly displacing the trachea to the right side. Most goitres, however, do not show calcification. Calcified goitres are usually benign but may be malignant.

Fig. 20.42 Goitre: deviation and narrowing of the trachea. This AP view of the thoracic inlet shows marked displacement of the trachea to the right by a large left-sided goitre which extends inferiorly to just below the sternal notch. The trachea is slightly narrowed in its transverse diameter just above the level of the thoracic inlet. No calcification can be seen within the goitre. Although any displacement or narrowing of the trachea in the AP plane can be readily assessed on a lateral view of the thoracic inlet, it may be difficult to determine whether or not there is any significant extension of a cervical goitre into the mediastinum.

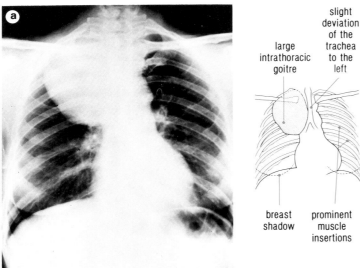
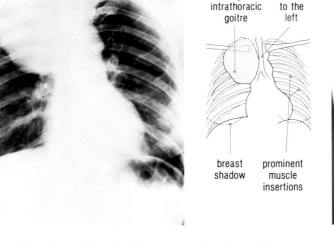

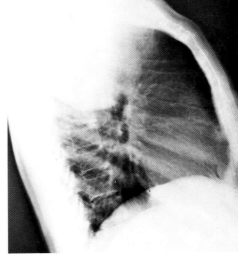
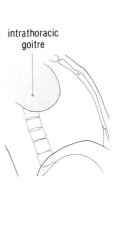

Fig. 20.43 Intrathoracic goitre in acromegaly: chest films. The PA chest film (a) shows a large mass in the right upper chest which is confluent with the mediastinum medially and has a well-defined lateral margin. The mass does not contain any obvious calcification and is only slightly displacing the trachea to the left. The right lateral view (b) shows a clearly defined mass lying posteriorly. The patient had presented with a goitre and had noticed some enlargement of the hands and feet. There were no symptoms of dysphagia or of thyrotoxicosis. The mass in the chest was subsequently shown on isotope and CT scans to be in

continuity with the cervical goitre (see Figs. 20.44 and 20.45). The patient was also found to have a pituitary tumour and acromegaly. Prominent muscle insertions can be seen on the PA chest film at the lower borders of the ribs but no bony changes of acromegaly are present in the dorsal spine (see Fig. 20.7). At the combined surgical approach of cervical incision and a right posterolateral thoracotomy, the large mass in the right side of the mediastinum was confirmed to be continuous with an enlarged right lobe of the thyroid gland and was removed. Histological examination showed that the mass was a large colloid goitre.

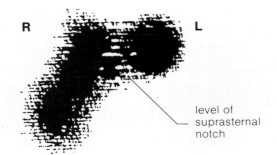

Fig. 20.44 Intrathoracic goitre: radionuclide scan. This anterior isotope scan of the same patient as in Fig. 20.43 shows uptake in the cervical thyroid and in the large intrathoracic extension. The activity was higher on the posterior scan indicating the posterior position of the mediastinal extension. Intrathoracic thyroids do not always contain functioning tissue in which case they will not take up the isotope.

level of suprasternal notch

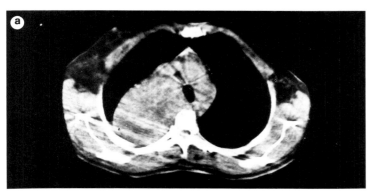

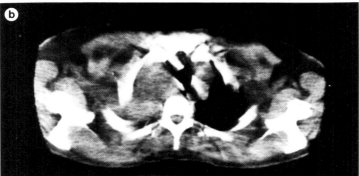

Fig. 20.45 Intrathoracic goitre: CT scans. On the CT scan of the same patient as in Figs. 20.43 and 20.44, the goitre is shown as a well-defined mass in the posterior mediastinum compressing and deviating the trachea to the left (upper picture). On a higher scan at the level of the sternal notch (lower picture) the mass is seen to be in continuity with the right lobe of the thyroid. The attenuation (density) of thyroid tissue on CT is usually slightly higher than that of other soft tissues because of the iodine content of the gland. This is not, however, obvious in this patient.

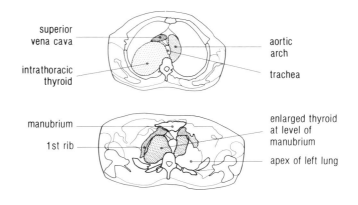

superior vena cava

intrathoracic thyroid

aortic arch

trachea

manubrium

1st rib

enlarged thyroid at level of manubrium

apex of left lung

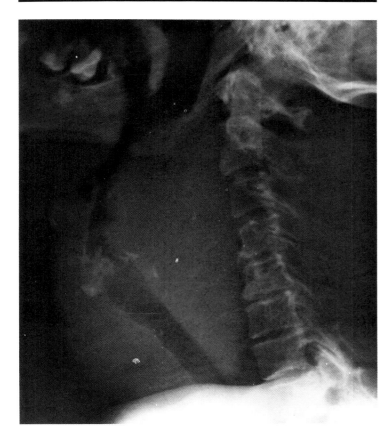

Fig. 20.46 Carcinoma of the thyroid: retrotracheal extension of tumour. This lateral view of the neck shows massive soft tissue swelling with marked anterior displacement of the trachea which is compressed in its anteroposterior diameter. The displacement is due to gross retrotracheal extension of the thyroid and is indicative of malignancy. This patient had an anaplastic carcinoma of the thyroid.

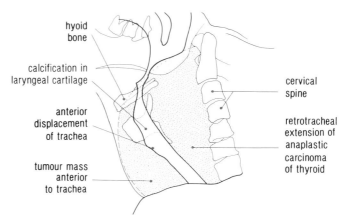

hyoid bone

calcification in laryngeal cartilage

anterior displacement of trachea

tumour mass anterior to trachea

cervical spine

retrotracheal extension of anaplastic carcinoma of thyroid

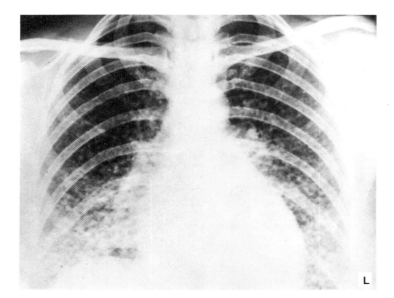

L

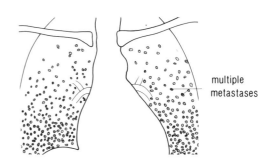

multiple
metastases

Fig. 20.47 Carcinoma of the thyroid: 'snow storm' appearance of pulmonary metastases. This PA chest film shows multiple small nodular opacities throughout both lungs, most marked at the bases, the characteristic 'snow storm' appearance of pulmonary metastases from carcinoma of the thyroid. Such metastatic deposits may remain unchanged over a long period of time due to a very low grade of malignancy and may take up and be treated with [131]I.

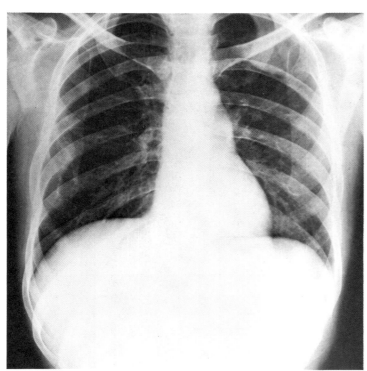

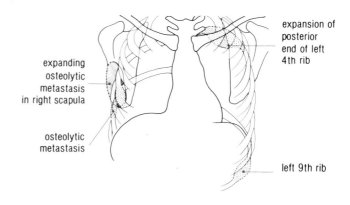

expanding
osteolytic
metastasis
in right scapula

osteolytic
metastasis

expansion of
posterior
end of left
4th rib

left 9th rib

Fig. 20.48 Carcinoma of the thyroid: chest radiograph showing expanded bony metastases. This PA chest film shows multiple osteolytic bony metastases. Those involving the right scapula and the left 4th and 9th ribs show marked expansion of bone. Carcinoma of the thyroid characteristically gives rise to osteolytic metastases, sometimes accompanied by marked expansion of bone, as in this patient. The appearance is, however, not diagnostic because metastatic renal cell carcinoma, multiple myeloma, and occasionally metastatic carcinoma of the breast may also cause similar bone expansion. Such thyroid carcinoma metastases may, but do not necessarily, show up on routine radionuclide bone scanning.

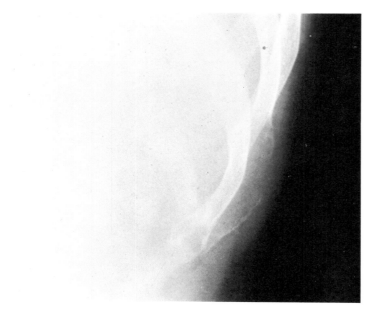

Fig. 20.49 Carcinoma of the thyroid: close-up view of an expanded rib metastasis. This coned view of the left 9th rib of the same patient as in Fig. 20.48 clearly shows the medullary destruction and expansion with thinning of the overlying cortex.

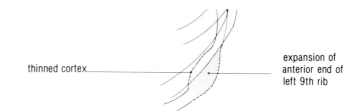

thinned cortex

expansion of
anterior end of
left 9th rib

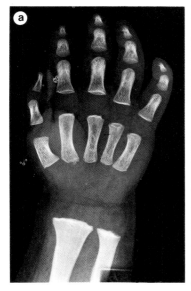
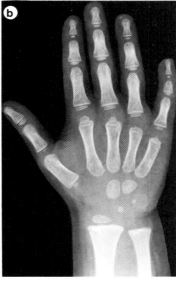

Fig. 20.50 Hypothyroidism in childhood: delay in skeletal maturation (with normal hand for comparison). This PA film (a) of the hand of a 3-year-old hypothyroid boy demonstrates the characteristic retardation of skeletal growth. The bones of the hand are smaller than normal reflecting the generalised delay in growth that occurs and ossification has not yet started in any of the carpal bones or secondary epiphyses. Irregularity and increased density of the metaphyses occurs and, in this view, these changes are best seen in the distal radius and ulna. The appearances should be compared with those of the hand of a normal boy of similar age (b).

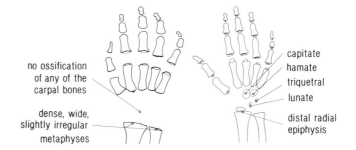

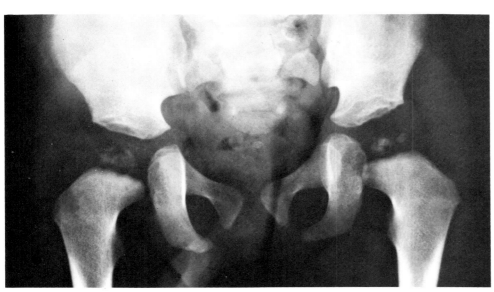

Fig. 20.51 Hypothyroidism in childhood: fragmentation of the femoral capital epiphyses. This AP view of the pelvis shows delay in ossification, with fragmentation and hypoplasia of the femoral capital epiphyses. Fragmentation of the ossification centres of the femoral heads might suggest the diagnosis of bilateral Perthes' disease; however, symmetrical involvement would be excessively rare in that condition.

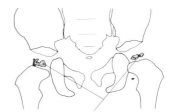

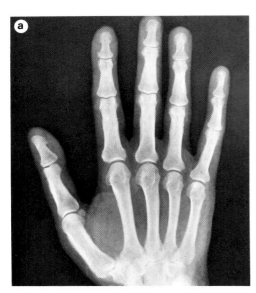
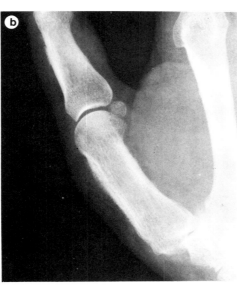

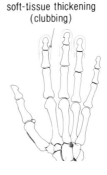
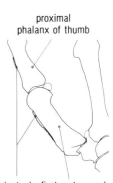

Fig. 20.52 Thyroid acropachy: hand radiograph showing periosteal reaction and clubbing. Thyroid acropachy occurs as part of Graves' disease and consists of clubbing of the fingers and toes, usually associated with exophthalmos and pretibial myxoedema. Bone changes are not necessarily part of the syndrome although they are frequently present. The PA film (a) of a hand shows the characteristic periosteal reaction of thyroid acropachy along the radial aspect of the shaft of the first metacarpal, the typical site. Soft tissue thickening is evident around some of the distal phalanges. The coned view (b) of the thumb and first metacarpal better demonstrates the characteristic lace-like appearance of the periosteal reaction. Besides the typical involvement of the first metacarpal, periosteal new bone formation may also occur along the shafts of the other metacarpals and the proximal phalanges. In this patient a slight periosteal reaction is also present along the shaft of the proximal phalanx of the thumb.

20.21

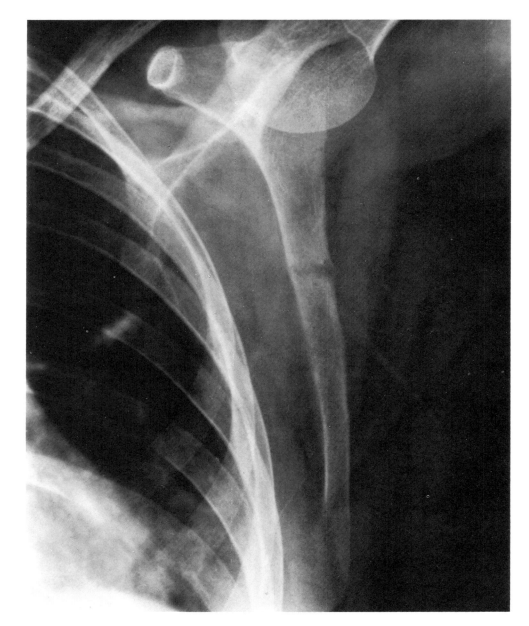

Fig. 20.53 Osteomalacia: Looser zone in the scapula. Osteomalacia is the term used to describe inadequate osteoid mineralisation in the adult. Stress fractures of the weakened bones are common and the resultant seams of osteoid are known as Looser's zones. This film of the left scapula of a woman with vitamin D deficiency illustrates the typical appearance of a Looser zone. There is little or no evidence of healing. Because Looser's zones are due to stress induced by normal activity they tend to occur at constant symmetrical sites: these include the ribs, the scapulae, the obturator rings of the pelvis, the metatarsal shafts, and the femoral necks (see Fig. 20.54). Osteomalacia results in generalised demineralisation of the bones but this may be evident radiologically only when the disease is severe. When gross osteomalacia is present deformities of the weakened bones may occur: these include triradiate pelvis, kyphosis, bowing of the limbs, 'hourglass' shaped thoracic cage, and basilar invagination of the skull.

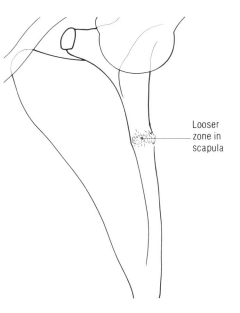

Looser zone in scapula

Fig. 20.54 Osteomalacia: Looser zone in the femoral neck. This coned AP view of the upper part of the right femur shows a linear lucency in the medial aspect of the femoral neck, a typical site for a Looser zone.

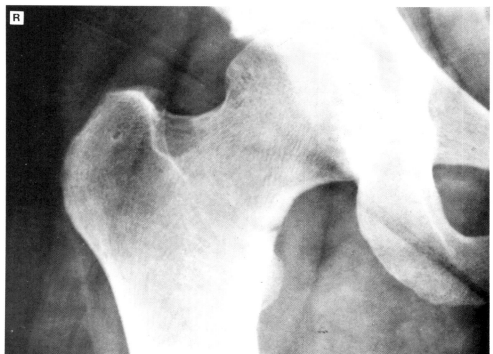

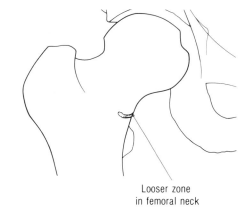

Looser zone in femoral neck

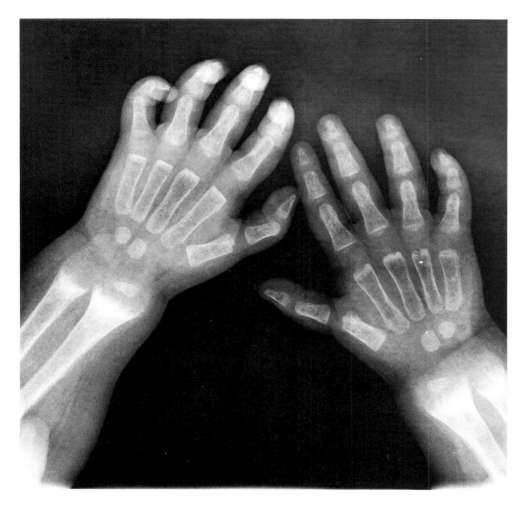

Fig. 20.55 Nutritional rickets: characteristic radiological appearance of the hands. Rickets is the term used when inadequate osteoid mineralisation affects the growing skeleton. This PA film of the hands of a 2-year-old boy illustrates the characteristic appearance of nutritional rickets. Gross demineralisation of the bones is present and ossification of the secondary epiphyseal centres is delayed. Wide bands of translucency in the metaphyses and irregularity of the metaphyseal margins are characteristic. The distal radial metaphyses are cupped or splayed due to the effects of weight bearing (i.e. crawling) on the weakened bones.

generalised loss of bone density

poor cortical definition | splaying of metaphyses | increased distance between epiphysis and metaphysis

Fig. 20.56 Nutritional rickets: bowing of the femora and genu vara. Gross demineralisation of the bones is seen in this AP film of the femora and knees of the same child as in Fig. 20.55. Bowing of the femora and genu vara result from the effects of weight bearing on the weakened bones. The film also shows typical splaying and irregularity of the metaphyses and poorly ossified epiphyseal centres.

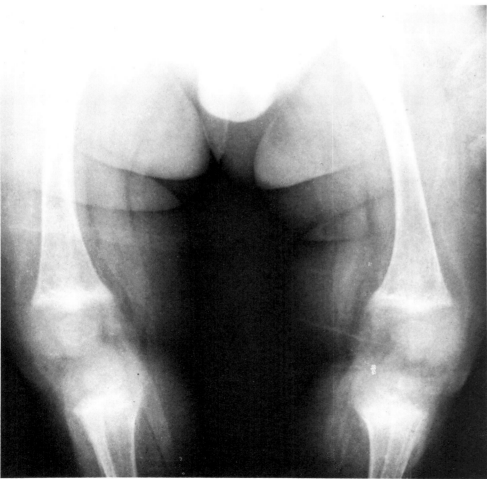

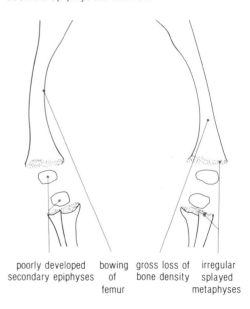

poorly developed secondary epiphyses | bowing of femur | gross loss of bone density | irregular splayed metaphyses

20.23

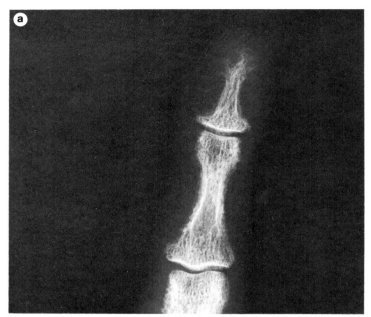

(a)

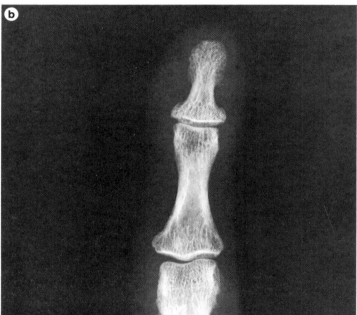

(b)

Fig. 20.57   Primary hyperparathyroidism: phalanges showing gross subperiosteal bone resorption (with appearance after healing for comparison). Bony changes are evident radiologically in 25 to 35 per cent of patients with primary hyperparathyroidism. Subperiosteal bone resorption is the earliest radiological sign and is specific for hyperparathyroidism. Generalised skeletal demineralisation is a late finding. The film (a) of the middle and distal phalanges of the index finger shows gross subperiosteal bone resorption of the shafts of the phalanges and also of the tip of the distal phalanx. The bone density is decreased and the texture of the cortex shows a 'basket-work' pattern with loss of definition of the normal corticomedullary junction. These appearances of gross hyperparathyroidism should be compared with those in (b), where healing had occurred following removal of a parathyroid adenoma . Although subperiosteal bone resorption classically involves the phalanges, it may also occur at many other sites. These include the outer ends and under-surface of the clavicles, the metaphyseal regions of the growing ends of the long bones, the ischial tuberosities, the pubic bones at the symphysis, the sacroiliac joints, and the inner wall of the dorsum sellae.

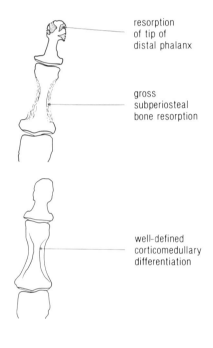

resorption
of tip of
distal phalanx

gross
subperiosteal
bone resorption

well-defined
corticomedullary
differentiation

Fig. 20.58   Primary hyperparathyroidism: magnification film of the index finger showing early subperiosteal bone resorption. This magnified film of the middle and distal phalanges of the index finger shows the early bony changes of hyperparathyroidism. Slight subperiosteal bone resorption is present along the radial aspect of the middle phalanx, the characteristic site for early change. There is also poor definition of the cortical outline of the tip of the distal phalanx. The technique of magnification radiography using a fine-focus X-ray tube is helpful in identifying these subtle appearances.

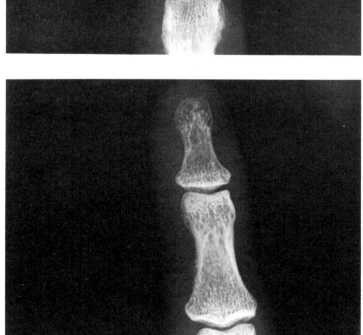

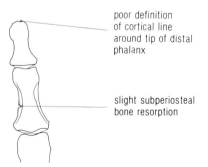

poor definition
of cortical line
around tip of distal
phalanx

slight subperiosteal
bone resorption

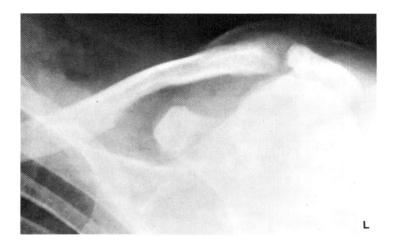

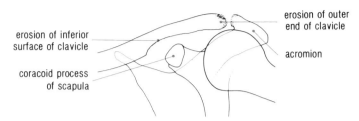

Fig. 20.59 Primary hyperparathyroidism: erosion of the outer end of the clavicle. This coned AP view of the lateral half of the left clavicle shows subperiosteal bone resorption of the outer end of the clavicle with slight widening of the acromioclavicular joint. There is also erosion of the under-surface of the clavicle above the coracoid process of the scapula.

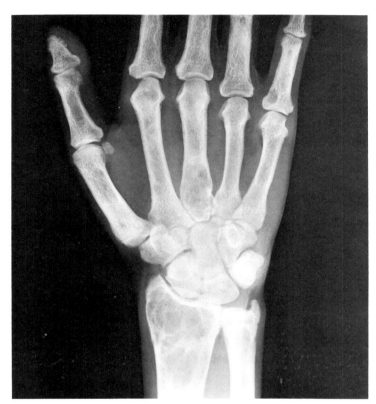

Fig. 20.60 Primary hyperparathyroidism: brown tumours.
Brown tumours sometimes occur in primary hyperparathyroidism but are relatively uncommon in secondary hyperparathyroidism. This PA film of the wrist shows the typical appearance of brown tumours. Osteolucent bony defects are present in the distal radius and ulna, the base of the third metacarpal and the proximal phalanx of the little finger. The bone density is generally decreased. After parathyroidectomy brown tumours fill slowly with new bone from the periphery. Incomplete healing results in an appearance which may closely resemble that of fibrous dysplasia.

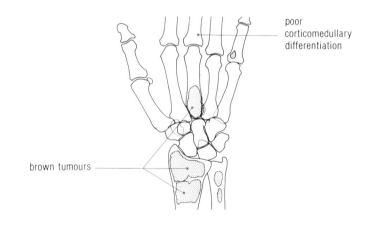

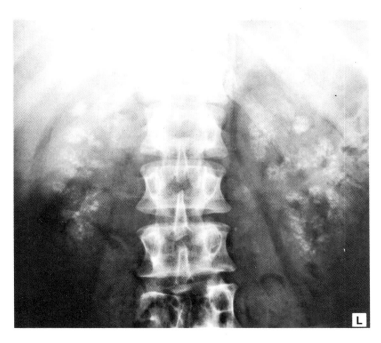

Fig. 20.61 Primary hyperparathyroidism: nephrocalcinosis and a brown tumour. Although pathologically about 60 per cent of patients with primary hyperparathyroidism have renal calculi or nephrocalcinosis, the radiological demonstration of such abnormalities is far less common. This coned abdominal film shows extensive nephrocalcinosis of the fine type seen in primary hyperparathyroidism. Generalised loss of bone density is present and a brown tumour has resulted in the partial collapse of the body of the fourth lumbar vertebra.

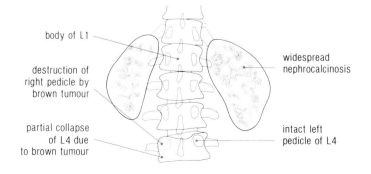

20.25

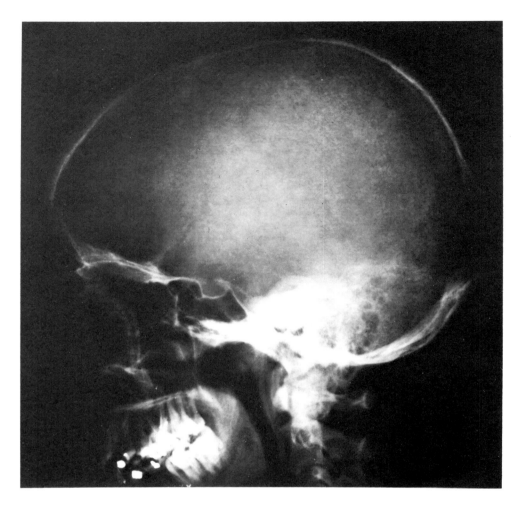

Fig. 20.62 Primary hyperparathyroidism: 'pepper pot' skull. This lateral film shows the classical changes in the skull vault of primary hyperparathyroidism. Generalised skeletal demineralisation is reflected by diffuse porotic mottling of the calvarium giving a granular or 'pepper pot' appearance. The vascular grooves are poorly defined and there is absence of the lamina dura of the teeth. The latter appearance is, however, not specific because it may occur in other demineralising disorders such as osteoporosis and osteomalacia. In some patients with primary hyperparathyroidism the dorsum sellae may be eroded and in those with polyglandular adenomatosis and an associated pituitary tumour there may be enlargement of the pituitary fossa.

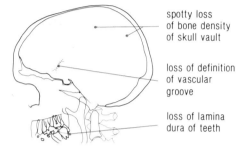

spotty loss of bone density of skull vault

loss of definition of vascular groove

loss of lamina dura of teeth

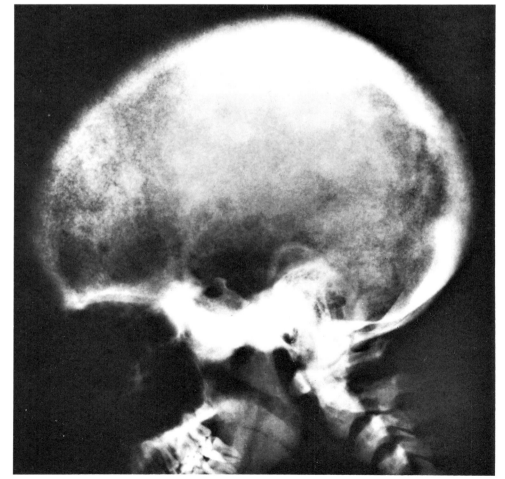

Fig. 20.63 Renal osteodystrophy: skull changes. The radiological appearances of renal osteodystrophy consist of areas of both demineralisation and sclerosis. These changes are thought to be due to a combination of osteomalacia, secondary hyperparathyroidism and a calcitonin effect. This lateral film of the skull of a 17-year-old girl with chronic renal failure shows marked calvarial thickening with considerable mottling. Sometimes such change may resemble Paget's disease. The skull base and the cervical spine are dense and there is loss of the lamina dura of the teeth.

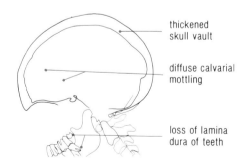

thickened skull vault

diffuse calvarial mottling

loss of lamina dura of teeth

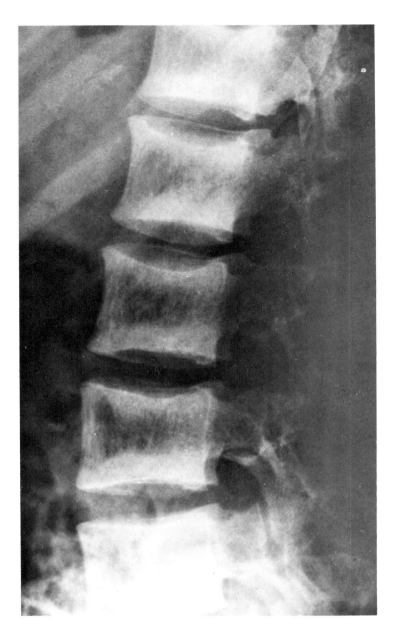

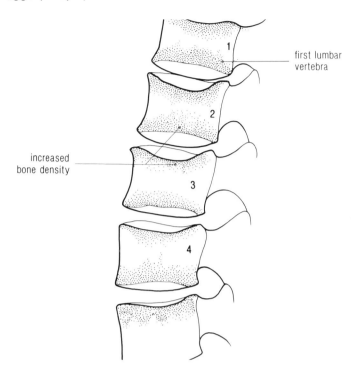

Fig. 20.64 Renal osteodystrophy: 'rugger jersey' spine. This lateral film of the lumbar spine shows central demineralisation and linear bands of subarticular density at the superior and inferior margins of the vertebral bodies – the classical appearance of a 'rugger jersey' spine.

first lumbar vertebra

increased bone density

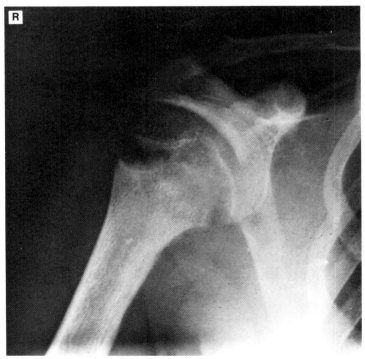

Fig. 20.65 Renal rickets: characteristic radiological appearance of the shoulder. This AP view of the right shoulder of a 16-year-old boy with chronic renal failure shows marked widening of the epiphyseal plate of the humerus with irregularity and splaying of the metaphysis - characteristic features of rickets. Subperiosteal erosion of the outer end of the clavicle and of the acromion with widening of the acromioclavicular joint indicate secondary hyperparathyroidism. The bone density is generally decreased and the humeral shaft in particular demonstrates thinning of the cortex and poor definition of the corticomedullary junction. The bone age is delayed.

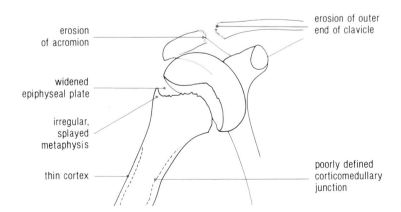

erosion of acromion

erosion of outer end of clavicle

widened epiphyseal plate

irregular, splayed metaphysis

thin cortex

poorly defined corticomedullary junction

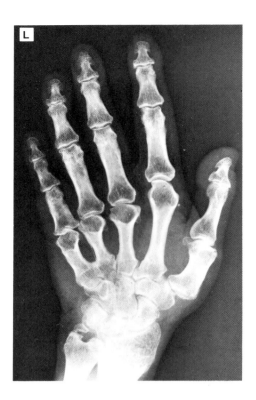
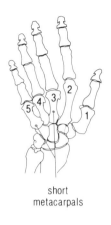

short
metacarpals

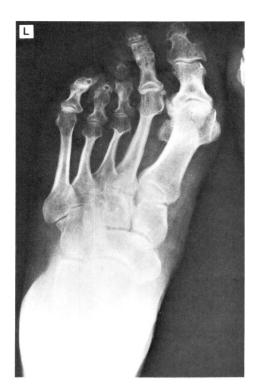
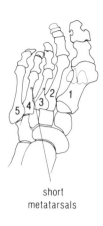

short
metatarsals

Fig. 20.66 Pseudohypoparathyroidism: short metacarpals.
This PA view of the hand shows short, rather broad metacarpals, an appearance seen in pseudohypoparathyroidism. In this patient, all the metacarpals except the second are rather short but the number involved may be variable.

Fig. 20.67 Pseudohypoparathyroidism: short metatarsals.
This AP view of the foot shows a similar appearance to that of the hand, with shortening of the third and fourth metatarsals.

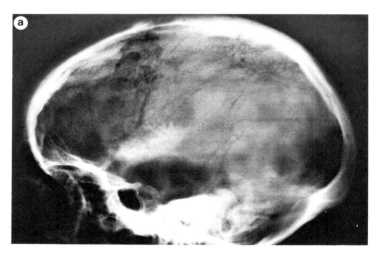
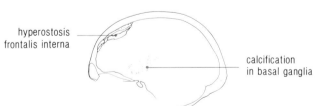

hyperostosis
frontalis interna

calcification
in basal ganglia

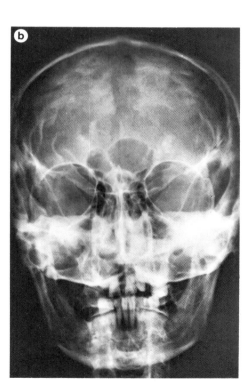
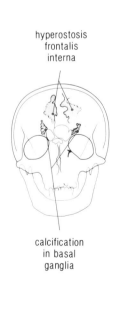

hyperostosis
frontalis
interna

calcification
in basal
ganglia

Fig. 20.68 Pseudohypoparathyroidism: calcification in the basal ganglia. In pseudohypoparathyroidism heterotopic deposits of calcium phosphate occur in the soft tissues and most commonly affect the basal ganglia. The lateral (a) and PA (b) skull films show characteristic symmetrical punctate calcification in the basal ganglia. Similar calcification, however, also occurs in hypoparathyroidism. In this patient, slight hyperostosis frontalis interna is also present.

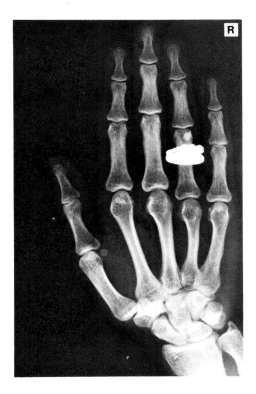
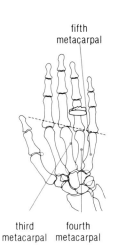

Fig. 20.69 Gonadal dysgenesis (Turner's syndrome): short fourth metacarpal. The fourth metacarpal is often short in gonadal dysgenesis, as in this patient. Normally a line tangential to the distal ends of the third and fifth metacarpals will transect the head of the fourth. If the fourth metacarpal is short, it will touch or lie below such a line. In gonadal dysgenesis the fifth metacarpal is often also short and occasionally the third metacarpal may be similarly affected. Premature fusion of the ossification centres of the involved metacarpals may be seen in young patients.

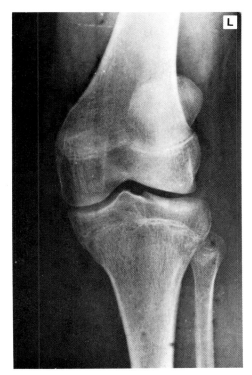
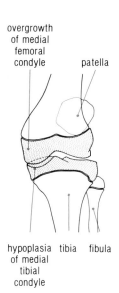

Fig. 20.70 Gonadal dysgenesis (Turner's syndrome): impaired development of the medial tibial condyle. This AP film of the knee shows hypoplasia of the medial tibial condyle which is often a feature of gonadal dysgenesis. The medial tibial condyle appears depressed and there is corresponding overgrowth of the medial femoral condyle.

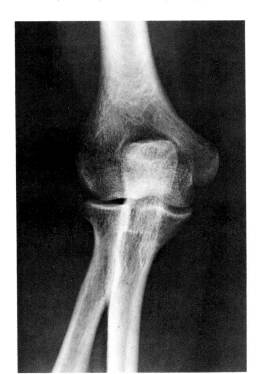
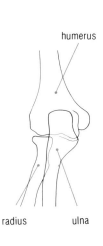

Fig. 20.71 Gonadal dysgenesis (Turner's syndrome): cubitus valgus. Bilateral cubitus valgus is frequently present in gonadal dysgenesis and this AP film of the elbow demonstrates the increase in the carrying angle, as shown by lateral deviation of the radius and ulna.

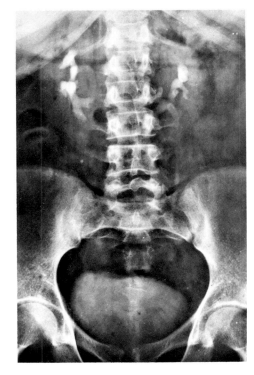
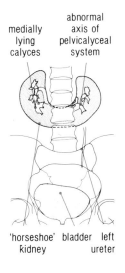

Fig. 20.72 Gonadal dysgenesis (Turner's syndrome): fused or 'horse-shoe' kidney. This full length film of an intravenous urogram shows a fused or 'horse-shoe' kidney, one of the commonest associated anomalies in gonadal dysgenesis. The lower poles of the kidneys are joined in the midline and this results in abnormal orientation of the pelvicalyceal systems and medially lying calyces. Other renal anomalies, in particular those involving rotation and ectopia, are also common in gonadal dysgenesis.

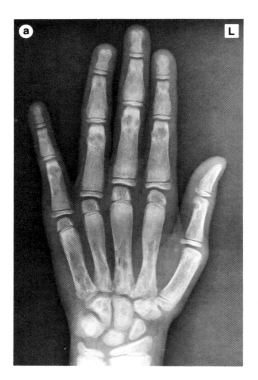
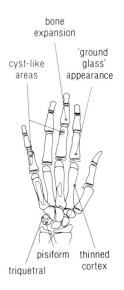
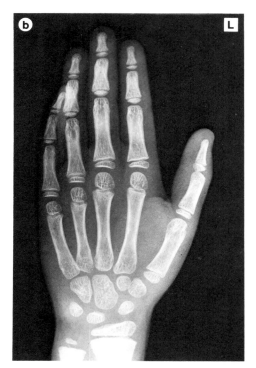
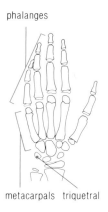

Fig. 20.73 Albright's syndrome: hand with normal for comparison. (a) This PA film of the hand of a 6-year-old girl with skin pigmentation and precocious puberty shows the characteristic appearances of polyostotic fibrous dysplasia. Both bone replacement and new bone formation are evident. The affected spongiosa has an amorphous appearance resembling that of 'ground glass' and the bones show areas of expansion with thinning of the overlying cortex. Small cyst-like lesions are also present with reactive sclerosis around some of their margins. The carpal bones and secondary epiphyses are well developed and the pisiform bone, which normally starts to ossify at about nine years in the female, is seen superimposed on the triquetral. The bone age is advanced to ten years and this film should be compared with (b), that of a normal 6-year-old girl, which shows the degree of bony development which usually occurs by that age.

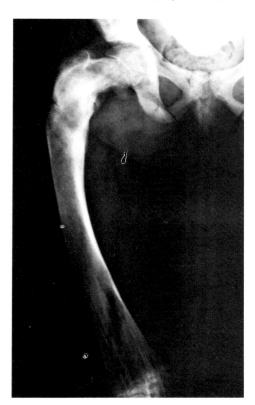
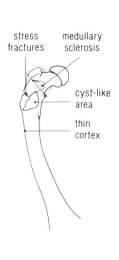
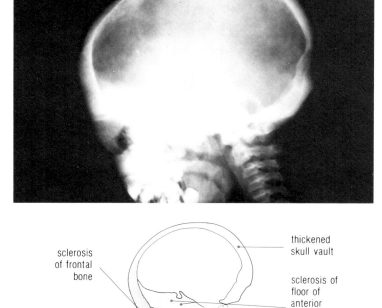

Fig. 20.74 Albright's syndrome: deformity of the femur. This AP film shows marked coxa vara and bowing of the shaft. The cyst-like lesions and areas of medullary sclerosis are typical of fibrous dysplasia. The cortex is thin, particularly at the lateral margin and stress fractures are present in the proximal femoral shaft. Such changes often progress and may result in a 'shepherd's crook' deformity of the upper femur.

Fig. 20.75 Albright's syndrome: skull showing leontiasis ossea. Involvement of the skull by fibrous dysplasia is usually manifest by extensive new bone formation and this lateral film of the same girl as in Fig. 20.73 shows the characteristic appearance of leontiasis ossea. The convexity of the calvarium is thickened and there is considerable sclerosis of the floor of the anterior fossae, the base of the skull, the maxillae and the frontal bones, making the radiograph features indistinct.

21 Neuroradiology of the Pituitary and Hypothalamus

Derek P E Kingsley, FRCS, DMRD, FRCR

The four main reasons for radiological investigation of the pituitary region are summarised in Figure 21.1. Although a number of neuroradiological techniques are now available each provides slightly different information, so that frequently a combination of procedures is necessary to establish the nature of the lesion.

SKULL RADIOGRAPHY AND PITUITARY TOMOGRAPHY

Since disease processes originating within the cranium at a distance from the pituitary fossa may result in an abnormal pituitary fossa, a full lateral skull radiograph should always be taken. Minor abnormalities of contour of the fossa can only be appreciated if the film is a true lateral, that is, with the two orbital rooves superimposed. Rotation and canting of the head may cause difficulty in interpretation.

Routine views of the pituitary fossa consist of lateral and frontal projections. Half axial (Towne's) and submentovertical (base) views may be used to augment these two. The lateral projection, to which may be added a coned view, is best taken with the median sagittal plane parallel to, and the interorbital line at right angles to, the film. The central ray of the tube is aligned at right angles to the centre of the film, and the patient positioned so that the central ray is 2.5cm above and in front of the external auditory meatus.

The frontal projection is taken with the brow and nose against the film and with the median sagittal plane and radiographic base line at right angles to the film. The tube is angled 10°–20° towards the feet with the central ray projected through the glabella. However, this angulation is best judged from the lateral so that the beam is tangential to the floor of the fossa. Although easily seen on the lateral view, the sella is often obscured on the frontal projection by the sphenoid bone and skull base. The frontal projection is used to assess the floor of the pituitary fossa and undercutting of the anterior clinoid processes.

Aims of Neuroradiological Investigations in Region of Pituitary
to document state of sella and extrasellar extension before treatment
to exclude an aneurysm
to assess the effects of treatment
to evaluate complications

Fig. 21.1 Table showing the main reasons for neuroradiological investigation.

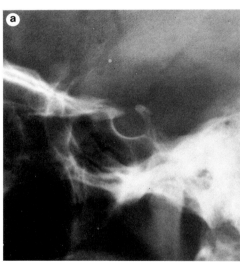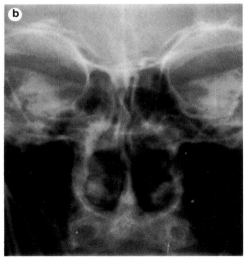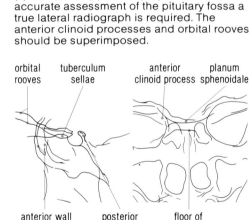

Fig. 21.2 Normal plain skull radiograph: (a) lateral and (b) frontal projections. For accurate assessment of the pituitary fossa a true lateral radiograph is required. The anterior clinoid processes and orbital rooves should be superimposed.

orbital rooves — tuberculum sellae — anterior clinoid process — planum sphenoidale

anterior wall of middle fossa — posterior clinoid process — floor of pituitary fossa

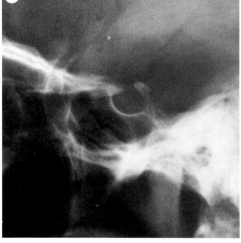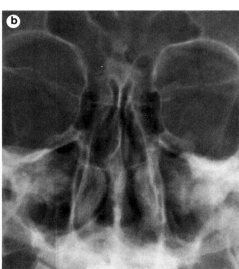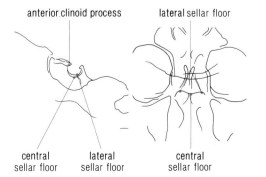

Fig. 21.3 Normal variant of skull radiograph: (a) lateral and (b) frontal projections. An incidental finding in an asymptomatic patient. The lateral projection suggests a double floor to the pituitary fossa, but this is due to a slight central depression confirmed by the frontal projection.

anterior clinoid process — lateral sellar floor

central sellar floor — lateral sellar floor — central sellar floor

There is great variation in the size of the normal sella and measurement of its volume is of little practical value since minor changes of contour may indicate significant pathology. There is therefore no substitute for good radiological technique and an experienced observer.

Although frequently used, pituitary tomography rarely adds to the information provided by good quality plain radiographs. Its value lies in: (i) confirming the extent of a downward or forward bulge in the sellar wall into the sphenoid sinus or clivus, (ii) confirming a grossly asymmetrical sellar floor not readily apparent on plain radiographs,(iii) demonstrating undercutting of the anterior clinoid processes and (iv) confirming equivocal changes on plain radiographs.

Tomography is best performed using complex motion, either trispiral or hypocycloidal, although high quality linear tomography is often satisfactory. Lateral tomograms are usually sufficient provided that the interval between sections taken from one anterior clinoid process to the other is 2 mm or less. Antero-posterior (AP) tomography is rarely required and should be discouraged since with it the eyes are exposed to more radiation than in lateral tomography. It should only be used where lateral tomography is uninformative and where access to modern computed tomography (CT) is not available.

The centre of the sella is first identified on the tomographic section halfway between the two anterior clinoid processes, so that minor differences in the size and shape of the two halves of the sella can be appreciated.

Although tomography is sometimes used to confirm minor sellar abnormalities, this practice should be discouraged since it is of little clinical value either in management of the disease or for follow-up.

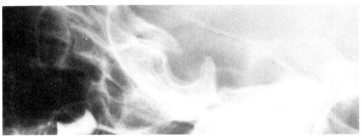
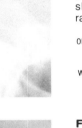

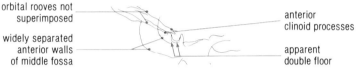

Fig. 21.4   Double floor artefact caused by rotation and canting of the head: lateral skull radiograph. The difficulty of assessing a pituitary fossa unless the radiograph is true lateral is shown. This is the commonest cause of misdiagnosis in pituitary radiology.

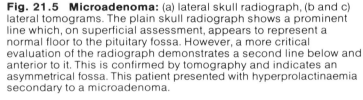

orbital rooves not superimposed — anterior clinoid processes

widely separated anterior walls of middle fossa — apparent double floor

Fig. 21.5   Microadenoma: (a) lateral skull radiograph, (b and c) lateral tomograms. The plain skull radiograph shows a prominent line which, on superficial assessment, appears to represent a normal floor to the pituitary fossa. However, a more critical evaluation of the radiograph demonstrates a second line below and anterior to it. This is confirmed by tomography and indicates an asymmetrical fossa. This patient presented with hyperprolactinaemia secondary to a microadenoma.

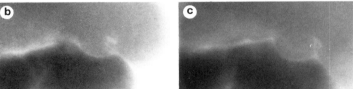

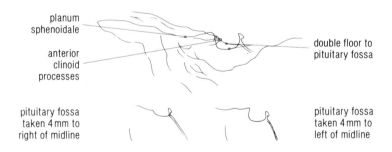

planum sphenoidale

anterior clinoid processes — double floor to pituitary fossa

pituitary fossa taken 4 mm to right of midline

pituitary fossa taken 4 mm to left of midline

Fig. 21.6   'Empty' sella: (a) lateral skull radiograph and (b) axial CT scan. The sella is deeper than usual, although retaining its normal configuration, and its volume greater. The appearances on the radiograph alone do not exclude a pituitary adenoma, but the low density within the sella on computed tomography (CT) is consistent with an 'empty' sella confirmed by contrast cisternography (cf. Figs. 21.47 and 21.48).

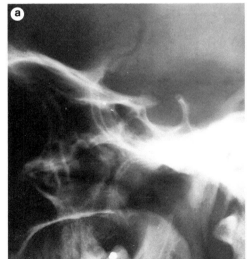
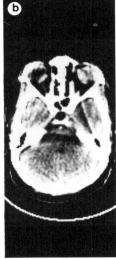

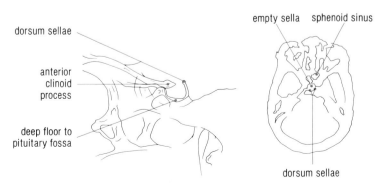

dorsum sellae

empty sella   sphenoid sinus

anterior clinoid process

deep floor to pituitary fossa

dorsum sellae

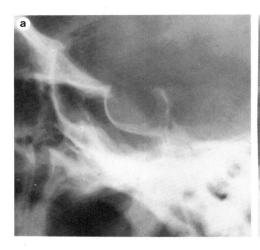
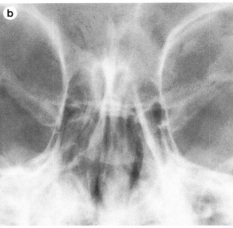
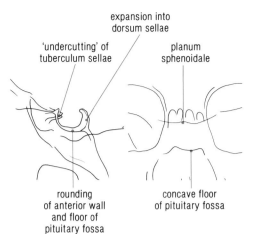

Fig. 21.7   Pituitary tumour: skull radiograph, (a) lateral and (b) frontal projections. The pituitary fossa is large. There is general expansion in all directions, particularly forwards with undercutting of the tuberculum sellae and backwards into the base of the dorsum sellae. The sella is not particularly deep (cf. Fig. 21.6) which suggests a tumour rather than an empty sella. CT is used to differentiate the two conditions.

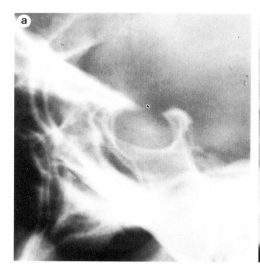
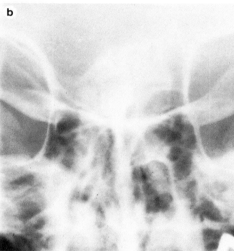
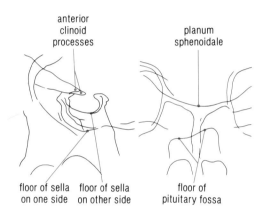

Fig. 21.8   Asymmetrical sellar enlargement with grossly sloping floor: skull radiograph, (a) lateral and (b) frontal projections. Minor degrees of variation in contour of the sellar floor are often easy to appreciate but a marked slope may be misinterpreted. Whenever there is doubt, tomography may be required; the true situation, however, is usually revealed on the frontal view.

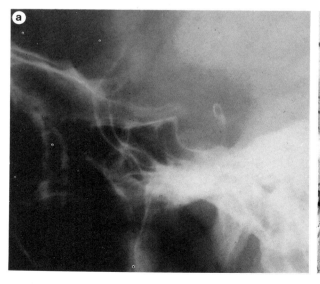
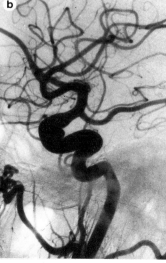
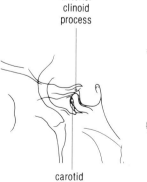
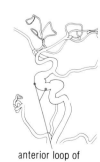

Fig. 21.9   Prominent carotid sulcus: (a) lateral skull radiograph and (b) subtraction carotid angiogram. The position of the anterior bend of the intracavernous segment of an ectatic carotid syphon is shown producing the prominent carotid sulcus. This should not be confused with an asymmetrically enlarged pituitary fossa.

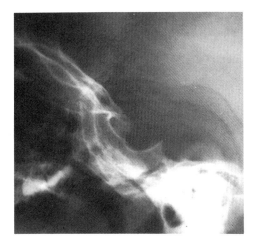
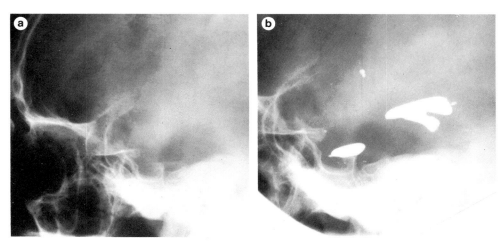

Fig. 21.10 Glioma of the optic chiasm:
lateral skull radiograph. Enlargement of the
sulcus chiasmaticus is a feature of tumours
of the optic chiasm in children. This
appearance has been referred to as the
omega-shaped sella.

Fig. 21.11 Truncation of dorsum sellae with J-shaped sella:
(a) lateral skull radiograph and (b) ventriculogram. Truncation may
be caused by any solid or cystic mass pressing on it from above (for
instance, a craniopharyngioma or dilated third ventricle). In this
example, due to long-standing aqueduct stenosis, the floor of the
dilated third ventricle is 'wafer thin'.

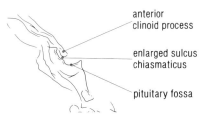

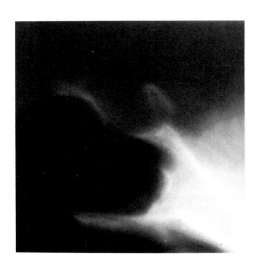
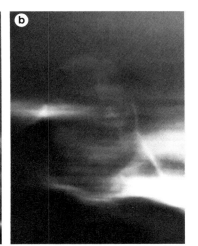

Fig. 21.12 Microadenoma: lateral
tomogram. A localised bulge with thinning of
the cortex in the antero-inferior wall of the
pituitary fossa can be seen. Such an
appearance strongly suggests an intrasellar
microadenoma although the tumour may be
some distance from the blistered wall. This
patient had grossly raised prolactin levels.

**Fig. 21.13 Intrasellar craniopharyngioma demonstrating
erosion of the clivus:** (a) lateral skull radiograph and (b) tomogram.
The extent of clival involvement is not apparent on the plain skull
radiograph. Tomography demonstrates that, although the tumour
extends through the floor of the fossa, the base of the clivus remains
intact.

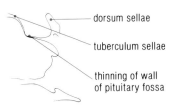
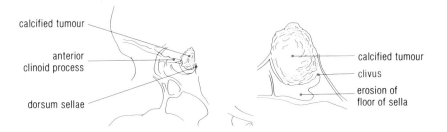

COMPUTED TOMOGRAPHY (CT)

CT should always be preceded by plain skull radiographs. When using 'second generation' (rotate/translate) scanners with a minimum slice width of 5mm, only significant sellar enlargement or extrasellar extensions (suprasellar masses greater than 1cm, or significant extensions into the cavernous sinus and temporal fossa) can be appreciated. Pre- and post-contrast scans are therefore usually necessary.

The most informative and efficient way to examine the pituitary fossa, both for primary diagnosis and follow-up is, however, by using more advanced (rotate/rotate and rotate/stationary) scanners with a thin slice capability (1–2mm). There are two equally satisfactory sequences which are commonly used after an intravenous injection of contrast containing 40–60 Gm of iodine. The first sequence involves contiguous 1.0 or 1.5mm thick axial slices from below the floor of the pituitary fossa to the inferior margin of the

anterior horns of the lateral ventricles. A special software program aligns each axial slice in the vertical plane, which enables lateral and frontal reformatted images to be produced (see Fig. 21.14a and b). These are used to produce lateral and frontal reformatted sections through the pituitary fossa. The second sequence involves direct axial and coronal scanning using 4–5 mm thick slices with the gantry angled to avoid the teeth during the latter.

The thin axial slice sequence with coronal, sagittal and oblique (along the pituitary stalk) reconstructions probably allows the most complete examination to be undertaken; however, it takes longer to perform and results in higher radiation to the globes. The normal cerebral and vascular anatomy and the presence and relationship of these structures to any intra- or parasellar mass, as well as the nature of the sellar contents, are usually revealed using this sequence.

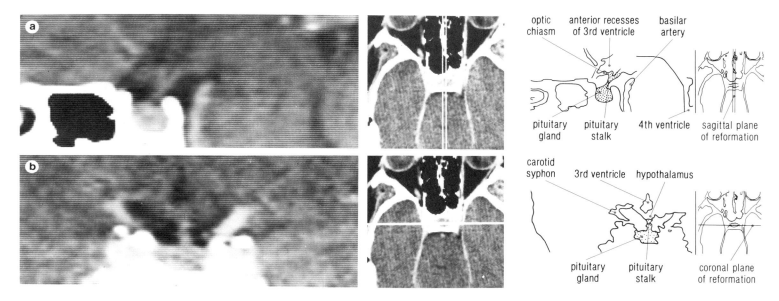

Fig. 21.14 Normal appearances: enhanced, reformatted 1.5mm thick axial CT scans after contrast, (a) lateral and (b) frontal projections together with their respective axial scans. The normal anatomy is well demonstrated.

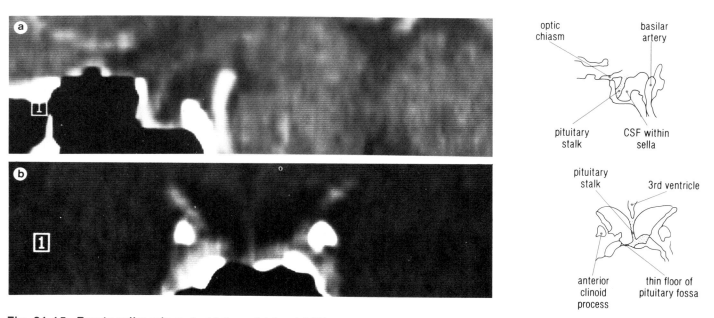

Fig. 21.15 Empty sella: reformatted 1.5 mm thick axial CT scans, (a) lateral and (b) frontal projections. The enhancing pituitary stalk projects into the sella on both lateral and frontal projections.

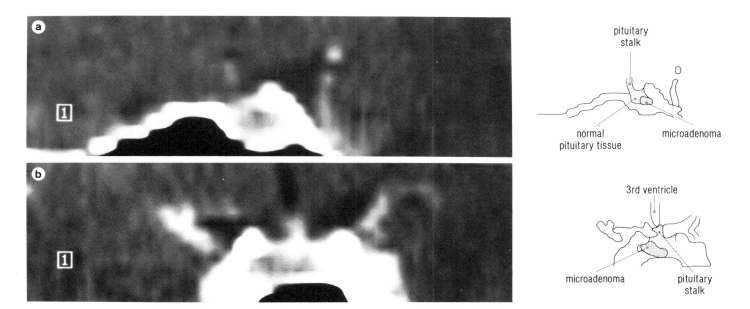

Fig. 21.16 Microadenoma: reformatted 1.5 mm thick axial CT scans after contrast, (a) lateral and (b) frontal projections. The typical prolactin-secreting microadenoma is of low density within the surrounding enhancing pituitary tissue. The upper margin of the gland is usually convex upwards and the pituitary stalk displaced to the opposite side (cf. Fig. 21.14). There may also be a depression in the floor of the fossa.

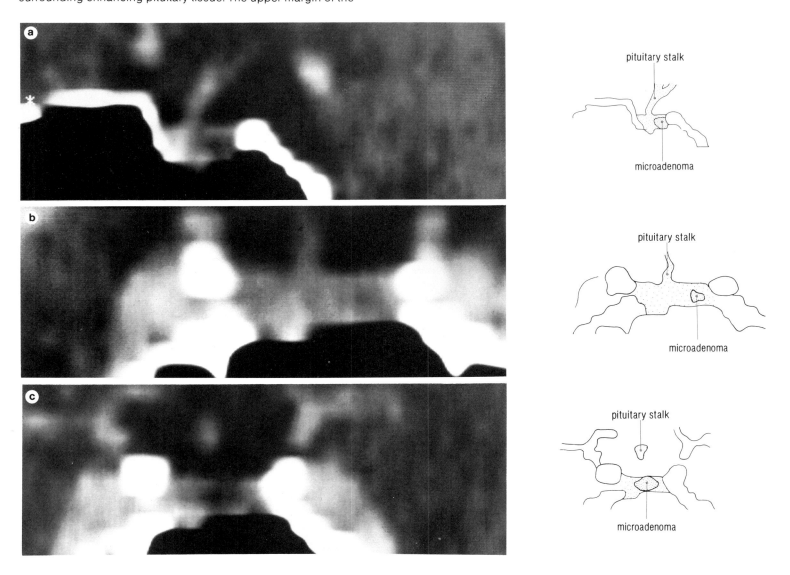

Fig. 21.17 Microadenoma: reformatted 1.5 mm thick axial CT slices after contrast, (a) lateral, (b and c) frontal projections. A small low-density microadenoma is demonstrated within the pituitary fossa. The pituitary stalk is displaced away from the adenoma. The floor of the sella slopes downwards and is deeper on the side opposite to the adenoma, demonstrating that the position of the microadenoma is not necessarily related to the bulge in the floor of the fossa.

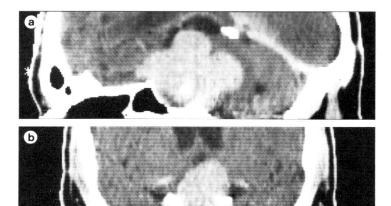

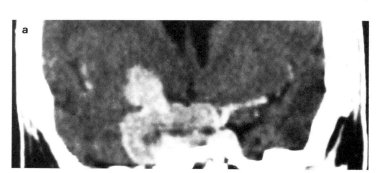

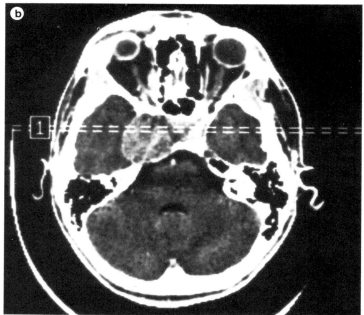

Fig. 21.18 Pituitary adenoma with huge extrasellar component: reformatted 1.5 mm thick axial CT scans after contrast, (a) lateral and (b) frontal projections. The relation between the suprasellar extension and the third ventricle is usually well demonstrated, and the distortion and elevation of the anterior recesses of the third ventricle are particularly marked on this examination. The optic chiasm may not be seen but its position can be inferred from the third ventricular recesses.

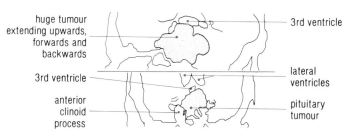

Fig. 21.19 Lateral extension of pituitary adenoma: reformatted 1.5 mm thick axial CT scans, (a) frontal projection from coronal plane reformation and (b) axial scan. Small lateral extensions are difficult to detect using any of the conventional methods of investigation currently available. Larger extensions widen the carotid syphon or displace it laterally (cf. Figs. 21.27 and 21.28). CT with reformatted thin axial slices usually provides the most information about the extent of the tumour, but may still not differentiate the tumour from the normal cavernous sinus.

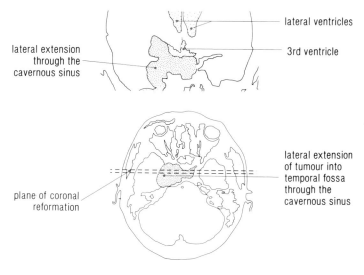

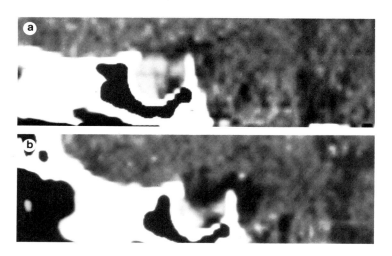

Fig. 21.20 Shrinkage of pituitary tumour in response to treatment with bromocriptine: reformatted 1.5mm thick axial CT scans, (a) before treatment and (b) six months later. The response of pituitary tumours to bromocriptine is most easily followed using reformatted thin axial slices, but where this is not available small changes are well demonstrated by positive contrast cisternography.

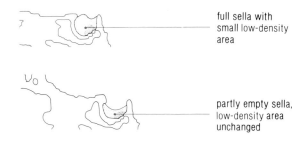

CONVENTIONAL POSITIVE CONTRAST CISTERNOGRAPHY

Conventional contrast cisternography (CCC) is a simple and safe procedure with a relatively low incidence of side-effects. It allows excellent demonstration of the perisellar anatomy except in the presence of very large suprasellar masses. CCC is of particular value in the assessment and follow-up of small suprasellar extensions where thin slice CT scanning is not available. It is also occasionally useful when there is doubt about the contents of a fossa on CT scanning, and discrimination between an empty sella and non-enhancing pituitary cyst may be made using this technique.

Cisternography is performed under image intensification (screening) with the patient in the prone position on any table with a moveable head support to enable the patient's head to be flexed or extended.

Approximately 3–6ml of isotonic, water soluble, intrathecal contrast agent (such as metrizamide, iohexol and iopamidol) is injected into the cerebrospinal fluid (CSF) through a lateral C1/2 puncture; the head is flexed to allow the contrast to flow along the clivus and into the suprasellar cistern. The patient's head is then extended so that the contrast remains within the cistern. Radiographs and tomograms are taken in the lateral and AP positions. The normal structures within and around the sella, particularly the carotid and basilar arteries, the optic chiasm and the pituitary stalk are usually well demonstrated, and their relation to any suprasellar extension can be seen. This technique can be combined to advantage with CT scanning when additional information is required or when, occasionally, the concentration of the contrast has become too dilute for conventional radiographs. Severe headaches may occur after intrathecal contrast administration. These may be alleviated by giving 1–2mg dexamethasone eight-hourly for forty-eight hours.

Conventional contrast cisternography is of limited value in large suprasellar extensions greater than 1.5cm. This is because contrast flows around the side of the mass and does not cap it. Since CCC does not define the anterior recesses of the third ventricle, the superior aspect of the mass cannot usually be appreciated.

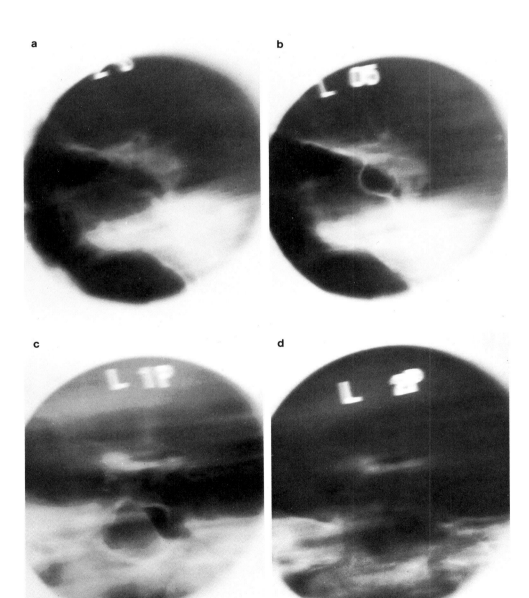

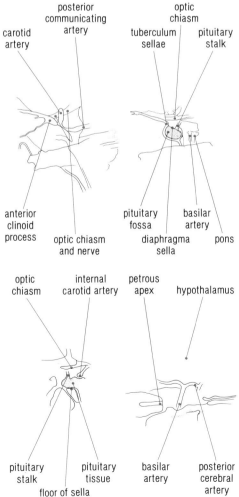

Fig. 21.21 Normal anatomy: lateral tomograms, (a) at level of anterior clinoid process and (b) in the midline; frontal tomograms, (c) through midsellar region and (d) at the level of the interpeduncular fossa.

posterior communicating artery

carotid artery

optic chiasm

tuberculum sellae

pituitary stalk

anterior clinoid process

optic chiasm and nerve

pituitary fossa

basilar artery

diaphragma sella

pons

optic chiasm

internal carotid artery

petrous apex

hypothalamus

pituitary stalk

pituitary tissue

basilar artery

posterior cerebral artery

floor of sella

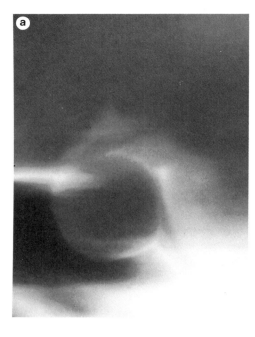

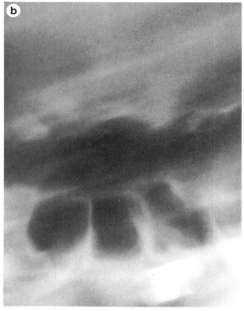

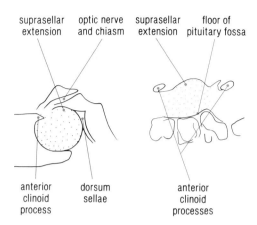

Fig. 21.22 Small suprasellar extension: tomogram, (a) lateral and (b) frontal projections. This examination, after intrathecal contrast, provides the most detailed information about the relationship of the pituitary tumour to the optic chiasm and anterior recesses of the third ventricle when the suprasellar extension is less than 1cm above the interclinoid line.

suprasellar extension optic nerve and chiasm suprasellar extension floor of pituitary fossa

anterior clinoid process dorsum sellae anterior clinoid processes

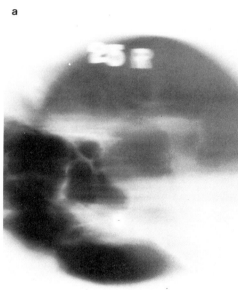

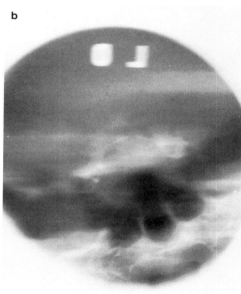

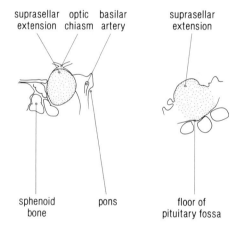

Fig. 21.23 Moderate suprasellar extension: tomogram, (a) lateral and (b) frontal projections. There is a large pituitary tumour with a significant suprasellar extension reaching the optic chiasm. The anterior end of the third ventricle is demonstrated in negative contrast.

suprasellar extension optic chiasm basilar artery suprasellar extension

sphenoid bone pons floor of pituitary fossa

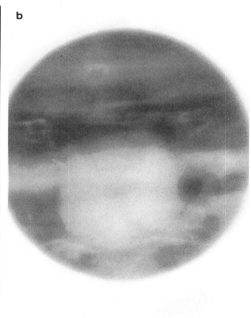

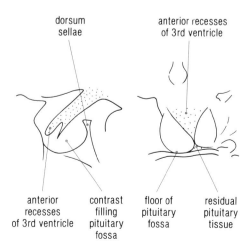

Fig. 21.24 Empty sella: tomogram, (a) lateral and (b) frontal projections. The anterior recesses of the third ventricle lie low in the pituitary fossa. This patient with acromegaly had previously been treated with radiotherapy.

dorsum sellae anterior recesses of 3rd ventricle

anterior recesses of 3rd ventricle contrast filling pituitary fossa floor of pituitary fossa residual pituitary tissue

21.10

ANGIOGRAPHY

The main functions of cerebral angiography in the pituitary are to exclude the possibility of an aneurysm, either as the main mass or as an associated finding, and to demonstrate the vascular anatomy prior to surgery. Bilateral carotid arteriograms are usually undertaken by catheter using the femoral approach. AP and lateral sequences demonstrate the vascular anatomy to best advantage. When an associated aneurysm is found, further views are used to demonstrate its neck.

Venous digital subtraction angiography may also be used to advantage where available. An intravenous injection of contrast is given by pump injection through a cannula in the basilic vein or by insertion of a catheter into the vena cava or right atrium. Imaging of the carotid vessels is usually sufficient to exclude a significantly-sized aneurysm and demonstrates the anatomy well. The technique is simple and quick. Other abnormal features which may be demonstrated are listed in Figure 21.33.

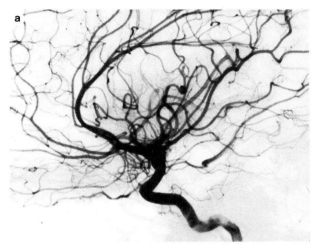
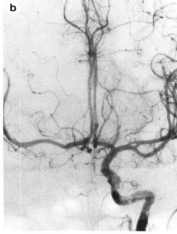

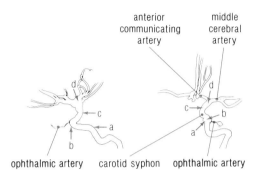

Fig. 21.25   Normal carotid syphon: angiogram, (a) lateral and (b) frontal projections. The segments of the carotid syphon labelled a to d indicate the same point on each view respectively.

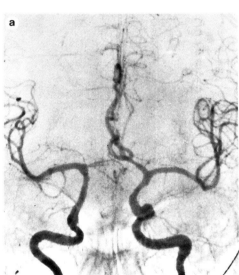
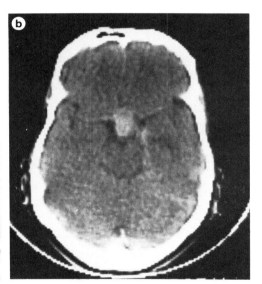

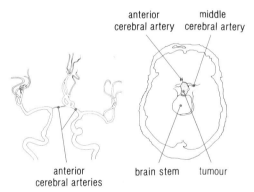

Fig. 21.26   Suprasellar extension on arterial angiography: (a) carotid angiogram frontal projection and (b) axial CT scan. The arterial phase of the bilateral carotid angiogram demonstrates that the anterior cerebral artery is bowed upwards by the suprasellar extension of a pituitary tumour (cf. Fig. 21.30).

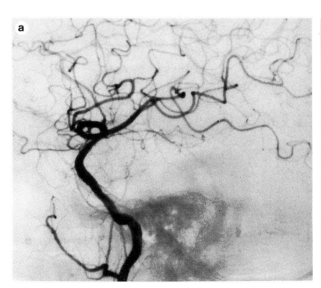
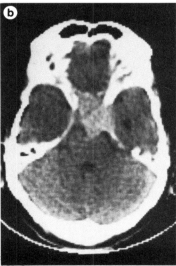

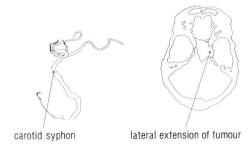

Fig. 21.27   Lateral extension on arterial angiography: (a) carotid angiogram lateral projection and (b) axial CT scan. The carotid syphon is sometimes opened by extension of a pituitary tumour into both the cavernous sinus and medial part of the temporal fossa. The corresponding axial CT slice demonstrates the lateral extension of the tumour.

21.11

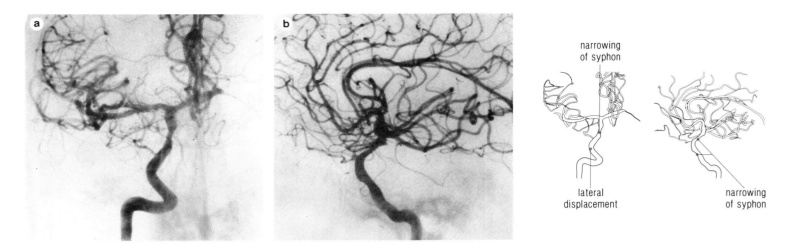

Fig. 21.28 Lateral extension on arterial angiography: carotid angiograms, (a) frontal and (b) lateral projections. The carotid syphon may be displaced laterally by tumours extending into the cavernous sinus, and may also become narrowed or occluded by an encircling tumour.

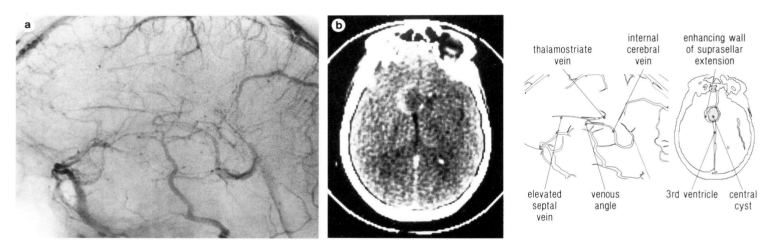

Fig. 21.29 Suprasellar extension on venous angiography: (a) venous phase lateral angiogram and (b) axial CT scan. There is elevation of the septal vein caused by the large, partly cystic, suprasellar extension of a pituitary tumour shown on the enhanced CT scan.

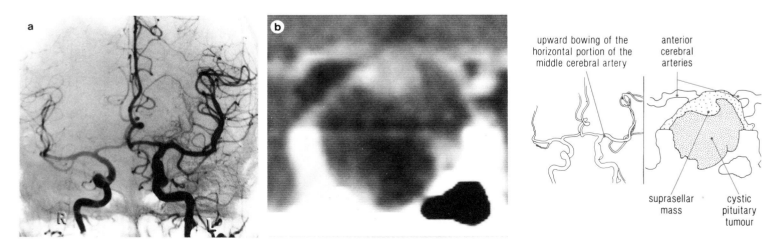

Fig. 21.30 Suprasellar extension on arterial angiography: (a) carotid angiogram frontal projection and (b) CT scan, frontal projection. There is suprasellar extension without displacement of the anterior cerebral arteries. Usually extensions of greater than 1 cm cause upward bowing of the horizontal portion of the anterior cerebral arteries. This may not occur, however, if either the carotid syphons are unfolded or the tumour projects upwards and backwards.

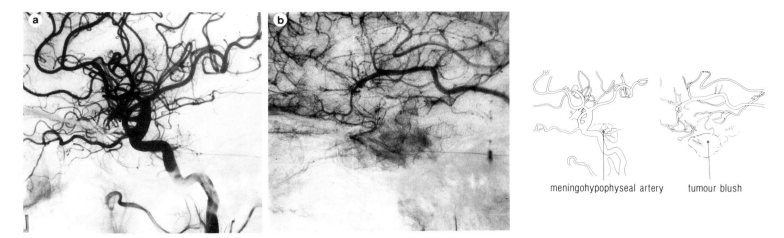

Fig. 21.31 Enlargement of the meningohypophyseal trunk with tumour blush: carotid angiogram (a) arterial and (b) venous phases. A pituitary tumour supplied by the hypophyseal branch of the meningohypophyseal artery is shown. Although most frequently supplied by this particular vessel, a tumour may take its blood supply from any meningeal branch in the neighbourhood into which the tumour enlarges. Large pituitary adenomas commonly 'blush' in the capillary and venous phases of a carotid arteriogram.

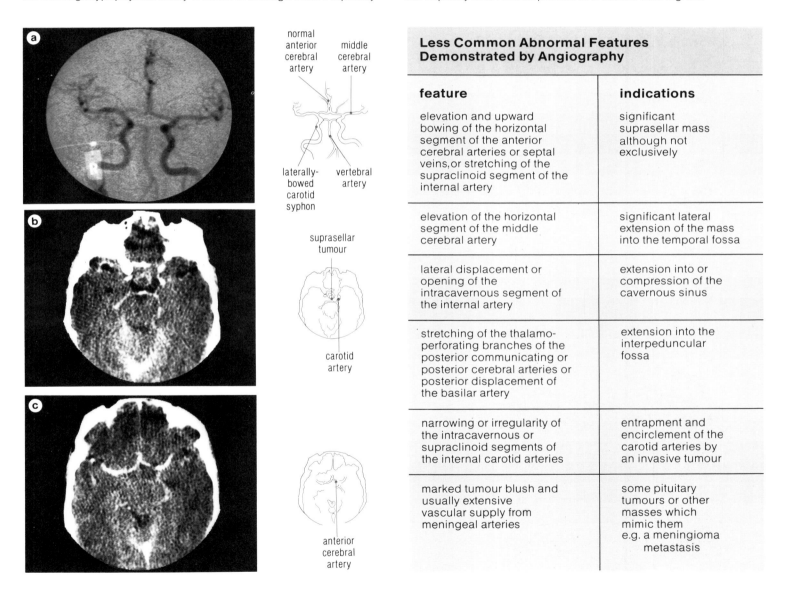

Fig. 21.32 Suprasellar tumour: (a) digital subtraction angiogram, frontal projection, (b and c) post-contrast intravenous axial CT scans. There is good filling of both internal carotid and also anterior and middle cerebral arteries. The cavernous portion of the internal carotid arteries are bowed laterally but there is no elevation of the anterior cerebral arteries since they lie anterior to the suprasellar extension. The angiogram excludes an aneurysm.

Fig. 21.33 Table of abnormal features, other than aneurysms, which may be demonstrated by angiography.

Less Common Abnormal Features Demonstrated by Angiography

feature	indications
elevation and upward bowing of the horizontal segment of the anterior cerebral arteries or septal veins, or stretching of the supraclinoid segment of the internal artery	significant suprasellar mass although not exclusively
elevation of the horizontal segment of the middle cerebral artery	significant lateral extension of the mass into the temporal fossa
lateral displacement or opening of the intracavernous segment of the internal artery	extension into or compression of the cavernous sinus
stretching of the thalamo-perforating branches of the posterior communicating or posterior cerebral arteries or posterior displacement of the basilar artery	extension into the interpeduncular fossa
narrowing or irregularity of the intracavernous or supraclinoid segments of the internal carotid arteries	entrapment and encirclement of the carotid arteries by an invasive tumour
marked tumour blush and usually extensive vascular supply from meningeal arteries	some pituitary tumours or other masses which mimic them e.g. a meningioma metastasis

21.13

PNEUMOENCEPHALOGRAPHY

Pneumoencephalography (PEG) is rarely required nowadays since most of the information obtained by this method is achieved either by lateral and frontal reformatted axial CT scans, or by water-soluble contrast cisternography. However, where CT scanning is not available, PEG is the only examination which outlines the margins of large suprasellar and lateral extensions and which shows distortions of the normal anatomy, especially of the third ventricle.

The standard technique is modified by limiting it to the examination of the sellar region only. It is preferably performed under general anaesthesia or neuroleptanalgesia. Air (10ml) is injected into the spinal canal by lumbar puncture, with the patient upright and the neck flexed to fill the ventricular system. A further 10–15ml is then injected with the neck extended so that air enters the cisterns. Plain radiographs and tomograms are taken in the erect and supine positions (the latter being required to visualise the anterior recesses of the third ventricle). The temporal horns are filled with air after performing a forward 360° somersault.

The side-effects of PEG, particularly headache and vomiting which can be severe, may also be mitigated by the administration of dexamethasone (see Conventional Positive Contrast Cisternography).

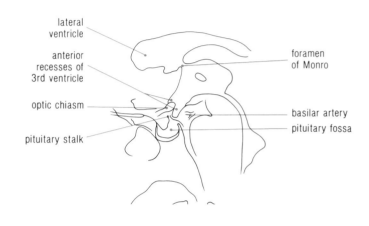

Fig. 21.34 Normal study: pneumoencephalogram, lateral projection. Tomogram taken through the midline in the 'brow up' position demonstrates the normal anatomy of the suprasellar region and also the relationship of the anterior recesses of the third ventricle to the pituitary fossa.

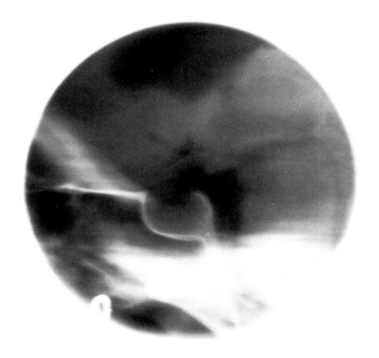

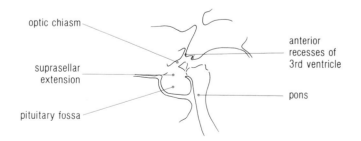

Fig. 21.35 Small suprasellar extension: pneumoencephalogram, lateral projection. There is a slight, generalised enlargement of the pituitary fossa. Although the position and shape of the anterior recesses of the third ventricle are normal, the suprasellar extension projects anteriorly to the chiasm between the optic nerves.

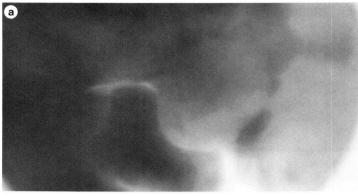

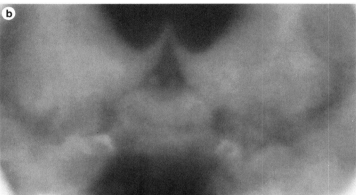

Fig. 21.36 Large suprasellar extension: pneumoencephalogram, (a) lateral and (b) frontal projections. There is gross expansion of the pituitary fossa with erosion of the dorsum sellae and a large suprasellar extension distorting the anterior recesses of the third ventricle (cf. Fig. 21.38). With conventional contrast cisternography, suprasellar masses of this size are poorly demonstrated since the contrast frequently does not 'cap' the tumour: the relationship of the tumour to the anterior recesses of the third ventricle cannot therefore be appreciated.

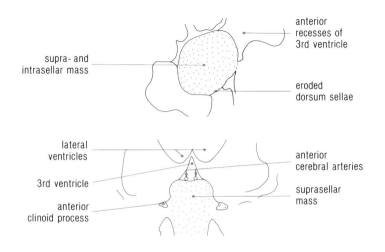

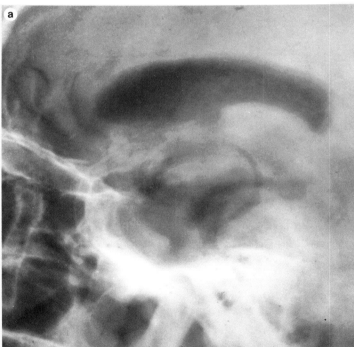

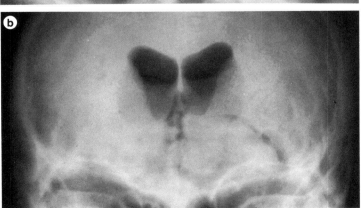

Fig. 21.37 Lateral extension: pneumoencephalogram, (a) lateral and (b) frontal projections. There is a large, left, temporal extension with elevation and lateral displacement of the temporal horn. There is also some suprasellar extension to the left of the midline displacing the third ventricle to the right.

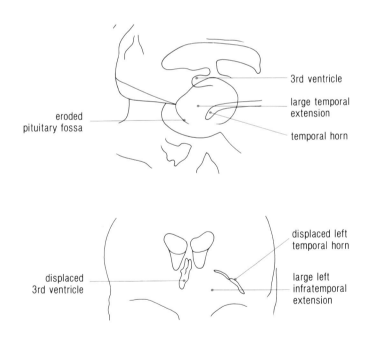

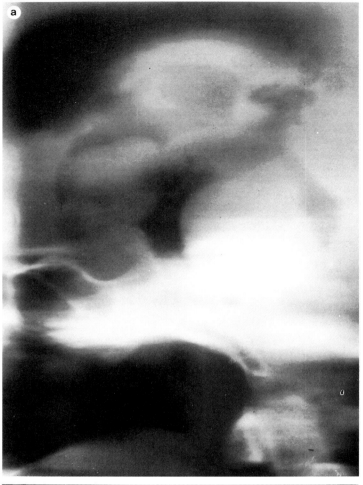

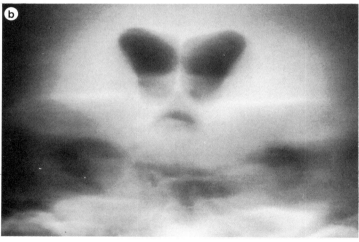

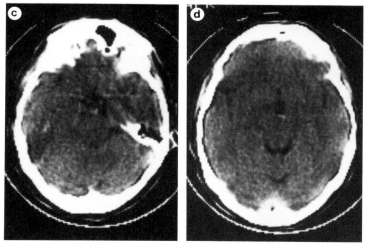

Fig. 21.38 Craniopharyngioma: tomograms,(a) lateral and (b) frontal projections; (c and d) axial CT scans. A large craniopharyngioma is compressing the anterior recesses and elevating the floor of the third ventricle. The pituitary fossa is slightly enlarged and, in the absence of calcification, a pituitary tumour is the most likely diagnosis on pneumoencephalography. However, axial CT slices, demonstrating a non-enhancing suprasellar mass, suggest the correct diagnosis. This tumour was not calcified.

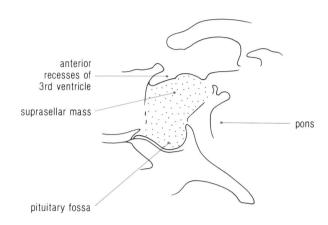

anterior recesses of 3rd ventricle

suprasellar mass

pons

pituitary fossa

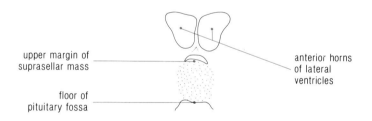

upper margin of suprasellar mass

anterior horns of lateral ventricles

floor of pituitary fossa

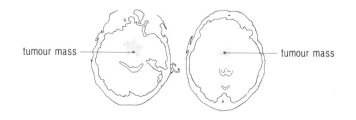

tumour mass

tumour mass

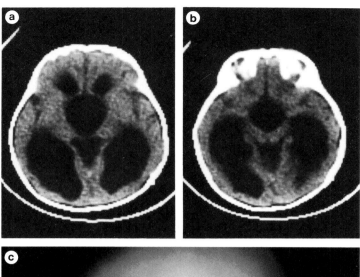

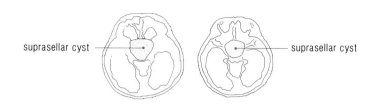

Fig. 21.39 Suprasellar arachnoid cyst: (a and b) axial CT scans and (c and d) pneumoencephalogram. The CT scans demonstrate a large mass of CSF density in the suprasellar cistern which extends from the pituitary fossa and compresses the body of the third ventricle. There is marked hydrocephalus. The pneumoencephalogram demonstrates a large suprasellar mass with air in the basal cisterns and ventricles. There is also truncation of the tip of the dorsum sellae (cf. Fig. 21.11).

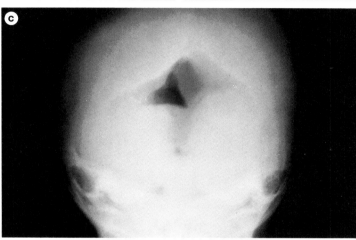

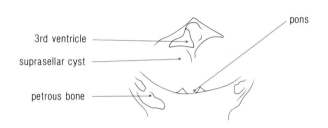

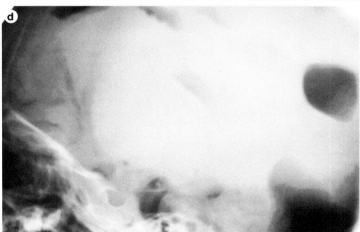

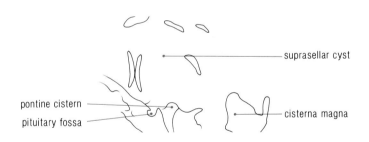

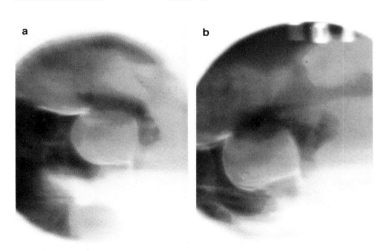

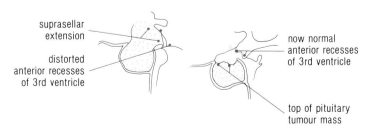

Fig. 21.40 Tumour response to treatment with bromocriptine: pneumoencephalograms, (a) before treatment and (b) 15 months later. There has been a marked reduction in tumour bulk with elimination of the suprasellar extension and restoration of the normal appearance of the anterior recesses of the third ventricle.

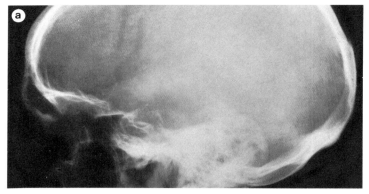

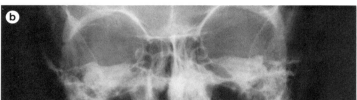

Fig. 21.41   Calcification of carotid artery and petroclinoid ligament: skull radiograph, (a) lateral and (b) frontal projections. Calcification of carotid syphon occurs frequently, but is usually less marked than in this case. It is seen as a linear calcification crossing the pituitary fossa and follows the course of the carotid artery. It is best appreciated on the lateral projection. If there is marked calcification, however, it may also be visible on the frontal projection. Calcification of the petroclinoid ligament is common and may appear as a linear streak or sometimes as a more amorphous mass on the posterior aspect of the dorsum sellae. The margins of the pituitary fossa are normal.

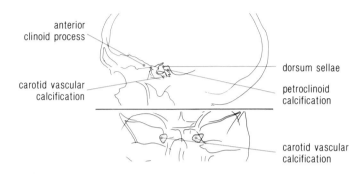

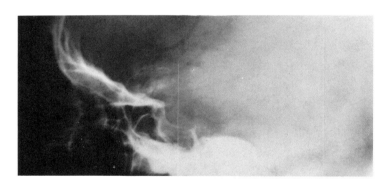

Fig. 21.42   Bilateral perisellar aneurysms: lateral skull radiograph. Calcification occurs most commonly in the wall of an aneurysm and is usually curvilinear. Occasionally, a more amorphous density indicates calcification of the contained clot.

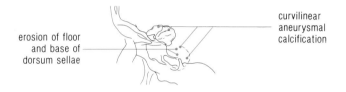

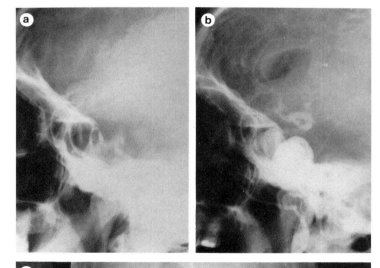

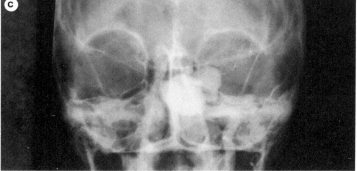

Fig. 21.43   Intrasellar aneurysm: (a) lateral skull radiograph demonstrating the absence of the floor of the pituitary fossa and also showing the curvilinear calcification overlying it, typical of an aneurysm; (b) lateral carotid angiogram and (c) frontal carotid angiogram demonstrating the filling of a large intrasellar aneurysm. Intrasellar aneurysms frequently produce erosion of the pituitary fossa which is usually unilateral (Sosman and Vogt, 1926).

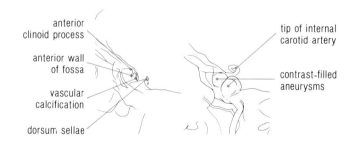

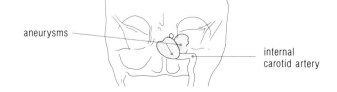

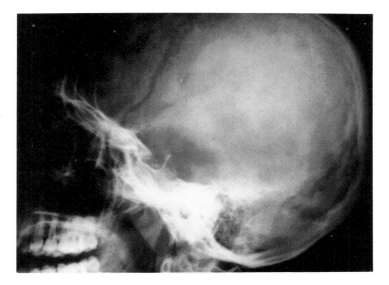

Fig. 21.44 Intrasellar craniopharyngioma: lateral skull radiograph. The pituitary fossa has an abnormal shape with a 'double bubble' to the anterior wall and floor of the dorsum sellae (omega shape) and there is punctate calcification lying within it. The patient suffered from hypopituitarism but did not exhibit any visual field defect. The intrasellar calcification was confirmed by CT but no further information was provided. The diagnosis was subsequently made at operation.

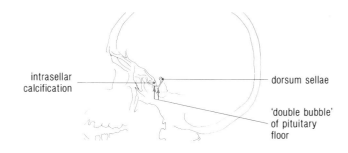

Fig. 21.45 Large suprasellar craniopharyngioma: lateral skull radiograph. There is also truncation of the tip of the dorsum sellae and posterior clinoid processes. There is a mass of amorphous calcification extending upwards from the tip of the dorsum sellae – an appearance typical of a craniopharyngioma (cf. Fig. 21.46).

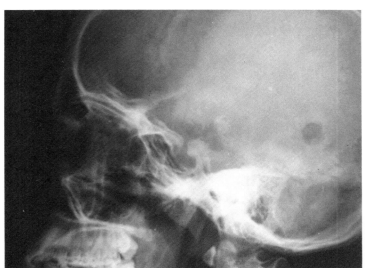

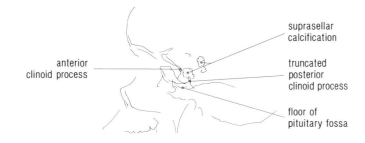

Fig. 21.46 Chordoma: (a) reformatted 1.5 mm thick axial CT slice, frontal projection and (b) lateral skull radiograph. There is extensive calcification within the pituitary fossa and in the suprasellar cistern. On the CT scan the calcification is shown to lie within the tumour. Approximately 40% of chordomas arise in the sphenoid region but account for only 1% of all intracranial tumours. Calcification occurs in approximately one third (Kendall and Lee, 1977).

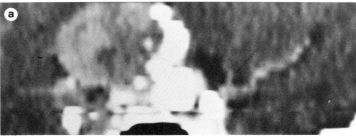

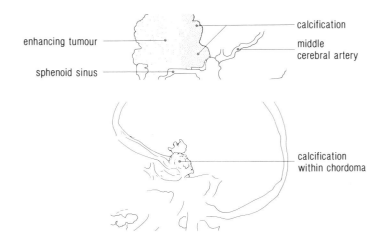

21.19

THE DIFFERENTIAL DIAGNOSIS OF CYSTIC LESIONS

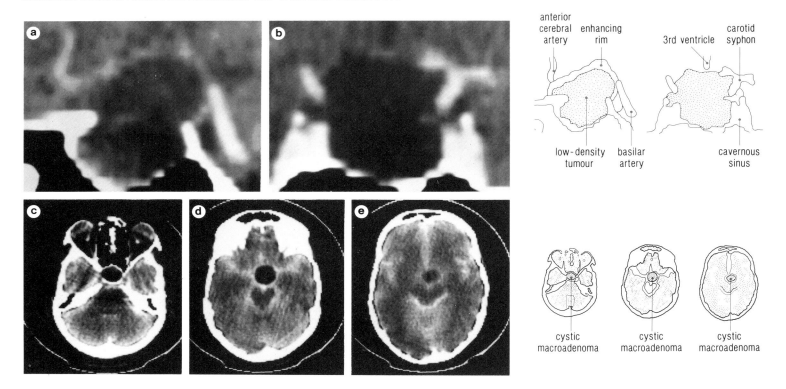

Fig. 21.47 Large, mainly 'cystic' prolactin-secreting macroadenoma: reformatted 1.5mm thick axial CT scans after contrast, (a) lateral, (b) frontal projections, (c, d and e) positive contrast CT cisternograms. This large tumour is mainly of low density with a thin enhancing rim. Positive contrast CT cisternography demonstrates contrast in the basal cisterns around the suprasellar extension; however, none has entered the cyst four hours after intrathecal contrast injections.

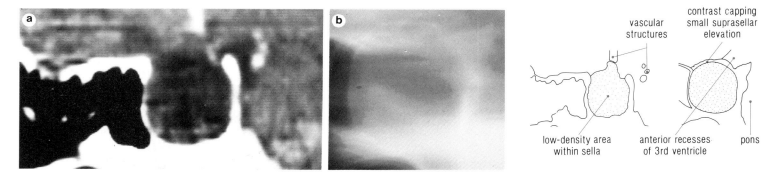

Fig. 21.48 Differentiation of pituitary cyst from empty sella: (a) lateral reformatted CT scan and (b) cisternogram. The low-density area within the enlarged pituitary fossa on CT scan is consistent with either CSF or a cystic tumour. Differentiation is difficult even on reformatted CT scans although the inability to visualise the pituitary stalk within the sella suggests a cyst. On conventional cisternography, contrast does not fill the pituitary fossa but caps a small suprasellar extension, indicating an intrasellar cyst (cf. Figs. 21.6 and 21.47).

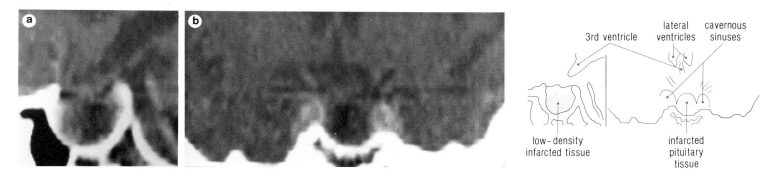

Fig. 21.49 Pituitary infarct: reformatted 1.5mm thick axial CT scans, (a) lateral and (b) frontal projections. Acromegalic patient with previously documented pituitary tumour and suprasellar extension presented with one week's history of headache and photophobia of sudden onset. Clinically diagnosed as pituitary infarction, or apoplexy, the CT appearances are consistent. The enlarged pituitary fossa contains low-density 'necrotic' tissue and there is no longer evidence of a suprasellar mass. Pituitary apoplexy is a haemorrhage into the pituitary and sometimes into the CSF. Pituitary infarction is a slower death of part or all of the pituitary and occurs most commonly in tumours.

THE DIFFERENTIAL DIAGNOSIS OF SUPRASELLAR LESIONS

Many suprasellar 'tumour' masses enhance after contrast. They may arise from the hypothalamus, optic chiasm, pituitary stalk or fossa or the neighbouring vessels, but when large the origin of the lesion is often impossible to establish. The basal meninges are also the site of metastases and granulomas. The nature of the pathological process is frequently indicated by the clinical features and radiology, but biopsy is usually necessary to establish the diagnosis where doubt exists.

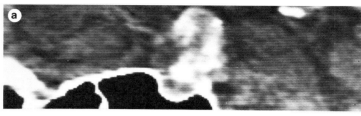

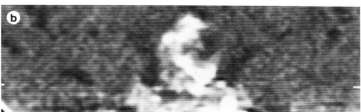

Fig. 21.50 Calcified craniopharyngioma: reformatted 1 mm thick axial CT scans after contrast, (a) lateral and (b) frontal projections. There is extensive patchy calcification throughout the enhancing tumour both within the sella and in the suprasellar extension. Although calcification may occur in pituitary tumours it is rare, and such an appearance makes a diagnosis of craniopharyngioma almost certain.

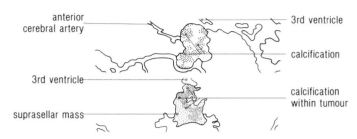

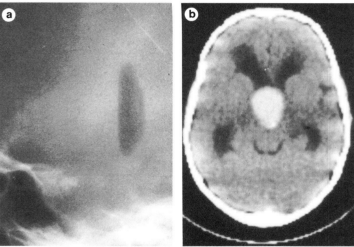
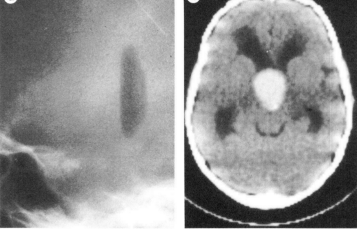

Fig. 21.51 High-density cystic craniopharyngioma: (a) cystogram and (b) axial CT scan. On the radiograph the destruction of the floor of the pituitary fossa and dorsum sellae and the calcification within the fossa can be seen. The plain CT scan demonstrates a high-density rounded mass projecting up and compressing the foramina of Monro, thus producing hydrocephalus. The cystic nature of the high-density area was established by stereotactic CT puncture demonstrating air in the cyst.

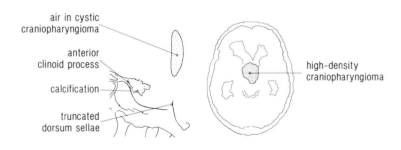

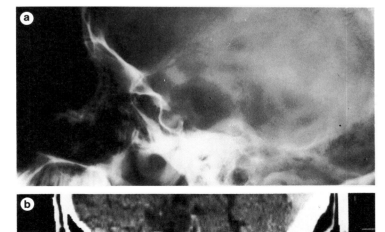

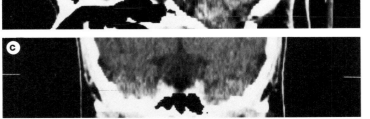

Fig. 21.52 Suprasellar epidermoid cyst: (a) lateral skull radiograph, (b and c) reformatted 1.5 mm thick axial CT scans. There is a large low-density, non-enhancing suprasellar mass which has truncated the dorsum sellae and distorted the anterior recesses of the third ventricle. The density of the mass is higher than the CSF in this ventricle but lower than that of the surrounding brain. The differential diagnosis lies between an epidermoid cyst and a non-calcified craniopharyngioma.

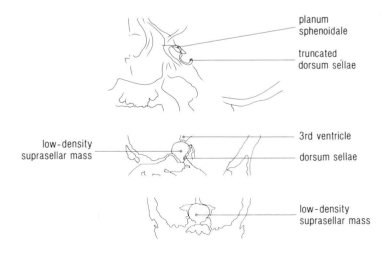

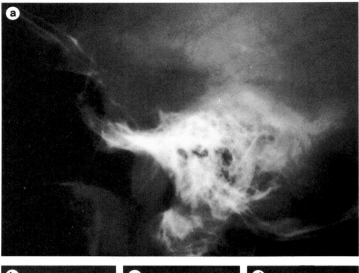

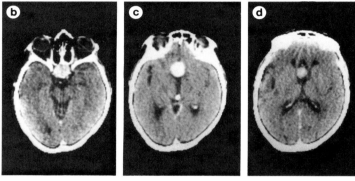

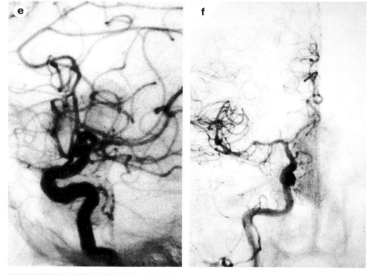

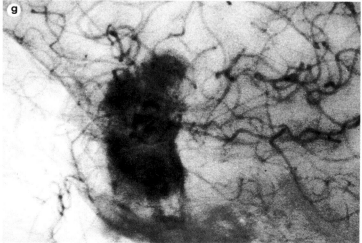

Fig. 21.53 Intra- and suprasellar meningioma: (a) plain skull radiograph showing expansion of the fossa and undercutting of the anterior clinoid process with thinning of the lamina dura and loss of the dorsum sellae; (b to d) axial CT scans showing a rounded, enhancing, partly intra- and partly suprasellar mass consistent with a pituitary adenoma; (e) lateral angiogram and (f) frontal angiogram demonstrating upward bowing of the anterior cerebral artery and the tumour supplied by the meningohypophyseal trunk; (g) the late arterial phase showing a large densely-staining intra- and suprasellar tumour. Pituitary tumours may 'blush' delicately but the staining is rarely marked. Such pronounced staining is typical of meningioma and occasionally of metastases, and, whilst the pituitary is commonly the site of metastases, intrasellar meningiomas are rare. Associated bone destruction differentiates metastases from meningiomas (which are more often associated with sclerosis and hyperostosis).

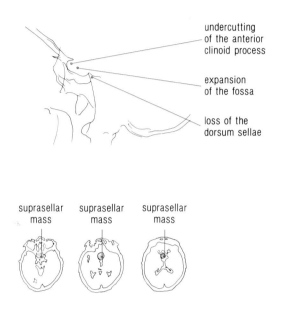

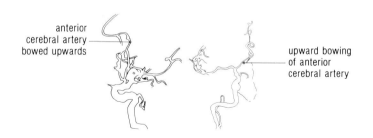

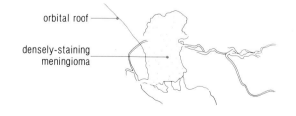

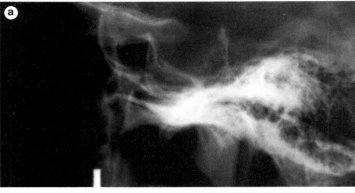

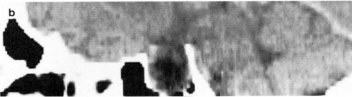

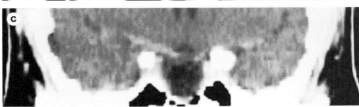

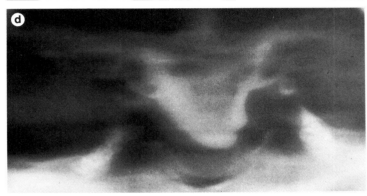

Fig. 21.54 Empty sella: (a) skull radiograph demonstrating an enlarged pituitary fossa with a double floor caused by ballooning of the anterior wall and floor of the fossa Reformatted 1.5mm thick axial CT slices, (b) lateral and (c) frontal projections and also (d), positive contrast cisternogram frontal projection, demonstrate CSF within the enlarged fossa. The anterior recesses of the third ventricle lie at the interclinoid line, thus excluding a suprasellar mass. An intrasellar cyst is excluded by the positive contrast cisternogram (d) which shows contrast within the pituitary fossa. Normal pituitary tissue is also present in the fossa (cf. Fig. 21.47).

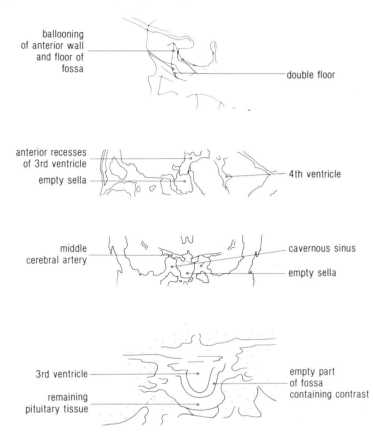

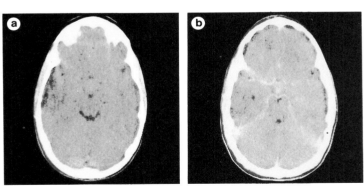

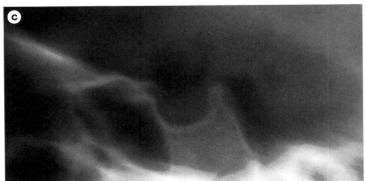

Fig. 21.55 Hamartoma of the hypothalamus: (a) pre-contrast and (b) post-contrast axial CT scans and (c) pneumoencephalogram. The axial CT scans demonstrate a rounded, isodense mass which has enhanced slightly after contrast injection. The pneumoencephalogram shows the mass arising from the hypothalamus and projecting into the suprasellar cistern surrounded by air. This radiology is of a male patient, aged 10 years, with neurofibromatosis who presented with precocious puberty.

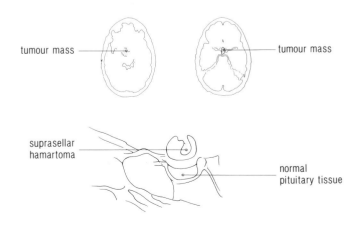

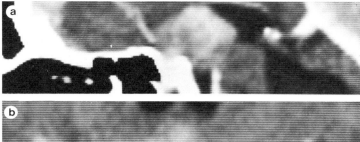

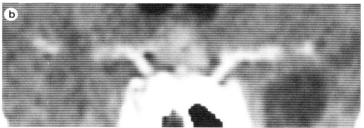

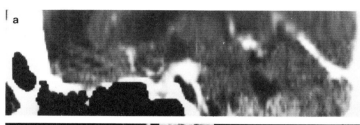

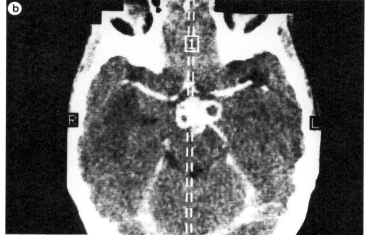

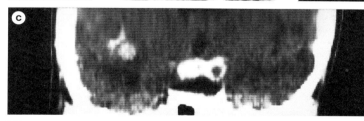

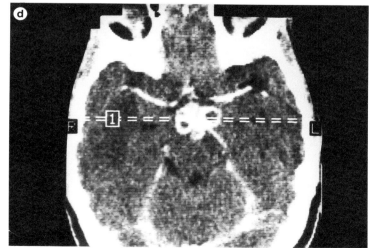

Fig. 21.56 Suprasellar and interpeduncular metastasis: reformatted 1.5 mm thick axial CT slices, (a) lateral and (b) frontal projections. There is a large enhancing suprasellar mass. Surgical removal of a posterior fossa medulloblastoma had been undertaken one year previously. Although the diagnosis was not established by biopsy, the nature of the mass was indicated by its good response to radiotherapy.

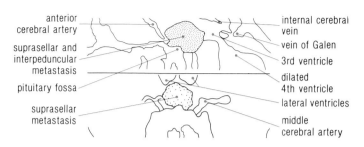

Fig. 21.57 Suprasellar tuberculomas: reformatted 1.5 mm thick axial CT slices, (a) lateral and (c) frontal projections; (b and d) corresponding axial scans. While on treatment the patient had increasing visual failure. On the CT scan there are several typical tuberculous granulomata in the suprasellar cistern, and at operation they were found to be surrounding and involving the optic chiasm and nerves and the basal arteries of the circle of Willis. Tuberculous granulomata, although not uncommon, calcify in less than 10% of cases (Ramamurthi and Varadarajan, 1961). They frequently involve the basal cisterns and may develop while on adequate therapy.

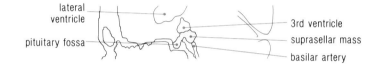

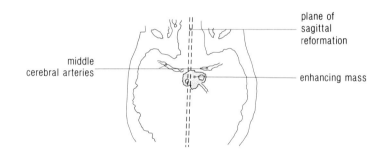

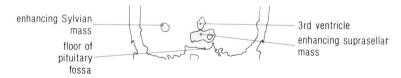

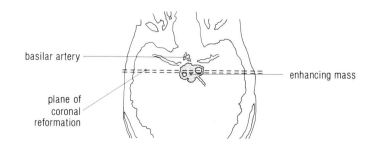

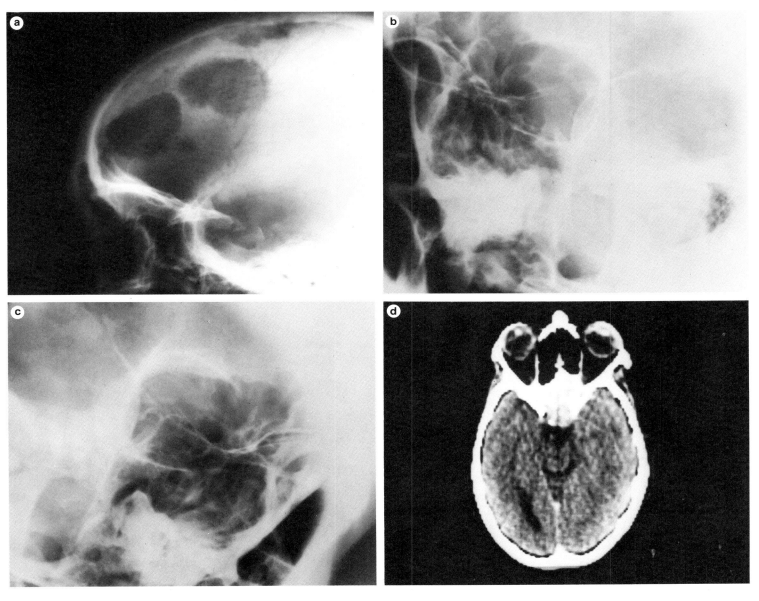

Fig. 21.58 Metastasis from carcinoma of the breast: (a) lateral skull radiograph, (b and c) radiographs of the optic foramina and (d) axial CT scan. The skull radiograph and views of the optic foramina demonstrate destruction of the boundaries of the pituitary fossa and presellar sphenoid with vault metastases. The left optic foramen is missing and there is erosion of the optic strut of the right foramen. The CT scan demonstrates an enhancing mass involving the sphenoid and pituitary fossa. Only malignant tumours will produce such extensive destruction and the presence of the other vault lesions indicates a metastasis.

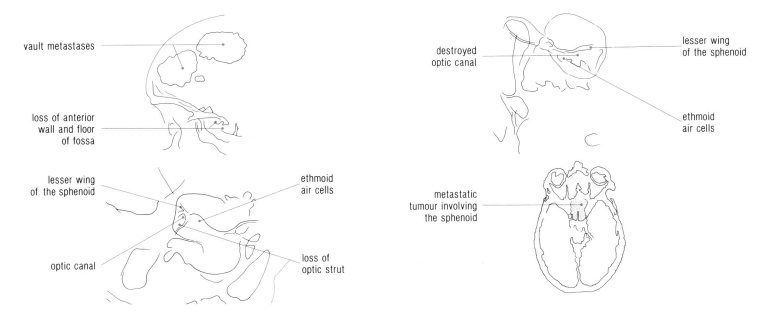

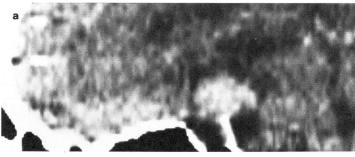

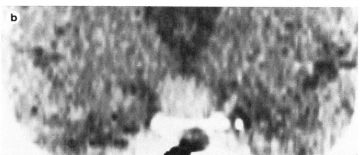

Fig. 21.59   Sarcoid granuloma: reformatted 1.5 mm thick axial slices, (a) lateral and (b) frontal projections demonstrating an enhancing suprasellar mass. The features of the lesion are non-specific. The patient presented with unilateral proptosis and increasing visual loss. Biopsy of the enlarged optic nerve demonstrated typical sarcoid granulomata. Granulomata involving the meninges occur in up to 14% of autopsy cases and are clinically evident in 3–5% of cases of systemic sarcoidosis (Kendall and Tatler, 1978).

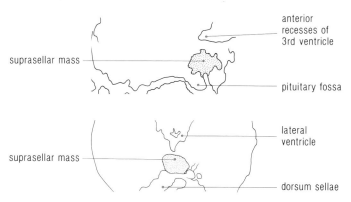

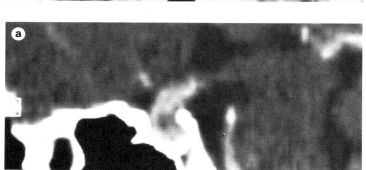

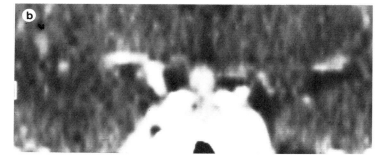

Fig. 21.60   Dysgerminoma of the pituitary stalk: reformatted 1.5 mm thick axial scans, (a) lateral and (b) frontal projections. The pituitary stalk is enlarged and enhances markedly. The third ventricle is displaced slightly to the left. This patient presented with diabetes insipidus and the diagnosis was established on biopsy. There was no definite tumour in the pituitary region.

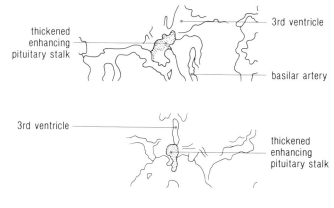

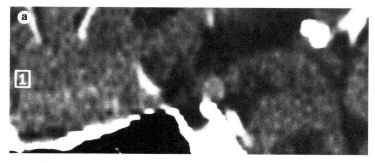

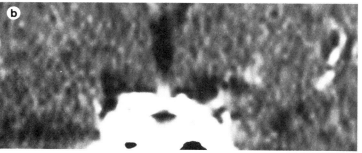

Fig. 21.61   Histiocytosis of the hypothalamus: reformatted 1.5 mm thick CT slices, (a) lateral and (b) frontal projections. Adult female patient with diabetes insipidus and a skin biopsy diagnosis of histiocytosis. There is an enhancing mass in the infundibulum and hypothalamus distorting the infundibular recess. The appearance is non-specific and can easily be confused with any cause of a small suprasellar mass. Diagnosis can only be established by biopsy. Although the triad of proptosis, diabetes insipidus and skull lesions is classical, histiocytic granulomata may occur anywhere in the cranial cavity, and may even exist without evidence of visceral or skeletal lesions (Kepes and Kepes, 1969).

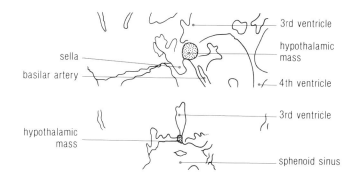

Acknowledgements

1 NEUROENDOCRINE CONTROL OF PITUITARY FUNCTION

Figure 1.1 redrawn from Reichlin S, *Introduction*. In: Reichlin S, Baldessarini RJ, Martin JB eds., *The Hypothalamus*. 1977: 1-14. Courtesy of Raven Press, New York.

Figure 1.2 redrawn from Gay VL, *The hypothalamus: physiology and clinical use of releasing factors*. Fertility and Sterility 1972; **23**: 50-63. Courtesy of the American Fertility Society, Baltimore.

Figures 1.3a and 1.3b reproduced from Lechan RM, Nestler JL, Jacobson S, *The tuberoinfundibular system of the rat as demonstrated by immunohistochemical localization of retrogradely transported wheat germ agglutinin (WGA) from the median eminence*. Brain Research 1982; **245**: 1-15. Courtesy of Elsevier Biomedical Press BV, Amsterdam.

Figure 1.4b reproduced from Reichlin S, *Neuroendocrinology*. In: Williams RH ed., *Textbook of Endocrinology*. 6th edition. 1981: 589-645. Courtesy of WB Saunders Company, Philadelphia.

Figures 1.9 and 1.15 redrawn from Reichlin S, *Neuroendocrinology*. In: Wilson JD, Foster DW eds., *Williams – Textbook of Endocrinology*. 7th edition. 1985: 492-567. Courtesy of WB Saunders Company, Philadelphia.

Figure 1.12 redrawn from Crowley WF Jr, McArthur JW, *Simulation of the normal menstrual cycle in Kallman's syndrome by pulsatile administration of luteinizing hormone-releasing hormone (LHRH)*. Journal of Clinical Endocrinology and Metabolism 1980; **51**: 173-175. Courtesy of Williams and Wilkins Company, Baltimore.

Figure 1.13 redrawn from Belchetz PE, Plant TM, Nakai Y, Keogh EJ, Knobil, E, *Hypophysial responses to continuous and intermittent delivery of hypothalamic gonadotropin-releasing hormone*. Science 1978; **202**: 631-633. Courtesy of the American Association for the Advancement of Science, Washington.

Figure 1.14 redrawn from Thorner MO, Rivier J, Spiess J, Borges JL, Vance ML, Bloom SR, Rogol AD, Cronin MJ, Kaiser DL, Evans WS, Webster JD, MacLeod RM, Vale W, *Human pancreatic growth-hormone-releasing factor selectively stimulates growth-hormone secretion in man*. Lancet 1983; **1**: 24-28. Courtesy of Lancet Ltd., London.

Figure 1.17 redrawn from Grossman A, Kruseman ACN, Perry L, Tomlin S, Schally AV, Coy DH, Rees LH, Comaru-Schally A-M, Besser GM, *New Hypothalamic hormone, corticotropin-releasing factor, specifically stimulates the release of adrenocorticotropic hormone and cortisol in man*. Lancet 1982; **1**: 921-922. Courtesy of Lancet Ltd., London.

Figures 1.18 and 1.19 redrawn from Martin JB, Reichlin S, Brown GM, *Clinical Neuroendocrinology*. 1977: 410pp. Courtesy of FA Davis Company, Philadelphia.

For kind provision of slides: Dr RM Lechan, Dr L Alpert and Dr JC King.

2 HYPOPITUITARISM

For kind provision of slides: Professor I Doniach.

3 ACROMEGALY

Figures 3.3 and 3.21 reproduced from Wass JAH, *Acromegaly*, and *Treatment of massive tumours: medical treatment*. In: Belchetz PE ed., *Management of Pituitary Disease*. 1984: 123-140 and 415-423. Courtesy of Chapman and Hall Ltd., London.

Figure 3.13 redrawn from Laws ER, Piepgras DG, Randall RV, Abboud CF, *Neurosurgical management of acromegaly*. Journal of Neurosurgery 1979; **50**: 454-461. Courtesy of the American Association of Neurological Surgeons, Hanover.

Figure 3.16 redrawn from Besser GM, Wass JAH, *The medical management of acromegaly*. In: Black P McL, Zervas NT, Ridgeway EC, Martin JB eds., *Secretory Tumours of the Pituitary Gland*. Progress in Endocrine Research and Therapy 1984; **1**: 155-168. Courtesy of Raven Press, New York.

Figure 3.19 redrawn from Thorner MO, Chait A, Aitken M, Benker G, Bloom SR, Mortimer CH, Sanders P, Stuart Mason A, Besser GM, *Bromocriptine treatment of acromegaly*. British Medical Journal 1975; **1**: 299-303. Courtesy of the British Medical Journal, London.

4 HYPERPROLACTINAEMIA

Figure 4.23 reproduced from Thorner MO, Martin WH, Rogol AD, Morris JL, Perryman RL, Conway BP, MacLeod RM, *Rapid regression of pituitary prolactinomas during bromocriptine treatment*. Journal of Clinical Endocrinology and Metabolism 1980; **51**: 438-445. Courtesy of Williams and Wilkins, Baltimore.

For kind provision of slides: Dr G Tindall.

5 THE POSTERIOR PITUITARY

Secretarial assistance: Mrs SA Mishreki.

7 CUSHING'S SYNDROME

We thank our many colleagues, clinical, radiological and pathological, for their contributions to this work, and particularly to Professor GM Besser, Professor I Doniach, Dr FE White and Mr GM Rees for permission to use their slides.

8 ADDISON'S DISEASE

For kind provision of slides: Professor I Doniach.

10 THE TESTIS

Figure 10.7 redrawn from Hayashi H, Harrison RG, *The development of the interstitial tissue of the human testis*. Fertility and Sterility 1971; **22**: 351. Courtesy of The American Fertility Society, Baltimore.

Figure 10.14 redrawn from Imperato-McGinley J, Guerrero L, Gautier T, Peterson RE, *Steroid 5α-reductase deficiency in man: an inherited form of male pseudohermaphroditism*. Science 1974; **186**: 1213-1215. Courtesy of The American Association for the Advancement of Science, Washington.

For kind provision of slides: Professor I Doniach, Professor RHT Edwards and Dr WE Kenyon.

11 THE OVARY

For kind provision of slides: Professor I Doniach, Dr JW Keeling and Dr PR Wheater.

12 NORMAL AND ABNORMAL SEXUAL DEVELOPMENT AND PUBERTY

Figures 12.2, 12.3 and 12.5 reproduced from Tanner JM, *Growth at Adolescence*. 1962. Courtesy of Blackwell Scientific Publications, Oxford.

Figure 12.4 redrawn from Winter JSD, Faiman C, *Pituitary gonadal relations in male children and adolescents*. Pediatric Research 1972; **6**: 126-135. Courtesy of Williams and Wilkins Company, Baltimore.

Figure 12.6 redrawn from Marshall WA, Tanner JM, *Variations in the pattern of pubertal changes in girls*. Archives of Disease in Childhood 1969; **44**: 291-303. Courtesy of The British Medical Association, London.

Figure 12.7 redrawn from Marshall WA, Tanner JM, *Variations in the pattern of pubertal changes in boys*. Archives of Disease in Children 1970; **45**: 13-23. Courtesy of The British Medical Association, London.

Figure 12.8 redrawn from Tanner JM, *Growth and endocrinology of the adolescent*. In: Gardner LI ed., *Endocrine and Genetic Diseases of Childhood Vol II*. 1975. Courtesy of WB Saunders Company, Philadelphia.

Figure 12.9 redrawn from Frisch RE, McArthur JW, *Menstrual cycles: fatness as a determinant of minimum weight for height necessary for their maintenance or onset*. Science 1974; **185**: 949-951. Courtesy of the American Association for the Advancement of Science, Washington.

Figure 12.11 redrawn from Laron Z, Arad J, Gurewitz R, Grunebaum M, Dickerman Z, *Age at first conscious ejaculation: a milestone in male puberty*. Helvetica Paediatrica Acta 1980; **35**: 13-20. Courtesy of Schwabe and Company, Basel.

Figure 12.12 redrawn from Smith DW, *Growth and its disorders: basics and standards, approach and classifications, growth deficiency disorders, growth excess disorders, obesity*. Major Problems in Clinical Pediatrics 1977; **15**: 1-155. Courtesy of WB Saunders Company, Philadelphia.

Figures 12.16 and 12.17 redrawn from Winter JSD, Hughes IA, Reyes FI, Faiman C, *Pituitary-gonadal relations in infancy: 2. Patterns of serum gonadal steroid concentrations in man from birth to two years of age*. Journal of Clinical Endocrinology and Metabolism 1976; **42**: 679-686. Courtesy of Williams and Wilkins Company, Baltimore.

Figure 12.18 redrawn from Knorr D, Bidlingmaier F, Butenandt O, Fendel H, Ehrt-Wehle R, *Plasma testosterone in male puberty. I. Physiology of plasma testosterone*. Acta Endocrinologica 1974; **75**: 181-194. Courtesy of Periodica, Copenhagen.

Figure 12.19 redrawn from Reiter EO, Fuldauer VG, Root AW, *Secretion of the adrenal androgen, dehydroepiandrosterone sulfate, during normal infancy, childhood and adolescence, in sick infants, and in children with endocrinologic abnormalities*. Journal of Pediatrics 1977; **90**: 766-770. Courtesy of The CV Mosby Company, St. Louis.

Figure 12.20 redrawn from Weitzman ED, Boyar RM, Kapen S, Hellman L, *The relationship of sleep and sleep stages to neuroendocrine secretion and biological rhythms in man*. Recent Progress in Hormone Research 1975; **31**: 399-441. Courtesy of Academic Press, Orlando.

Figures 12.21 and 12.22 redrawn from Winter JSD, Faiman C, *The development of cyclic pituitary gonadal function in adolescent females*. Journal of Clinical Endocrinology and Metabolism 1973; **37**: 714-718. Courtesy of Williams and Wilkins Company, Baltimore.

Figure 12.27 redrawn from Conte FA, Grumbach MM, Kaplan SL, *A diphasic pattern of gonadotropin secretion in patients with the syndrome of gonadal dysgenesis*. Journal of Clinical Endocrinology and Metabolism 1975; **40**: 670-674. Courtesy of Williams and Wilkins Company, Baltimore.

Figure 12.29 redrawn from Grumbach MM, Richards HE, Conte FA, Kaplan SL, *Clinical disorders of adrenal function and puberty*. In: James VHT, Serio M, Giusti G, Martini L eds., *The Endocrine Function of the Human Adrenal Cortex*. Proceedings of the Serono Symposium 1978; **18**: 583-612. Courtesy of Academic Press, London.

Figure 12.30 redrawn from Grumbach MM, *The neuroendocrinology of puberty*. In: Krieger DT, Hughes JC eds., *Neuroendocrinology*. 1980: 249-258. Courtesy of Hospital Practice Publishing Company Inc., New York.

Figures 12.40 and 12.41 redrawn from Frisch RE, Gotz-Welbergen AV, McArthur JW, Albright T, Witschi J, Bullen B, Birnholz J, Reed RB, Hermann H, *Delayed menarche and amenorrhoea of college athletes in relation to age of onset of training*. Journal of the American Medical Association 1981; **246**: 1559-1563. Courtesy of the American Medical Association, Chicago.

Figures 12.42 and 12.43 redrawn from Warren MP, *The effects of exercise on pubertal progression and reproductive function in girls*. Journal of Clinical Endocrinology and Metabolism 1980; **51**: 1150-1157. Courtesy of Williams and Wilkins Company, Baltimore.

Figure 12.63 redrawn from Comite F, Cutler GB, Rivier J, Vale WW, Loriaux DL, Crowley WF, *Short-term treatment of idiopathic precocious puberty with a long-acting analogue of luteinizing hormone-releasing hormone*. New England Journal of Medicine 1981; **305**: 1546-1550. Courtesy of the New England Journal of Medicine, Massachusetts.

For kind provision of slides: Dr D Grant and Dr PHW Rayner.

13 THYROID PHYSIOLOGY AND HYPOTHYROIDISM

For kind provision of slides: Professor I Doniach.

15 HYPERTHYROIDISM AND GRAVES' DISEASE

For kind provision of slides: Dr F Clarke, Dr I Hughes, Professor GS Kilpatrick, Dr J Lazarus, Dr R Staughton, Department of Medical Illustration, University of Wales College of Medicine and Department of Medical Illustration, Westminster Hospital, London.

17 CALCIUM AND COMMON ENDOCRINE BONE DISORDERS

Figures 17.7 and 17.8 redrawn from Fisken RA, Heath DA, Bold AM, *Hypercalcaemia – A hospital survey*. Quarterly Journal of Medicine 1980; **49**: 405-418. Courtesy of Oxford University Press, Oxford.

Figure 17.21 redrawn from Marx SJ, Attie MF, Levine MA, Spiegel AM, Downs RW, Lasker RD, *The hypocalciuric or benign variant of familial hypercalcaemia: clinical and biochemical features in fifteen kindreds*. Medicine 1981; **60**: 397-412. Courtesy of Williams and Wilkins Company, Baltimore.

For kind provision of slides: Dr JD Hosking, Professor EL Jones and Dr KJ Shah.

20 RADIOLOGY OF ENDOCRINE DISEASE

Figures 20.19 and 20.22 reproduced from White FE, White MC, Drury PL, Kelsey Fry I, Besser GM, *Value of computed tomography of the abdomen and chest in the investigation of Cushing's syndrome*. British Medical Journal 1982; **284**: 771-774. Courtesy of the British Medical Journal, London.

21 NEURORADIOLOGY OF THE PITUITARY AND HYPOTHALAMUS

I would like to thank Miss Wendy Pidgeon for her secretarial assistance.

References

1 NEUROENDOCRINE CONTROL OF PITUITARY FUNCTION

Brazeau P, Vale W, Burgus R, Ling N, Butcher M, Rivier J, Guillemin R, *Hypothalamic polypeptide that inhibits the secretion of immunoreactive pituitary growth hormone*. Science 1973; **179**: 77-79.

Campbell HJ, Feuer G, Harris GW, *The effect of intrapituitary infusion of median eminence and other brain extracts on anterior pituitary gonadotrophic secretion*. Journal of Physiology 1964; **170**: 474-486.

Du Vigneaud V, Gish DT, Katsoyannis PG, Hess GP, *Synthesis of the pressor-antidiuretic hormone, arginine-vasopressin*. Journal of the American Chemical Society 1958; **80**: 3355.

Du Vigneaud V, Ressler C, Trippett S, *The sequence of amino acids in oxytocin, with a proposal for the structure of oxytocin*. Journal of Biological Chemistry 1953; **205**: 949-957.

Grossman A, Kruseman ACN, Perry L, Tomlin S, Schally AV, Coy DH, Rees LH, Comaru-Schally A-M, Besser GM, *New hypothalamic hormone, corticotropin-releasing factor, specifically stimulates the release of adrenocorticotropic hormone and cortisol in man*. Lancet 1982; **1**: 921-922.

Guillemin R, Brazeau P, Böhlen P, Esch F, Ling N, Wehrenberg WB, *Growth hormone-releasing hormone from a human pancreatic tumour that caused acromegaly*. Science 1982; **218**: 585-587.

Guillemin R, Burgus R, Vale W, *The hypothalamic hypophysiotropic thyrotropin-releasing factor*. Vitamins and Hormones 1971; **29**: 1-39.

Kamberi IA, Mical RS, Porter JC, *Hypophysial portal vessel infusion: in vivo demonstration of LRF, FRF and PIF in pituitary stalk plasma*. Endocrinology 1971; **89**: 1042-1046.

Krulich L, Dhariwal AP, McCann SM, *Stimulatory and inhibitory effects of purified hypothalamic extracts on growth hormone release from rat pituitary* in vitro. Endocrinology 1968; **83**: 783-790.

McCann SM, Taleisnik S, Friedman HM, *LH-releasing activity in hypothalamic extracts*. Society for Experimental Biology: Medical Proceedings 1960; **104**: 432-434.

Martin JB, Reichlin S, Brown GM, *Clinical Neuroendocrinology*. 2nd edition. FA Davis, Philadelphia 1986: in Press.

Meites J, *Control of mammary growth and lactation*. In: Martini L, Ganong WF eds., *Neuroendocrinology*. Volume I. Academic Press, New York 1966: 669-707.

Reichlin S, *Neuroendocrinology*. In: Wilson JD, Foster DW eds., *Williams-Textbook of Endocrinology*. 7th edition. WB Saunders Company, Philadelphia 1985: 492-567.

Saffran M, Schally AV, Benfrey BG, *Stimulation of the release of corticotropin from the adenohypophysis by neurohypophysial factor*. Endocrinology 1955; **57**: 439-444.

Schally AV, Kastin AJ, Arimura A, *Hypothalamic follicle-stimulating hormone (FSH) and luteinizing hormone (LH)-regulating hormone: structure, physiology and clinical studies*. Fertility and Sterility 1971; **22**: 703-721.

Scharrer E, Scharrer B, *Neuroendocrinology*. Columbia University Press, New York 1963.

Thorner MO, Rivier J, Spiess J, Borges JL, Vance ML, Bloom SR, Rogol AD, Cronin MJ, Kaiser DL, Evans WS, Webster JD, MacLeod RM, Vale W, *Human pancreatic growth-hormone-releasing factor selectively stimulates growth-hormone secretion in man*. Lancet 1983; **1**: 24-28.

Vale W, Spiess J, Rivier C, Rivier J, *Characterization of a 41-residue ovine hypothalamic peptide that stimulates secretion of corticotropin and beta-endorphin*. Science 1981; **213**: 1394-1397.

White WF, *On the identity of the LH- and FSH-releasing hormones*. In: Gibian H, Plotz EJ eds., *Mammalian Reproduction*. Springer Verlag, Berlin 1970: 84-87.

2 HYPOPITUITARISM

Besser GM ed., *The Hypothalamus and Pituitary*. Clinics in Endocrinology and Metabolism 1977; **6**: 1-281.

Edwards CRW, Besser GM, *Diseases of the hypothalamus and pituitary gland*. Clinics in Endocrinology and Metabolism 1974; **3**: 475-505.

Nabarro JDN, *Pituitary surgery for endocrine disorders*. Clinical Endocrinology 1980; **13**: 285-298.

3 ACROMEGALY

Belchetz PE ed., *Management of Pituitary Disease*. Chapman and Hall, London 1984: 123-140 and 343-376.

Christy NP, Warren MP, *Disease syndromes of the hypothalamus and anterior pituitary*. In: Degroot LJ ed., *Endocrinology*. Grune and Stratton Inc., New York 1979: 215-252.

Davidoff LM, *Studies in acromegaly III. The anamnesis and symptomatology in one hundred cases*. Endocrinology 1926; **10**: 461-483.

Eastman RC, Gorden P, Roth J, *Conventional supervoltage irradiation is an effective treatment for acromegaly*. Journal of Clinical Endocrinology and Metabolism 1979; **48**: 931-940.

Laws ER, Piepgras DG, Randall RV, Abboud CF, *Neurosurgical management of acromegaly*. Journal of Neurosurgery 1979; **50**: 454-461.

Wass JAH, Thorner MO, Morris DV, Rees LH, Stuart Mason A, Jones AE, Besser GM, *Long-term treatment of acromegaly with bromocriptine*. British Medical Journal 1977; **1**: 875-878.

Wass JAH, Williams J, Charlesworth M, Kingsley DPE, Halliday AM, Doniach I, Rees LH, McDonald WI, Besser GM, *Bromocriptine in management of large pituitary tumours*. British Medical Journal 1982; **284**: 1908-1911.

4 HYPERPROLACTINAEMIA

Chiodini P, Liuzzi A, Cozzi R, Verde G, Oppizzi G, Dallabonzana D, Spelta B, Silvestrini F, Borghi G, Luccarelli G, Rainer E, Horowski R, *Size reduction of macroprolactinomas by bromocriptine or lisuride treatment*. Journal of Clinical Endocrinology and Metabolism 1981; **53**: 737-743.

Hardy J, *Le Prolactinome (prolactinoma)*. Neurochirurgie 1981; **27** (suppl. 1): 1-110.

Thorner MO, Evans WS, MacLeod RM, Nunley WC Jr, Rogol AD, Morris JL, Besser GM, *Hyperprolactinaemia: current concepts of management including medical therapy with bromocriptine*. In: Goldstein G, Calne DB, Leiberman A, Thorner MO eds., *Ergot Compounds and Brain Function – Neuroendocrine Aspects*. Raven Press, New York 1980: 165-189.

Thorner MO, Martin WH, Rogol AD, Morris JL, Perryman RL, Conway BP, Howards SS, Wolfman MG, MacLeod RM, *Rapid regression of pituitary prolactinomas during bromocriptine treatment*. Journal of Clinical Endocrinology and Metabolism 1980; **51**: 438-445.

Thorner MO, Perryman RL, Rogol AD, Conway BP, MacLeod RM, Login IS, Morris JL, *Rapid changes of prolactinoma volume after withdrawal and reinstitution of bromocriptine*. Journal of Clinical Endocrinology and Metabolism 1981; **53**: 480-483.

5 THE POSTERIOR PITUITARY

Bie P, *Osmoreceptors, vasopressin and control of renal water excretion*. Physiological Reviews 1980; **60**: 962-1048.

Brownstein MJ, Russell JT, Gainer H, *Synthesis, transport and release of posterior pituitary hormones*. Science 1980; **207**: 373-378.

Hays RM, *Antidiuretic hormone*. New England Journal of Medicine 1976; **295**: 659-665.

Roberts JS, *Oxytocin*. Annual Research Reviews, Churchill Livingstone, Edinburgh 1977.

Robertson GL, Shelton RL, Athar S, *The osmoregulation of vasopressin*. Kidney International 1976; **10**: 25-37.

6 ADRENAL CORTEX PHYSIOLOGY

Brown MS, Kovanen PT, Goldstein JL, *Receptor-mediated uptake of lipoprotein-cholesterol and its utilisation for steroid synthesis in the adrenal cortex*. Recent Progress in Hormone Research 1979; **35**: 215-257.

Chester Jones I, Henderson IW eds., *General, Comparative and Clinical Endocrinology of the Adrenal Cortex. Volume 2*. Academic Press, London 1978: 670pp.

Gower DB, *Modifiers of steroid-hormone metabolism: a review of their chemistry, biochemistry and clinical applications*. Journal of Steroid Biochemistry 1974; **5**: 501-523.

Gray CH, James VHT eds., *Hormones in Blood. Volumes 4 and 5*. 3rd edition. Academic Press, London 1983: 510pp and 316pp.

James VHT ed., *Comprehensive Endocrinology. The Adrenal Gland*. Raven Press, New York 1979: 332pp.

Kellier-Wood ME, Dallman MF, *Corticosteroid inhibition of ACTH secretion*. Endocrine Reviews 1984; **5**: 1-24.

Lieberman S, Greenfield NJ, Wolfson A, *A heuristic proposal for understanding steroidogenic processes*. Endocrine Reviews 1984; **5**: 128-148.

Makin HJL, *Biochemistry of Steroid Hormones*. 2nd edition. Blackwell Scientific Publications, Oxford 1984: 714pp.

Vinson GP, Pudney JA, Whitehouse BJ, *The mammalian adrenal circulation and the relationship between adrenal blood flow and steroidogenesis*. Journal of Endocrinology 1985; **105**: 285-294.

7 CUSHING'S SYNDROME

Beardwell C, Robertson GL eds., *The Pituitary*. Butterworth's International Medical Reviews, London 1981: 337pp.

Crapo L, *Cushing's syndrome: a review of diagnostic tests*. Metabolism 1979; **28**: 955-977.

Faiman C, *The etiology and management of Cushing's syndrome*. In: Anderson DC, Winter JSD eds., *Adrenal Cortex*. Butterworth's International Medical Reviews, London 1985: 154-168.

Howlett TA, Rees LH, Besser GM, *Cushing's syndrome*. Clinics in Endocrinology and Metabolism 1985; **14**: 911-945.

Krieger DT, *Physiopathology of Cushing's disease*. Endocrine Reviews 1983; **4**: 22-43.

Ross EJ, Linch DC, *Cushing's syndrome – killing disease: discriminatory values of signs and symptoms aiding early diagnosis*. Lancet 1982; **2**: 646-649.

8 ADDISON'S DISEASE

Bondy PK, *Disorders of the adrenal cortex*. In: Wilson JD, Foster DW eds., *Williams – Textbook of Endocrinology*. 7th edition. WB Saunders Company, Philadelphia 1985: 816-890.

Gilkes JJH, Rees LH, Besser GM, *Plasma immunoreactive corticotrophin and lipotrophin in Cushing's syndrome and Addison's disease*. British Medical Journal 1977; **1**: 996-998.

Hornsby PJ, *The regulation of adrenocortical function by control of growth and structure*. In: Anderson DC, Winter JSD eds., *Adrenal Cortex*. Butterworth's International Medical Reviews, London 1985: 1-31.

Irvine WJ, Toft AD, Feek CM, *Addison's disease*. In: James VHT ed., *Comprehensive Endocrinology. The Adrenal Gland*. Raven Press, New York 1979: 131-164.

Takahashi H, Teranishi Y, Nakanishi S, Numa S, *Isolation and structural organization of the human corticotropin-beta-lipotropin gene*. FEBS Letters 1981; **135**: 97-102.

Whitfeld PL, Seeburg PH, Shine J, *The human pro-opiomelanocortin gene: organization, sequence and interspersion with repetitive DNA*. DNA 1982; **1**: 133-143.

9 ENDOCRINE HYPERTENSION

Biglieri EG, Herron MA, Brust N, *17-hydroxylation deficiency in man*. Journal of Clinical Investigation 1966; **45**: 1946-1954.

Breslin DJ, Swinton NW, Libertino JA, Zinman L eds., *Renovascular Hypertension*. Williams and Wilkins Company, Baltimore 1982: 210pp.

Edwards CRW, Carey RM eds., *Essential Hypertension as an Endocrine Disease*. Butterworth's International Medical Reviews, London 1985: 380pp.

Mantero F, Biglieri EG, Edwards CRW eds., *Endocrinology of Hypertension*. Proceedings of the Serono Symposium, Volume 50. Academic Press, London 1982: 434pp.

Vallotton MB, Favre L, *The adrenal cortex and hypertension*. In: Anderson DC, Winter JSD eds., *Adrenal Cortex*. Butterworth's International Medical Reviews, London 1985: 169-187.

10 THE TESTIS

Ahmad KN, Dykes JRW, Ferguson-Smith MA, Lennox B, Mack WS, *Leydig cell volume in chromatin-positive Klinefelter's syndrome*. Journal of Clinical Endocrinology and Metabolism 1971; **33**: 517-520.

Anderson DC, *Sex-hormone-binding globulin*. Clinical Endocrinology 1974; **3**: 69-96.

Anderson DC, *Endocrine function of the testis*. In: O'Riordan JLH ed., *Recent Advances in Endocrinology and Metabolism*. Churchill Livingstone, Edinburgh 1978; **1**: 111-136.

Chandley AC, *The chromosomal basis of human infertility*. British Medical Bulletin 1979; **35**: 181-186.

De Kretser DM, *Endocrinology of male infertility*. British Medical Bulletin 1979; **35**: 187-192.

Franchimont P, Chari S, Hazee-Hagelstein MT, Debruche ML, Duraiswami S, *Evidence for the existence of inhibin*. In: Troen P, Nankin HR eds., *The Testes in Normal and Infertile Men*. Raven Press, New York 1977: 253-270.

London DR, *Medical aspects of hypogonadism*. Clinics in Endocrinology and Metabolism 1975; **4**: 597-618.

Peterson RE, Imperato-McGinley J, Gautier T, Sturla E, *Male pseudohermaphroditism due to steroid 5α-reductase deficiency*. American Journal of Medicine 1977; **62**: 170-191.

Rifka SM, Sherins RJ, *Current concepts in evaluation of the infertile male*. Clinics in Obstetrics and Gynaecology 1978; **5**: 481-497.

11 THE OVARY

Chard T, Lilford R, *Basic Sciences for Obstetrics and Gynaecology*. Springer Verlag, London 1983: 80-103.

Edwards RG, *Conception in the Human Female*. Academic Press, London 1980: 271-385.

Jacobs HS ed., *Advances in Gynaecological Endocrinology*, Study Group Proceedings. Royal College of Obstetricians and Gynaecologists, London 1978: 1-34.

Jeffcoate SL ed., *Ovulation: Methods for its Prediction and Detection*. John Wiley and Sons, Chichester 1983: 126pp.

12 NORMAL AND ABNORMAL SEXUAL DEVELOPMENT AND PUBERTY

Eisenberg E, *Menarche: the transition from childhood to womanhood*. Advances in Pediatrics 1984; **31**: 359-369.

Frisch RE, Revelle R, Cook S, *Components of weight at menarche and the initiation of the adolescent growth spurt in girls: estimated total water, lean body weight and fat*. Human Biology 1973; **45**: 469-483.

Griffin JE, Wilson JD, *Disorders of the testes and male reproductive tract*. In: Wilson JD, Foster DW eds., *Williams – Textbook of Endocrinology*. 7th edition. WB Saunders Company, Philadelphia 1985: 259-311.

Grumbach MM, *True or central precocious puberty*. In: Krieger DT, Bardin CW eds., *Current Therapy in Endocrinology and Metabolism 1985-1986*. BC Decker Inc., Toronto 1985: 4-8.

Reiter EO, Grumbach MM, *Neuroendocrine control mechanisms and the onset of puberty.* Annual Review of Physiology 1982; **44**: 594-614.

Ross GT, *Disorders of the ovary and female reproductive tract.* In: Wilson JD, Foster DW eds., *Williams – Textbook of Endocrinology.* 7th edition. WB Saunders Company, Philadelphia 1985: 206-258.

Styne DM, Grumbach MM, *Puberty in the male and female: its physiology and disorders.* In: Yen SSC, Jaffe RB eds., *Reproductive Endocrinology.* 7th edition. WB Saunders Company, Philadelphia 1978: 189-240.

13 THYROID PHYSIOLOGY AND HYPOTHYROIDISM

Hall R, Anderson J, Smart GA, Besser GM, *Fundamentals of Clinical Endocrinology.* 3rd edition. Pitman Medical Ltd, Tunbridge Wells 1980: 94-207.

14 CARCINOMA OF THE THYROID

Hedinger Chr, *Histological Typing of Thyroid Tumours.* WHO International Histological Classification of Tumours, No. 11, Geneva 1974: 1-28.

Meissner WA, Supplement to *Tumours of the Thyroid Gland.* Fascicle 4, 2nd series of the *Atlas of Tumour Pathology.* Armed Forces Institute of Pathology, Washington DC 1984: 1-44.

15 HYPERTHYROIDISM AND GRAVES' DISEASE

Hall R, *Thyrotrophin receptor antibodies and Graves' disease.* Hospital Update 1981; **7**: 161-172.

Hall R, McGregor AM, McLachlan SM, Lazarus J, Rees Smith B, *The treatment of hyperthyroidism.* In: Tunbridge WMG ed., Newcastle Advanced Medicine. Pitman Medical Press, London 1981: 32-36.

Hall R, McLachlan SM, McGregor AM, Weetman AT, Rees Smith B, *Thyrotrophin receptor antibodies – clinicopathological correlations.* In: Evered DC, Whelan J eds., *Receptors, Antibodies and Diseases.* CIBA Foundation Symposium No. 90. Pitman Medical Press, London 1982: 133-144.

McGregor AM, Collins PN, Peterson MM, Rees Smith B, Bottazzo GF, Hall R, *Specificity of the immunosuppressive action of carbimazole in Graves' disease.* British Medical Journal 1982; **284**: 1750-1751.

McGregor AM, Rees Smith B, Hall R, *Hyperthyroid Graves' disease: predicting relapse.* Thyroid Today 1982; **5**: 1.

Scanlon MF, Peters J, Foord S, Dieguez C, Hall R, *The clinical relevance of TRH in diagnosis and investigation.* In: Griffiths EC, Bennett GW eds., *Thyrotropin-Releasing Hormone.* Raven Press, New York 1983: 303-314.

16 GROWTH DISORDERS

Brook CGD ed., *Clinical Paediatric Endocrinology.* Blackwell Scientific Publications, Oxford 1981: 684pp.

Brook CGD, *Growth Assessment in Childhood and Adolescence.* Blackwell Scientific Publications, Oxford 1982: 164pp.

17 CALCIUM AND COMMON ENDOCRINE BONE DISORDERS

Aitken M, *Osteoporosis: In Clinical Practice.* John Wright, Bristol 1984: 146pp.

Barnes AD, *The changing face of parathyroid surgery.* Annals of the Royal College of Surgeons of England 1984; **66**: 77-80.

Dent CE, *Some problems of hyperparathyroidism.* British Medical Journal 1962; **2**: 1419-1425 and 1495-1500.

Hamdy RC, *Paget's Disease of Bone: Assessment and Management.* Praeger, New York 1981: 203pp.

Heath D, Marx SJ eds., *Calcium Disorders.* Butterworth's International Medical Reviews, London 1982: 286pp.

Mundy GR, Cove DH, Fisken RA, Primary hyperparathyroidism: changes in the pattern of clinical presentation. Lancet 1980; **1**: 1317-1320.

Nordin BEC ed., *Metabolic Bone and Stone Disease.* Churchill Livingstone, Edinburgh 1984: 435pp.

O'Riordan JLH, *Hormonal control of mineral metabolism.* In: O'Riordan JLH ed., *Recent Advances in Endocrinology and Metabolism.* Churchill Livingstone, Edinburgh 1978; **1**: 189-217.

Pyrah LN, Hodgkinson A, Anderson CK, *Primary hyperparathyroidism.* British Journal of Surgery 1966; **53**: 245-316.

Watson L, *Primary hyperparathyroidism.* Clinics in Endocrinology and Metabolism 1974; **3**: 215-235.

18 HYPOGLYCAEMIA AND INSULINOMAS

Aynsley-Green A, *Hypoglycaemia.* In: Brook CGD ed., *Clinical Paediatric Endocrinology.* Blackwell Scientific Publications, Oxford 1981: 637-659.

Berger M, Bordi C, Cüppers HJ, Berchtold P, Gries FA, Münterfering H, Sailer R, Zimmerman H, Orci L, *Functional and morphologic characterization of human insulinomas.* Diabetes 1983; **32**: 921-931.

Charles MA, Hofeldt F, Shackelford A, Waldeck N, Dodson LE Jr, Bunker D, Coggins JT, Eichner H, *Comparison of oral glucose tolerance tests and mixed meals in patients with apparent idiopathic postabsorptive hypoglycemia: absence of hypoglycemia after meals.* Diabetes 1981; **30**: 464-470.

Friesen SR, *Tumours of the endocrine pancreas.* New England Journal of Medicine 1982; **306**: 580-590.

Gould VE, Memoli VA, Dardi LE, Gould NS, *Nesidiodysplasia and nesidioblastosis of infancy; ultrastructural and immunohistochemical analysis of islet cell alterations with and without associated hyperinsulinemic hypoglycemia.* Scandinavian Journal of Gastroenterology 1981; **16** (suppl. 70): 129-142.

Marks V, Rose FC, *Hypoglycaemia.* 2nd edition. Blackwell Scientific Publications, Oxford 1981: 521pp.

Service FJ ed., *Hypoglycemic Disorders: Pathogenesis, Diagnosis and Treatment.* GK Hall, Boston 1983: 187pp.

19 ECTOPIC HUMORAL SYNDROMES

Baylin SB, Mendelsohn G, *Ectopic (inappropriate) hormone production by tumours: mechanisms involved in the biological and clinical implications.* Endocrine Reviews 1980; **1**: 45-77.

Eipper BA, Mains RE, *Structure and biosynthesis of pro-adrenocorticotrophin endorphin and related peptides,* Endocrine Reviews 1980; **1**: 1-27.

Odell W, Wolfsen A, Yoshimoto Y, Weitzman R, Fisher D, Hirose F, *Ectopic peptide synthesis: a universal concomitant of neoplasia.* Transactions of the Association of American Physicians 1977; **90**: 204-227.

Roth J, LeRoith D, Shiloach J, Rosenzweig JL, Lesniak MA, Havrankova J, *The evolutionary origins of hormones, neurotransmitters and other extracellular chemical messengers: implications for mammalian biology.* New England Journal of Medicine 1982; **306**: 523-527.

Sherwood LM, Gould VE, *Ectopic hormone syndromes and multiple endocrine neoplasia.* In: DeGroot LJ ed., *Endocrinology.* Grune and Stratton Inc., New York 1979: 1733-1766.

Sherwood LM, *Ectopic hormone syndromes.* In: Ingbar SH ed., *Contemporary Endocrinology.* Plenum Press, New York 1979: 341-386.

Sherwood LM, *Ectopic hormone syndromes.* In: Ingbar SH ed., *Contemporary Endocrinology.* Plenum Press, New York 1985: 345-402.

Takahashi H, Teranishi Y, Nakanishi S, Numa S, *Isolation and structural organization of the human corticotropin-beta-lipotropin gene.* FEBS letters 1981; **135**: 97-102.

Whitfeld PL, Seeburg PH, Shine J, *The human pro-opiomelanocortin gene: organization, sequence and interspersion with repetitive DNA.* DNA 1982; **1**: 133-143.

20 RADIOLOGY OF ENDOCRINE DISEASE

Grainger RG, Allison DJ eds., *Diagnostic Radiology: an Anglo-American Textbook of Imaging.* Volumes 1, 2 and 3. Churchill Livingstone, Edinburgh 1986: 2234pp.

Ross EJ, Prichard BNC, Kaufman L, Robertson AIG, Harries BJ, *Preoperative and operative management of patients with phaeochromocytoma.* British Medical Journal 1967; **1**: 191-198.

Siegelman SS, Gatewood OMB, Goldman SM, *Computed Tomography of the Kidneys and Adrenals.* Churchill Livingstone, New York 1984: 288pp.

21 NEURORADIOLOGY OF THE PITUITARY AND HYPOTHALAMUS

Banna M, Baker HL, Houser JW, *Pituitary and parapituitary tumours on computed tomography. A review article based on 230 cases.* British Journal of Radiology 1980; **53**: 1123-1144.

Daniels DL, Williams AL, Thornton RS, Meyer GA, Cusick JF, Haughton VM, *Differential diagnosis of intrasellar tumours by computed tomography.* Radiology 1981; **141**: 697-701.

Doyle FH, *Radiology of the pituitary.* Recent Advances in Radiology and Medical Imaging 1979; **6**: 121-143.

Gado M, Bull JWD, *The carotid angiogram in suprasellar masses.* Neuroradiology 1971; **2**: 136-153.

Kendall BE, Lee BCP, *Cranial chordomas.* British Journal of Radiology 1977; **50**: 687-698.

Kendall BE, Tatler GLV, *Radiological findings in neurosarcoidosis.* British Journal of Radiology 1978; **51**: 81-92.

Kepes JJ, Kepes M, *Predominantly cerebral forms of histiocytosis-X.* Acta Neuropathologica 1969; **14**: 77-98.

Kier EL, *'J' and 'Omega' shape of the sella turcica. Anatomic clarification of radiological misconceptions.* Acta Radiologica; Diagnosis 1969; **9**: 91-94.

Ramamurthi B, Varadarajan MG, *Diagnosis of tuberculomas of the brain.* Journal of Neurosurgery 1961; **18**: 1-7.

Sosman MC, Vogt EC, *Aneurysms of the internal carotid artery and the circle of Willis, from a roentgenological viewpoint.* American Journal of Roentgenology 1926; **15**: 122-134.

Wakai S, Fukushima T, Teramoto A, Sano K, *Pituitary apoplexy: incidence and clinical significance.* Journal of Neurosurgery 1981; **55**: 187-193.

Endocrine Normal Ranges

These should be regarded as guidelines only since laboratories use different reagents and therefore may obtain somewhat different values in the same situations. Each laboratory must derive its own normal ranges.

	Conventional Units	SI Units

ADRENAL STEROIDS (serum or plasma)

Aldosterone		
upright, normal diet	5-20ng/dl	0.14-0.56nmol/l
supine, saline suppression	<8.5ng/dl	<0.24nmol/l

Cortisol		
0900hrs	11-25µg/dl	300-700nmol/l
1600hrs	3-10µg/dl	84-270nmol/l
2400hrs	0-5µg/dl	0-140nmol/l
low dose dexamethasone suppression test (2mg/day for 48 hrs)	<5µg/dl	<140nmol/l
after hypoglycaemia (blood glucose <2.2mmol/l or <40ng/dl)	≥21µg/dl	≥580nmol/l

Dehydroepiandrosterone (DHEA)	0.2-0.9µg/dl	7-31nmol/l

DHEA-sulphate		
women	110-468µg/dl	3-12.0µmol/l
men	75-370µg/dl	2-9.5µmol/l

PANCREATIC AND GUT HORMONES (serum or plasma)

Gastrin	<120pg/ml	<57pmol/l

Insulin		
overnight fasting	<16µu/ml	<16mu/l
after hypoglycaemia (blood glucose <2.2mmol/l or <40ng/dl)	<3µu/ml	<3mu/l

GONADAL STEROIDS (serum or plasma)

Androstenedione		
women and men	90-230ng/dl	3-8nmol/l

17-Hydroxyprogesterone	30-595ng/dl	0.9-17.8nmol/l

Oestradiol		
women: prepuberty	<27pg/ml	<100pmol/l
postmenopausal	<27pg/ml	<100pmol/l
basal adult (follicular phase)	55-110pg/ml	200-400pmol/l
ovulatory surge	110-330pg/ml	400-1200pmol/l
men	<50pg/ml	<180pmol/l

Progesterone		
women: follicular phase	1-4ng/ml	3-12 nmol/l
midcycle peak	0.3-3.5ng/ml	0.95-11nmol/l
postovulatory	>10ng/ml	>30nmol/l
men, prepubertal girls and postmenopausal women	<2ng/ml	<6nmol/l

Testosterone		
prepubertal boys and girls	<20ng/dl	<0.8nmol/l
women	14-87ng/dl	0.5-3.0nmol/l
men	260-1,010ng/dl	9-35nmol/l

Dihydrotestosterone (DHT)		
women	8.7-27.0ng/dl	0.3-0.93nmol/l
men	29.0-75.7ng/dl	1.0-2.6nmol/l

ANTERIOR PITUITARY HORMONES (serum or plasma)

Adrenocorticotrophic Hormone (ACTH)		
0800-0900hrs	10-80pg/ml	2.3-18.0pmol/l

Follicle Stimulating Hormone (FSH)		
women: follicular phase	1-10mu/ml	1-10u/l
midcycle	6-25mu/ml	6-25u/l
luteal phase	0.3-2.1mu/ml	0.3-2.1u/l
postmenopausal	>30mu/ml	>30u/l
men	1-7mu/ml	1-7u/l
prepubertal children	<5mu/ml	<5u/l

Growth Hormone (GH) after hypoglycaemia (blood glucose <2.2mmol/l or <40ng/l)		
normal	>10ng/ml	>20mu/l
equivocal	10-20ng/ml	20-40mu/l

Luteinising Hormone (LH)		
women: follicular phase	2.5-21mu/ml	2.5-21u/l
midcycle	25-70mu/ml	25-70u/l
luteal phase	<1-13mu/ml	<1-13u/l
postmenopausal	>30mu/ml	>30u/l
men	1-10mu/ml	1-10u/l
prepubertal children	<5mu/ml	<5u/l

Prolactin (PRL)	<18ng/ml	<360mu/l

Thyroid Stimulating Hormone (TSH)		
by radioimmunoassay	0.5-6µu/ml	0.5-6mu/l
by immunoradiometric assay	0.4-5.0µu/ml	0.4-5.0mu/l

THYROID HORMONES (serum or plasma)

Thyroxine (T$_4$)		
free	8.0-18.0pg/ml	10-22pmol/l
total	50-120ng/ml	60-150nmol/l

Triiodothyronine (T$_3$)		
free	3.5-6.5pg/ml	5-10pmol/l
total	0.65-1.7ng/ml	1.0-2.6nmol/l

CATECHOLAMINES (plasma)

(lying and with venous cannula in place)

Adrenaline (epinephrine)	0.01-0.19ng/ml	0.06-1.07nmol/l
Noradrenaline (norepinephrine)	0.07-0.56ng/ml	0.46-3.68nmol/l

URINARY VALUES

Aldosterone	5-19µg/day	14-53nmol/24hr
Calcium	<300mg/day	<7.5mmol/day
Cortisol	20-100µg/day	50-250nmol/24hr
5-Hydroxyindoleacetic Acid	2-9mg/day	10-45µmol/day
Metanephrins	<1.2mg/24hr	<6µmol/24hr

17-Oxosteroids (values vary with age)		
women	5-15mg/day	17-55µmol/24hr
men	5-20mg/day	17-70µmol/24hr

17-Oxogenic Steroids (values vary with age)		
women	5-15mg/day	17-55µmol/24hr
men	7-20mg/day	24-70µmol/24hr

Vanillyl Mandelic Acid (VMA)	1.0-7.0mg/24hr	5-35µmol/24hr

Index